Carcinoma of the Larynx and Hypopharynx

Sudhir Bahadur • Alok Thakar
Bidhu K. Mohanti
Editors

Carcinoma of the Larynx and Hypopharynx

BYWORD BOOKS™

Springer

Editors
Sudhir Bahadur
All India Institute of Medical Sciences
New Delhi
India

Alok Thakar
All India Institute of Medical Sciences
New Delhi
India

Bidhu K. Mohanti
Department of Radiation Oncology
Manipal Hospital
New Delhi
India

ISBN 978-981-13-3109-1 ISBN 978-981-13-3110-7 (eBook)
https://doi.org/10.1007/978-981-13-3110-7

Library of Congress Control Number: 2018963983

Co-publishing partnership between Byword Books Private Limited and Springer Nature India Private Limited.
This Springer imprint is published by the registered company Springer Nature Singapore Pte Ltd.
The registered company address is: 152 Beach Road, #21-01/04 Gateway East, Singapore 189721, Singapore

Preface

The incidence of cancer of the larynx and hypopharynx is high in India comprising of significant tumor load, and it may be largely attributed to consumption of tobacco and alcohol. Despite the availability of improved techniques for better assessment of disease such as the use of rigid and flexible telescopes and much improved imaging, less than 20% of patients are diagnosed in early stages. Unfortunately, most patients still present with advanced disease and thus pose considerable challenge in management. The tumor board consisting of multidisciplinary team including a head and neck surgeon and radiation and medical oncologists has become the standard practice to implement the treatment protocol after initial work-up and diagnosis. However, the decision-making is complex and demanding.

The prognosis of early lesions is good, and results of treatment whether by radiotherapy, by open partial laryngectomy, or by trans-oral laser surgery are generally excellent. Though, open partial laryngectomy, once extremely popular, is now seldom employed except in radiation-failed salvage setting. It has been mainly replaced by TOLS (trans-oral laser surgery), but the question of technical expertise and availability of equipment still persists.

However, the surgeon faces a major dilemma while treating advanced tumors, whether to sacrifice the larynx or make an effort to preserve the organ. Surgery with postoperative radiotherapy is still considered by many as the gold standard treatment. Though oncologic results in terms of survival are usually good, quality of life is significantly impaired because of the loss of speech and the presence of permanent tracheostomy. This has been partly overcome by the placement of tracheoesophageal prosthesis, though the cost of prosthesis and its frequent changes are important issues. There has been serious research undertaken since the 1990s using chemotherapy in combination with radiotherapy to improve the organ preservation and survival. Concurrent chemotherapy and radiotherapy has shown to produce excellent results, almost comparable to that of surgery while preserving the larynx in more than half of cases and keeping the possibility of salvage surgery in the remaining cases. However, some significant problems still remain.

1. Selection of patients
2. Toxicity reactions
3. Diagnosis of residual/recurrent disease, timing of salvage surgery, and its morbidity
4. Cost involved and follow-up of patient

The editors and other authors have combined efforts to produce this textbook to provide guidelines for the update management with appropriate radiology, pathology, surgery, radiotherapy, chemoradiation, and rehabilitation. This textbook should be of significant value to the residents as well as faculty staff of various specialities including otolaryngology, head and neck surgery, general surgery, radiation oncology, medical oncology, and radiology.

All the images of patients used in this textbook are original, and consent was taken from them, as part of the treatment that these images may be used for educational purposes. No image reveals the identity of a patient.

This book on the larynx and hypopharynx is dedicated to our patients.

New Delhi, India — Sudhir Bahadur
New Delhi, India — Alok Thakar
New Delhi, India — Bidhu K. Mohanti

Contents

Editors and Contributors

About the Editors

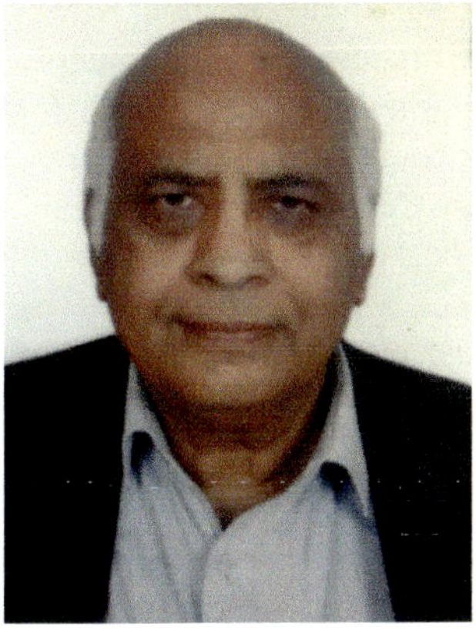

Sudhir Bahadur, MS, FAMS, PhD is a highly experienced cancer surgeon, trained in all types of complex head and neck cancer surgeries. Dr. Bahadur has worked at the All India Institute of Medical Sciences, New Delhi, as a faculty member for nearly 30 years. His areas of interest are head and neck surgery/oncology and surgery of the skull base. He is the past president of the Foundation for Head and Neck Oncology and Skull Base Surgery Society of India and has published 200 research papers and textbook chapters. Dr. Bahadur has received numerous honors, including from the Foundation for Head and Neck Oncology, Association of Otolaryngology of India, and ICMR, New Delhi.

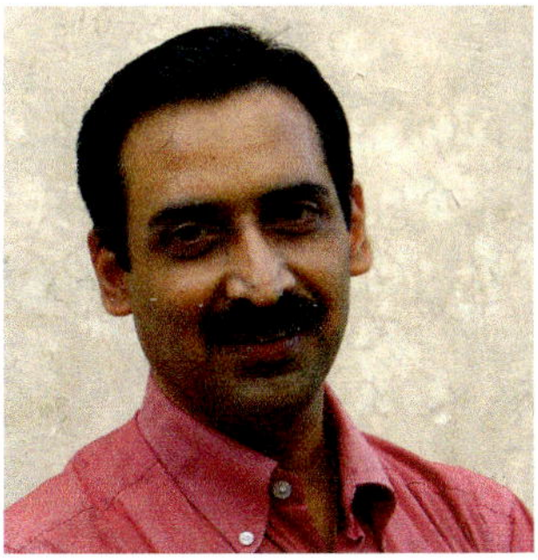

Alok Thakar, MS, FRCS is a professor of Otolaryngology and Head and Neck Surgery at the All India Institute of Medical Sciences, New Delhi. His clinical and research interests have been directed toward optimizing outcomes and minimizing the disability following treatment of head-neck and skull base lesions. He has been instrumental in the development of trans-oral laser surgery, as well as voice-conserving oncosurgery, minimally invasive skull base surgery, and techniques for rehabilitation of facial nerve and lower cranial nerve lesions. He has had a pioneering role in the introduction of trans-oral robotic surgery in the Indian subcontinent.

Professor Thakar has served in several prominent advisory positions including for the Task Force on Head-Neck Cancer Management, Indian Council of Medical Research. He was a recipient of the Shakuntala Amir Chand National Award by the

Indian Council of Medical Research and has served as honorable secretary of the Foundation for Head and Neck Oncology. He has authored over 200 research publications and was recently appointed as honorary consultant to the Armed Forces Medical Services.

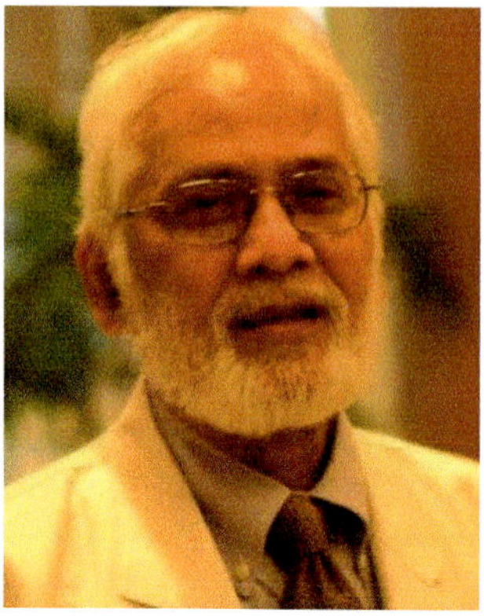

Bidhu K. Mohanti is an MBBS graduate from MKCG Medical College, Berhampur, and has an MD in Radiotherapy from PGIMER, Chandigarh. He is currently a consultant at Manipal Hospitals, Delhi. Dr. Mohanti has over 30 years of experience in oncology, covering academic, clinical, and research responsibilities. He has worked as a radiation oncologist and as faculty at Kidwai Memorial Institute of Oncology, Bangalore, and the AIIMS, New Delhi. He has also worked on an assignment for the Ministry of Health, Oman, to establish the first radiotherapy department and set up patient care at the National Oncology Center, Royal Hospital, Muscat. Dr. Mohanti has served as an expert for the IAEA, Vienna, and European Commission. He has been a member of numerous professional societies and has received several awards, including the Life Time Achievement Award from the Foundation for Head and Neck Oncology. He has published 165 peer-reviewed journal articles, international abstracts, book, and chapters. He is the editor of *Textbook of Radiation Oncology: Principles and Practice* (Elsevier) and has been invited to give many national and international presentations.

Contributors

S. S. Anand Department of Radiodiagnosis, Hamdard Institute of Medical Sciences and Research, Jamia Hamdard, New Delhi, India

Sudhir Bahadur Department of Otolaryngology and Head-Neck Surgery, Formerly at All India Institute of Medical Sciences, New Delhi, India

Shikha Halder Department of Radiation Oncology, BLK Super Specialty Hospital, New Delhi, India

Abhinav Jain Department of Radiodiagnosis, Hamdard Institute of Medical Sciences and Research, Jamia Hamdard, New Delhi, India

Anjali Kochhar Department of Anaesthesiology, Hamdard Institute of Medical Sciences and Research, Jamia Hamdard, New Delhi, India

Rajeev Kumar Department of Otolaryngology and Head-Neck Surgery, All India Institute of Medical Sciences, New Delhi, India

Junaid Malik Department of Otolaryngology and Head-Neck Surgery, Hamdard Institute of Medical Sciences and Research, Jamia Hamdard, New Delhi, India

Bidhu K. Mohanti Department of Radiation Oncology, Manipal Hospital, New Delhi, India

Tapaswani Pradhan Department of Surgical Oncology, BLK Super Speciality Hospital, Delhi, India

Prem Sagar Department of Otolaryngology and Head-Neck Surgery, All India Institute of Medical Sciences, New Delhi, India

Arun Sharma Department of Otolaryngology and Head-Neck Surgery, Hamdard Institute of Medical Sciences and Research, Jamia Hamdard, New Delhi, India

Kapil Sikka Department of Otolaryngology and Head-Neck Surgery, All India Institute of Medical Sciences, New Delhi, India

Alok Thakar Department of Otolaryngology and Head-Neck Surgery, All India Institute of Medical Sciences, New Delhi, India

Surgical Anatomy and Tumour Spread in the Larynx and Hypopharynx

1

Rajeev Kumar and Prem Sagar

1.1 Epidemiology

Laryngeal cancer is the ninth most common cancer in males in Asia. This is the seventh most common cancer in Indian males with an incidence of 1.26–8.18 per 100,000 population in India [1]. The incidence is strongly related to advanced age (fifth decade onwards) and uncommon before 40 years of age [2]. Laryngeal cancer is strongly associated with socioeconomic status, being less common in affluent population. Worldwide, the most common site of laryngeal cancer is glottis (approximately 49%), preceding supraglottis (16%). In India, the most common subsite of involvement is combined supraglottis and glottis followed by supraglottis and glottis alone, as most of the patients present in advanced stage of disease [3]. The most common type of neoplasia is squamous cell carcinoma (85%).

The two most common risk factors for laryngeal cancer are tobacco smoking and alcohol consumption. Smoking is related to glottis cancers and alcohol is associated with supraglottis cancers. These two risk factors act synergistically [4]. Hashibe et al. (2009) have found a population attributable risk of approximately 88% for laryngeal cancer: 52% due to tobacco alone, 3% due to alcohol alone and 33% due to combined tobacco and alcohol [5]. Other risk factors are long-term exposure to indoor pollution, spicy food and nonvegetarian food intake as mentioned in few Indian studies [6].

R. Kumar (✉) · P. Sagar
Department of Otolaryngology and Head-Neck Surgery, All India Institute of Medical Sciences, New Delhi, India

S. Bahadur et al. (eds.), *Carcinoma of the Larynx and Hypopharynx*,
https://doi.org/10.1007/978-981-13-3110-7_1

1.2 Surgical Anatomy of the Larynx

The larynx is an important organ in the upper airway which is functionally associated with speech, respiration and prevention of aspiration. As per UICC (1997), the larynx is anatomically divided into three subsites, namely, supraglottis, glottis and subglottis. This subsite division is based on embryological development. Though the laryngeal mucosa is continuous throughout, the submucosa is compartmentalized as per the subsites. Each subsite contains potential tissue spaces through which laryngeal cancer can spread across the subsites and beyond the laryngeal confines. Tumours in these anatomical and embryological distinct subunits of larynx have different modes of initial presentation. Also, the pattern of lymph node metastasis is distinct for malignancy of each subsite. This leads to various treatment modalities available for addressing laryngeal cancers as per the subsite and stage of disease. The different subsites have been diagramatically shown in Fig. 1.1.

1.2.1 Supraglottis

The supraglottic larynx arises from the buccopharyngeal anlage (arches III and IV). As per UICC (1997), the supraglottis is further subdivided into the suprahyoid epiglottis, aryepiglottic fold (laryngeal surface), arytenoids, infrahyoid epiglottis and false cords. Inferiorly ventricles separate the supraglottis from the glottis. The

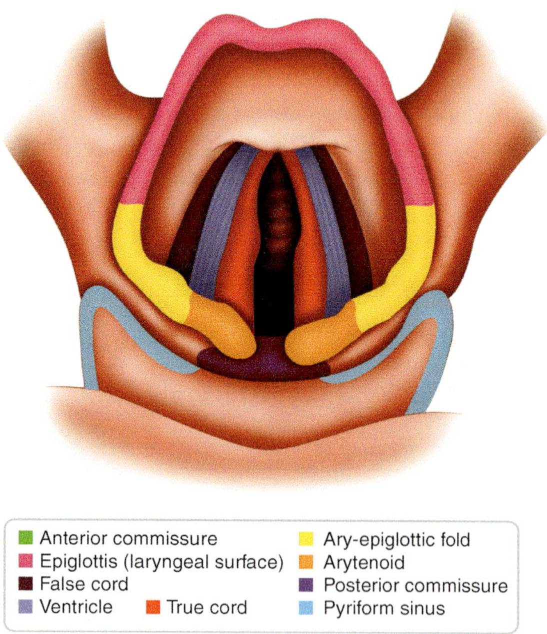

Fig. 1.1 Diagrammatic representation of the subsites of larynx

petiole is the small part of epiglottis that is attached in midline to the thyroid cartilage. Thyro-epiglottic ligament connects the epiglottis to the thyroid cartilage. The supraglottic larynx has rich lymphatic network accounting for early lymph node metastasis in supraglottic laryngeal cancer. Lymphatic vessels exit through thyrohyoid membrane along the superior laryngeal vascular pedicle and drain into deep cervical lymph nodes located at level II and III. The epiglottic cartilage has numerous small openings in its inferior part through which tumour can spread into fat-filled pre-epiglottic space.

1.2.2 Glottis

The glottis is embryologically derived from the pulmonary anlage (arch VI). As per UICC (1997), the glottic larynx is further subdivided into true vocal cords, anterior commissure and posterior commissure.

The right and left true vocal cords meet anteriorly in midline to form anterior commissure. Posteriorly the loose mucosa over anterior surface of arytenoids and vocal processes form posterior commissure. The space between two cords is called glottic chink which is narrow anteriorly and broader posteriorly. The anterior two-third of vocal cords are membranous, while posterior one-third is cartilaginous in origin. Vocal process of arytenoids cartilage contributes to posterior cartilaginous vocal cords. The vocal cords are histologically divided into five layers – stratified squamous epithelium, superficial lamina propria (Reinke's space), intermediate lamina propria, deep lamina propria and muscular layer of thyroarytenoid and vocalis muscle. The epithelium and superficial lamina propria forms the loose mucosal cover that lies over the vocal ligament (intermediate and deep lamina propria layers). The third zone is the muscular body consisting of thyroarytenoid and vocalis muscles. This histologic division is the basis of different types of laser cordectomy performed during transoral laser microsurgery for glottis cancers.

The lymphatic drainage of glottis is very sparse. Lymphatic vessels from the glottis and subglottis pass through the cricothyroid membrane and drain into prelaryngeal (Delphian) nodes and paratracheal and deep cervical lymph nodes (level IV).

1.2.3 Subglottis

Subglottic portion is derived from the pulmonary anlage (arch VI). The subglottic larynx extends till inferior border of the cricoid cartilage. The upper border of subglottis lies 1 cm below the level of true vocal cords. It is further subdivided into two parts. The anterior triangular part is fixed, and the mucosa is adherent to the cricoid cartilage. Its apex lies at the level of anterior commissure. It has foramina through which tumour can spread extralaryngeally. The lateral part is mobile and covers the conus elasticus.

1.3 Potential Tissue Spaces in Relation to Laryngeal Cancer Spread

The potential spaces in the larynx are compartmentalized by virtue of their embryological development. These spaces act as barriers against for early laryngeal cancers and form the basis for conservation laryngeal surgery. However, once breached by progressive cancer, the cancer spread occurs along the path of least resistance along these connective tissue planes and vascular pedicles.

1.3.1 Reinke's Space

It is a potential submucosal space along most of the length of free edge of true cord. It allows mucosa to slide over underlying tissue (vocal ligament and vocalis muscle). Very early glottic cancers limited to epithelial layer only present as voice change. These lesions can either be stripped off, or subepithelial cordectomy with CO_2 laser can be performed without significant voice worsening.

1.3.2 Paraglottic Space

It is another potential tissue space, which is present bilaterally between the glottis mucosa and the thyroid cartilage. The boundaries of paraglottic space are:

- Superior – vallecula and aryepiglottic fold
- Inferior – conus elasticus
- Lateral – thyroid cartilage
- Posterior – pyriform sinus
- Medial – vestibular fold and quadrangular membrane
  - The paraglottic space contains thyroarytenoid muscle; involvement of this muscle by lateral spread of laryngeal cancer leads to cord fixation. Also inferolaterally it is continuous with cartilaginous defect between cricoid and thyroid cartilage and can lead to extralaryngeal cancer spread.

1.3.3 Pre-epiglottis Space (Fig. 1.2)

Pre-epiglottic space is another potential tissue space present in supraglottic larynx. It is a fat-filled space, which communicates with bilateral paraglottic space deep to quadrangular membrane. The boundaries are described below:

(a) Superior – hyoepiglottic ligament
(b) Inferior – thyroepiglottic ligament
(c) Posterior – epiglottis
(d) Anterior – thyrohyoid membrane and thyroid cartilage

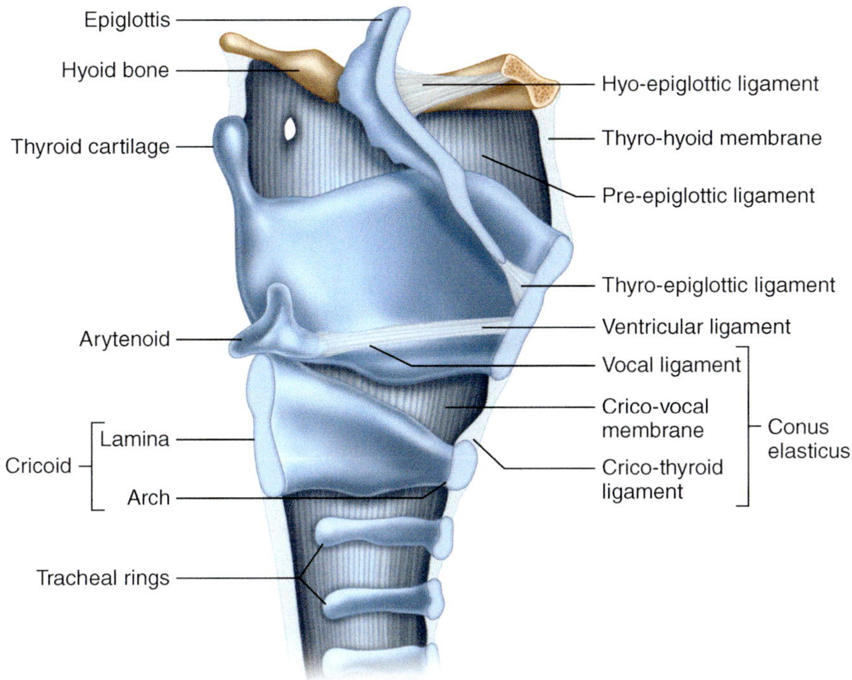

Fig. 1.2 Diagrammatic representation of the sagittal section across the larynx

1.3.4 Anterior Subglottic Wedge

It is a triangular-shaped zone with the apex just below the anterior commissure tendon.

Inferiorly it is limited by anterior arch of the cricoid cartilage. Anterior commissure growth tends to involve this space, which may lead to early extralaryngeal spread through cricothyroid ligament.

1.4 Natural Laryngeal Barriers to Cancer Spread

1.4.1 Quadrangular Membrane (Fig. 1.3)

Quadrangular membrane is one of the natural barriers present in the supraglottic larynx. It is composed of elastic fibrous tissue. Its extension is described below:

- Anterior – lateral border of epiglottis
- Posterior – medial surface of arytenoid
- Inferior – thickened lower part forms vestibular ligament

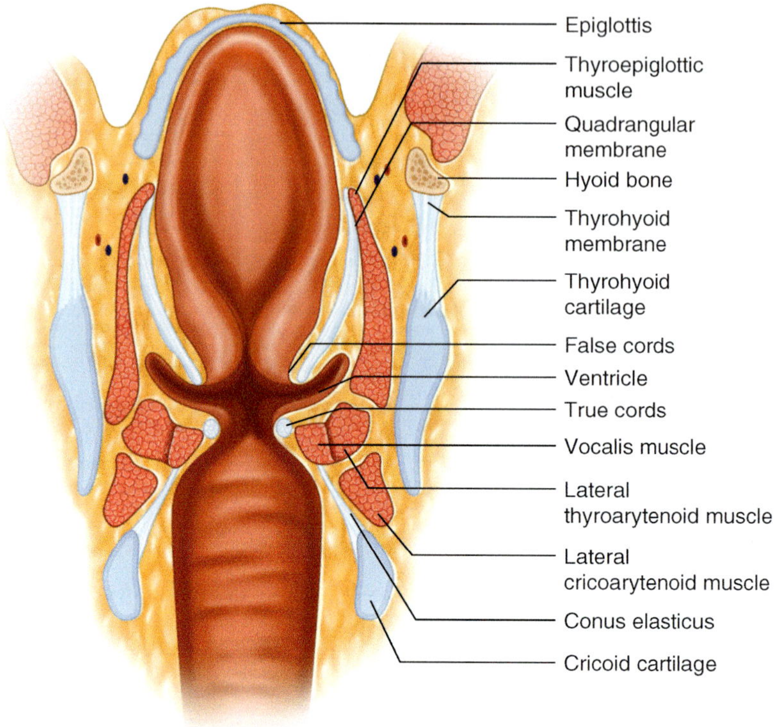

Fig. 1.3 Diagrammatic representation of the coronal section through the larynx

- Medially – covered by loose mucosa
- Laterally – paraglottic space
- Upper free margin – aryepiglottic fold

1.4.2 **Conus Elasticus** (Figs. 1.2 and 1.3)

The conus elasticus is one of the natural barriers present in glottic and subglottic larynx. Its extension is described below:

- Anterior – median cricothyroid ligament
- Posterior – vocal process
- Lateral – thyroid cartilage
- Superior – thickened upper end forms vocal ligament
- Inferior – lower border of cricoid cartilage

1.4.3 Anterior Commissure Tendon

It is formed by the fusion of vocal ligament of both true vocal cords anteriorly and attached to the thyroid cartilage.

1.4.4 Vocal Ligament

The thickened cricovocal membrane forms the vocal ligament. It is attached anteriorly at the level of anterior commissure and posteriorly to inferior border of vocal process of the arytenoid cartilage. It forms the body of the vocal cords over which mucosa is freely mobile.

1.5 Pattern of Spread of Laryngeal Cancers

Tumour invasion is generally along the path of least resistance into different potential spaces. Tumours spread along the nerves, blood vessels and lymphatics into loose connective tissue.

1.5.1 Spread Pattern of Glottic Carcinoma

The progression of glottic carcinoma is slow and predictable. The most common sites are anterior half of true vocal cord and anterior commissure. Its possible extension in different dimensions is described below:

- Glottic plane – radially (anterior–posterior)
- Vertical – anterior commissure to supraglottis or subglottic spread
- Deep – through the vocal ligament, conus elasticus and thyroarytenoid muscle into paraglottic space

Glottic lesion with mobile cord is superficial to conus elasticus, whereas glottic carcinoma with fixed cord may be due to either of the following:

- Thyroarytenoid muscle involvement (most common)
- Cricoarytenoid joint or vocal process of arytenoid involvement
- Subglottic extension
- Perineural spread (recurrent laryngeal nerve involvement) in massive tumours

Lymphatic spread is less common.

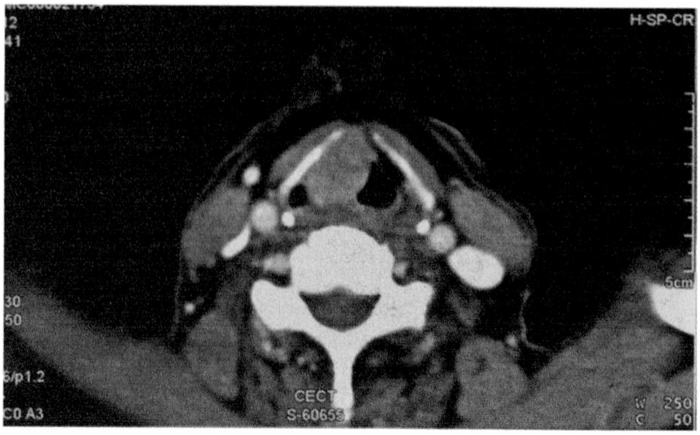

Fig. 1.4 CECT neck (axial cut) shows heterogeneously enhancing lesion of the right true cord and anterior commissure, infiltrating into the paraglottic space. Note the early extralaryngeal spread through the anterior commissure (*)

Thyroid cartilage invasion is common in ossified parts. Extralaryngeal spread in anterior midline is through thyroid cartilage or cricothyroid membrane. Laterally tumour spreads through cricothyroid space.

Anterior commissure tumours invade thyroid cartilage through Broyles ligament. Superiorly AC tumours invade the petiole of epiglottis and extend inferiorly to the subglottis by the cricothyroid membrane. This leads to early extralaryngeal spread in anterior commissure tumours (Fig. 1.4).

Clinically anterior commissure tumours may appear T1 lesion, but on radiology, it may be T4 because of thyroid cartilage involvement.

1.5.2 Pattern of Spread in Supraglottic Carcinoma

Supraglottic carcinoma usually remains localized to its subsites. Glottic spread is relatively late. This is because of anatomical/embryological barrier to downward spread of these tumours below ventricles. Tumour behaviour and spread is influenced by nature of the growth, i.e. exophytic or ulcerative. Supraglottic tumours with pushing margins are better differentiated, exophytic and less invasive. Exophytic tumours usually remain above the ventricle with fewer propensities for submucosal spread. On the other hand, ulcerative tumours have tendency for extension inferiorly to the anterior commissure, ventricle and thyroid cartilage. Thyroid cartilage involvement occurs through pre-epiglottic and paraglottic space spread. It predisposes to extralaryngeal spread.

Supraglottic carcinomas have frequent occult neck metastasis with high frequency for bilateral lymph node metastasis for lesions crossing midline. Regional metastasis occurs to level II, III and IV cervical lymph nodes.

1.6 Epiglottis Carcinoma

Suprahyoid epiglottic tumours spread to the vallecula and base of the tongue, whereas infrahyoid epiglottic carcinomas invade pre-epiglottic space through lacunae and may also involve the anterior glottis (Figs. 1.5 and 1.6).

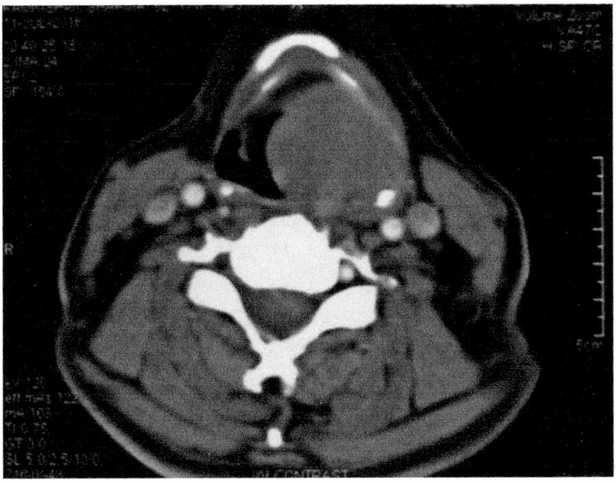

Fig. 1.5 CECT neck (axial cut) shows a bulky mildly enhancing tumour in the left side of epiglottis and aryepiglottic fold invading into the pre-epiglottic space and possible thyroid cartilage involvement

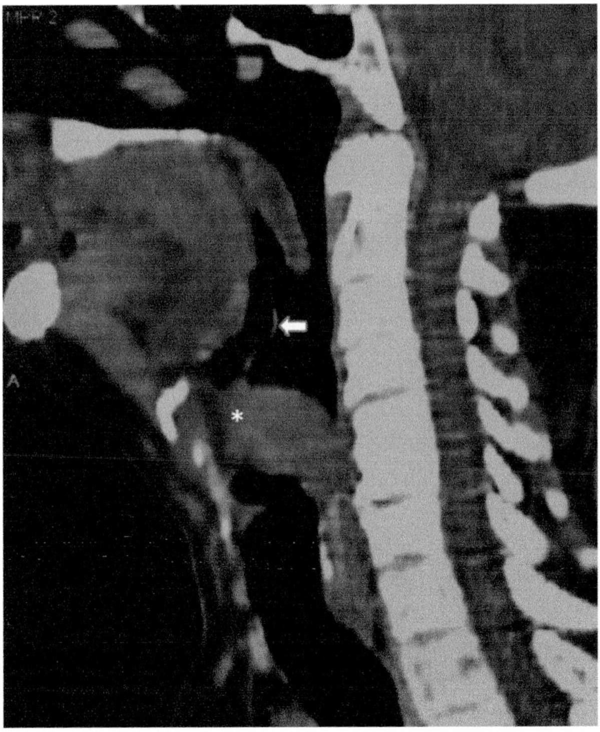

Fig. 1.6 CECT neck (sagittal cut) shows an enhancing tumour in the supraglottis arising from the infrahyoid epiglottis (arrow shows suprahyoid epiglottis) and infiltrating into the pre-epiglottic space through the epiglottis (*)

1.7 False Cord Carcinoma

Inferior spread is less common because of natural barrier by quadrangular membrane. It usually spreads upwards to the epiglottis, AE fold and arytenoid.

1.8 Ventricular Carcinoma

Ventricular carcinoma is usually transglottic at presentation, and pre-epiglottic space extension is more common.

1.9 Arytenoid and AE Fold Carcinoma

Tumours arising from these subsites usually extend to pyriform fossa sinus and post-cricoid area. Because of rich lymphatics, there is high incidence of bilateral occult lymph node metastasis.

1.10 Transglottic Carcinoma

Tumours, which cross the ventricle involving glottic and supraglottic region, are known as transglottic carcinoma. They are ventricular tumours that spread deeply upwards and downwards with relatively intact mucosa. They invade paraglottic space, lateral part of thyroid ala and cricothyroid membrane leading to extralaryngeal spread. Often there is very little mucosal involvement. Superficial biopsy may be negative for tumour and indicate the need for multiple deep biopsies from the ventricle for confirmation of malignancy.

1.11 Surgical Anatomy of Hypopharynx

The hypopharynx is a part of the pharynx which is funnel shaped with upper limit at the level of the floor of vallecula or hyoid bone and lower limit at the level of lower border of the cricoid cartilage. It is further divided into three subsites:

- Pyriform sinus
- Posterior pharyngeal wall
- Post-cricoid area

1.11.1 Pyriform Sinus (PFS)

PFS extends from the level of pharyngoepiglottic fold (PEF) to upper end of the oesophagus. The lateral wall of PFS is continuation of lateral pharyngeal wall. The medial wall is the lateral surface of aryepiglottic fold. AEF is the transitional zone from the supraglottic larynx to the hypopharynx and is also known as marginal zone. The apex of PFS is a narrow converging area situated at the level of the cricoid cartilage. PFS is bounded:

- Laterally: thyrohyoid membrane, thyroid cartilage
- Medially: hypopharyngeal surface of AEF, arytenoid and cricoid cartilages

1.11.2 Posterior Pharyngeal Wall

It extends from superior level of the hyoid bone to inferior border of the arytenoid cartilage and from the apex of one pyriform sinus to another pyriform sinus apex.

1.11.3 Post-cricoid Area (PCA)

PCA extends from level of arytenoid cartilages to inferior border of cricoid cartilages. It forms the anterior wall of hypopharynx. Inferiorly it becomes continuous with cervical oesophagus.

1.12 Pattern of Spread in Hypopharyngeal Cancers

1.12.1 Pattern of Spread in Pyriform Fossa Tumours

Tumours arising from the medial wall of the PFS can spread in the following patterns:

- Extend through AEF to invade paraglottic space and can fix the hemilarynx
- Extend into pre-epiglottic space
- Occasionally extend posteriorly into PCA leading cricoarytenoid joint fixation
  - Tumours arising from the lateral wall of the PFS can spread in the following patterns:
- Extend laterally through thyroid cartilage and through thyrohyoid membrane to produce palpable neck mass. It can be differentiated from neck node by its movement on deglutition. Tumour can involve carotid sheath and thyroid gland with extralaryngeal spread.
- Large tumour extends superiorly into the tongue base through PE ligament.

1.12.2 Pattern of Spread in Post-cricoid Area Tumours

PCA tumours extend downwards to the cervical oesophagus. Submucosal spread is commonly seen in this subsite. They usually spread circumferentially with dysphagia as a predominant symptom. Anteriorly tumour spread to involve party wall between the oesophagus and trachea. It also leads to recurrent laryngeal nerve involvement in trachea-oesophageal groove resulting in cord fixation. Laterally the tumour tends to involve the thyroid gland. Posterior spread into prevertebral muscles occurs following breach in the fascial barrier. Laryngeal crepitus (gritty sound on moving cricoid cartilage over vertebrae) becomes absent in PCA tumours. This is known as positive Boca's sign, which is indicative of PCA tumours or involvement of PCA, by other surrounding tumours.

1.12.3 Pattern of Spread in Posterior Pharyngeal Wall Tumours

Posterior pharyngeal wall tumours are relatively rare and usually involve prevertebral fascia. They attain large size before causing cord fixation. Nodal spread is bilateral into deep cervical nodes and retropharyngeal nodes.

1.13 Summary

Advancement in surgical refinements necessitates detailed knowledge of laryngeal and hypopharyngeal anatomy. Predetermined pathways help us to predict disease spread and design surgical plan especially in management of early laryngeal and hypopharyngeal cancers.

References

1. ICMR. Individual registry-wise annexure. In: Three-year report of population based cancer registries 2009–2011. Bangalore: National Cancer Registry Program (ICMR); 2013. p. 92–150.
2. Bobdey S, Jain A, Balasubramanium G. Epidemiological review of laryngeal cancer: an Indian prospective. Indian J Med PaediatrOncol. 2015;36:154–60.
3. Chadha S, Gupta B, Jatwani S, Gulati A. A study of patient factors and tumour characteristics in malignancy of larynx: a tertiary care centre experience. J Laryngol Voice. 2011;1:79–80.
4. Tyns AJ, Audigier JC. Double wave cohort increase for oesophageal and laryngeal cancer in France in relation to reduced alcohol consumption during second world war. Digestion. 1976;14:197–208.
5. Hashibe M, Brennan P, C Huang SC, et al. Interaction between tobacco and alcohol use and the risk of head and neck cancer: pooled analysis in the International Head and Neck Cancer Epidemiology Consortium. Cancer Epidemiol Biomarkers Prev. 2009;18:541–50.
6. Kapil U, Singh P, Bahadur S, et al. Assessment of risk factors in laryngeal cancer in India; A case control study. Asian Pacific J Cancer Prev. 2005;6:202–7.

Imaging in Carcinoma of the Larynx

2

Abhinav Jain and S. S. Anand

2.1 Overview

The advancements in cross-sectional imaging techniques have made pre- and post-surgical evaluation of carcinoma larynx more comprehensive and faster. Early diagnosis and treatment in laryngeal cancer not only impact the overall survival; it also augments the possibility of preserving voice and nasal respiration [1]. Clinical mirror examination and endoscopy are used to evaluate the larynx [2]. Integration of endoscopic findings with cross-sectional imaging, improves the T staging and precision which influences the treatment decisions in these patients. Imaging also contributes to information about the nodal disease, systemic metastases, any synchronous tumours and recurrent disease.

As with any cross-sectional technique, a comprehensive knowledge of laryngeal anatomy is crucial to understand the patterns of disease spread and the prognosis of laryngeal carcinoma. The next few images show labelled cross-sectional anatomy of the larynx as seen on CT scan, followed by brief description of normal anatomy and subsequent discussion of the disease spread and involvement of different anatomical divisions of the larynx (Figs. 2.1, 2.2, 2.3, 2.4, 2.5, 2.6, and 2.7).

A. Jain (✉) · S. S. Anand
Department of Radiodiagnosis, Hamdard Institute of Medical Sciences and Research, Jamia Hamdard, New Delhi, India

S. Bahadur et al. (eds.), *Carcinoma of the Larynx and Hypopharynx*,
https://doi.org/10.1007/978-981-13-3110-7_2

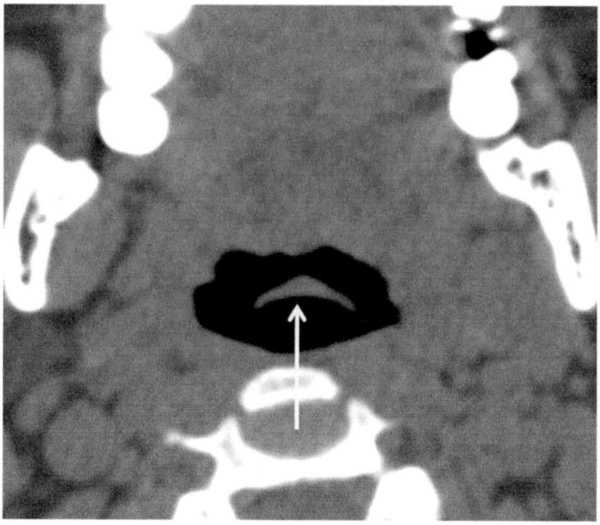

Fig. 2.1 Normal anatomy of the larynx on axial CT image of supraglottic region. The arrow shows the epiglottis in midline

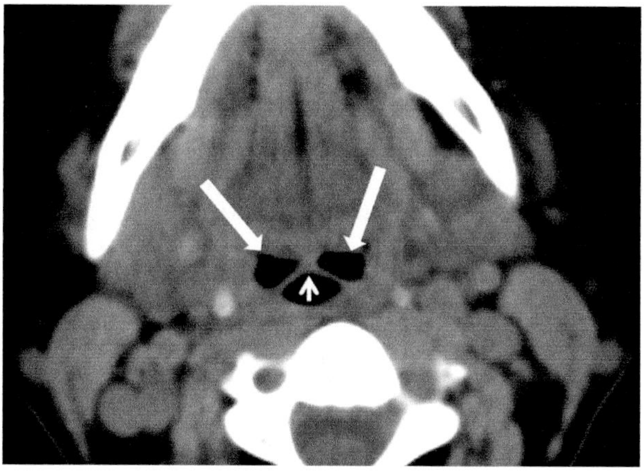

Fig. 2.2 Normal anatomy of the larynx on axial CT image of supraglottic region. The short arrow shows the epiglottis in midline. The long arrows show paired valleculae on either sides of hypoepiglottic ligament

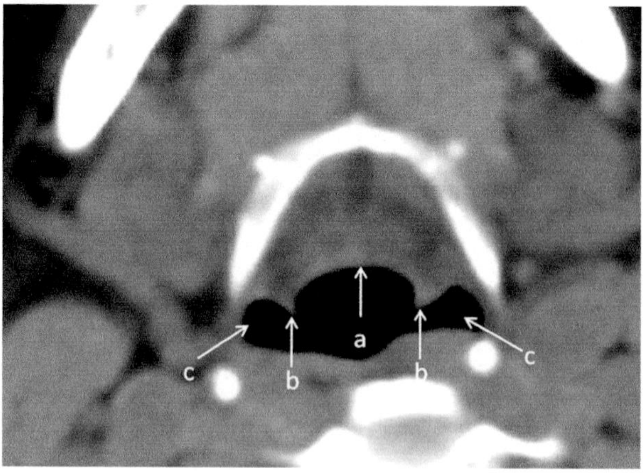

Fig. 2.3 Normal anatomy of the larynx on axial contrast CT image of supraglottic region. *a*, the epiglottis with space anterior to it representing pre-epiglottic space; *b*, aryepiglottic folds; and *c*, piriform sinus

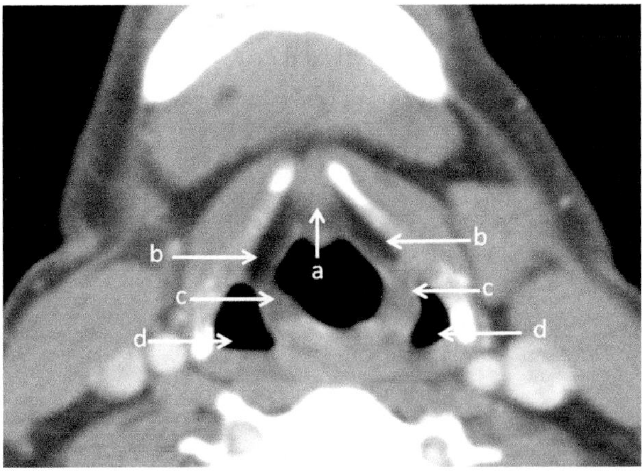

Fig. 2.4 Normal anatomy of the larynx on axial contrast CT image of supraglottic region. *a*, epiglottis attaching to the thyroid cartilage; *b*, paraglottic spaces; *c*, aryepiglottic folds; and *d*, piriform sinus

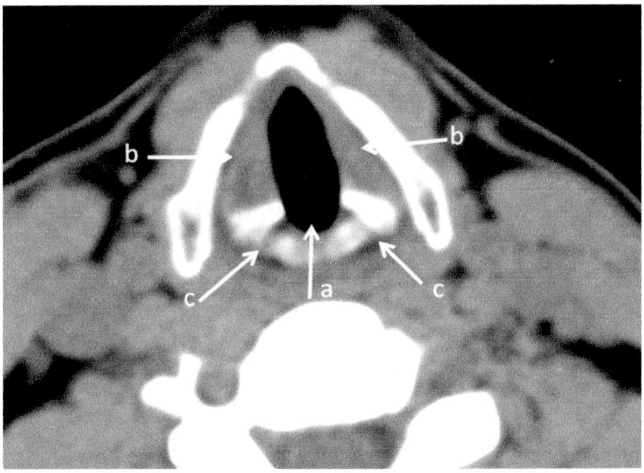

Fig. 2.5 Normal anatomy of the larynx on axial contrast CT image of glottic region. *a*, posterior commissure; *b*, vocal cords; and *c*, cricoarytenoid joints

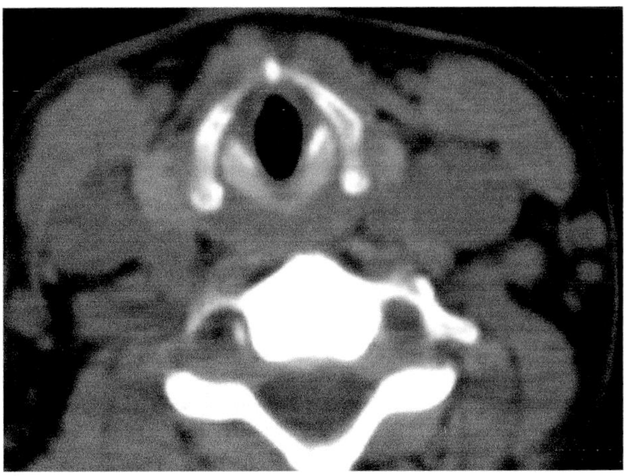

Fig. 2.6 Normal anatomy of the larynx on axial contrast CT images—subglottic region shows the cricoid ring

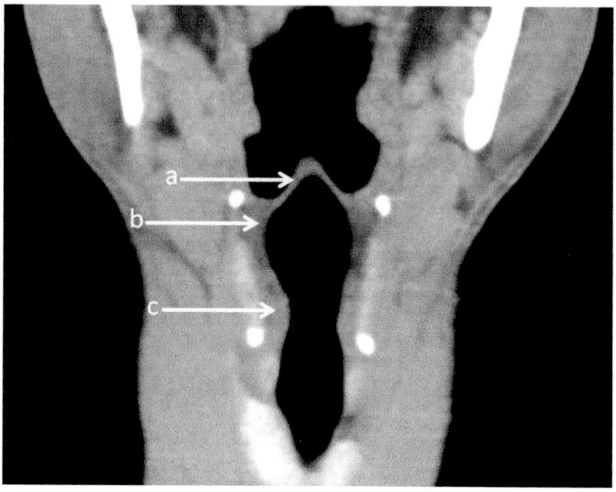

Fig. 2.7 Normal anatomy of the larynx. Coronal image shows the *a*, epiglottis; *b*, false cord; and *c*, true cord

2.2 Cartilages of the Larynx

On CT/MR scans the demarcation of glottic structures from supra- and subglottic structures is based on identification of the cricoarytenoid joint. The cartilaginous structures of the epiglottis, thyroid cartilage, arytenoid cartilage, and cricoid cartilage can be easily differentiated on imaging. The cricoid cartilage is the only intact ring of the larynx, having a complete posterior component. The inferior margin of the arytenoid cartilage with its vocal processes marks the border of the true vocal cord.

2.3 Spaces of the Larynx

MR imaging is highly effective (sensitivity, 100%; specificity, 84%; accuracy, 90%) for evaluating the pre-epiglottic space for tumour spread [3, 4].

The pre-epiglottic fat and paraglottic fat separate the paraglottic tissues. Therefore, on both CT scanning (where fat is dark) and T1-weighted MR imaging (where fat is bright), the separation of pre-epiglottic and paraglottic fat of the supraglottis can be discriminated from the muscular density (soft tissue on CT) or intensity (intermediate on T1-weighted MR imaging) of the thyroarytenoid muscle of the glottis. The differentiation between pre-epiglottic fat and paraglottic fat is pivotal from the standpoint of some of the T staging issues that require addressing the pre-epiglottic fat.

2.4 Muscles and Ligaments

Thyroarytenoid muscle makes the bulk of the true vocal cord.

An important obstacle to supraglottic and subglottic tumour spread is the conus-elasticus which is a membrane between the cricoid and cartilage that forms the free edge of the vocal cords.

2.5 Choice of Imaging Modality

2.5.1 Computed Tomography

Multislice CT allows the radiologist to evaluate almost all the relevant imaging concerns. A longitudinal field of view extends from the skull base to the sternoclavicular joints with the patient breathing quietly and not swallowing. It may be advantageous to perform an additional examination focused on the tumour with e-phonation (for better assessment of the laryngeal ventricle, anterior commissure and aryepiglottic folds) or modified valsalva (for better survey of the piriform sinus and post-cricoid regions) manoeuvres. In addition to soft tissue windows, the bone windows (reconstructed with a bony algorithm) should be routinely analysed if the tumour contacts ossified laryngeal cartilage. It should be ensured that axial images are reformatted in the plane of the larynx. Recent studies have explored the use of post-processing such as 'virtual endoscopy' which might be useful in evaluating features such as subglottic extension.

2.5.2 Magnetic Resonance Imaging

MRI is best performed with a high-field MRI scanner. An amalgamation of T2-w sequences with fat saturation, T1-w sequences and T1-w fat-saturated sequences with gadolinium should be used in axial and coronal planes. The sagittal plane is also fruitful to assess potential tongue base involvement. Patients are asked to refrain from coughing and swallowing during the acquisition and MRI may produce substandard results in the breathless or restless patient who is compromised by the tumour.

Since approach with both CT and MRI is acceptable, the choice in management depends on machine availability and local expertise as well as the ability of the patient to tolerate a prolonged MRI examination [5]. MR imaging is most commonly used if there is uncertainty in assessing cartilage involvement and when this is crucial for therapeutic decisions. It may also better delineate the margin between the tumour and thyroarytenoid muscle and involvement of the tongue base.

Ultrasound with FNA may be routinely used in some centres for the assessment of nodal metastasis. Although it may be used to visualise the anterior laryngeal structures, it is not sufficient for adequate primary tumour staging. Endolaryngeal high-frequency ultrasound has also been evaluated as a diagnostic tool [6].

2.5.3 Positron Emission Tomography (PET) and CT-PET

It may also be beneficial for the detection of recurrent tumour and in distinguishing this from post-radiotherapy change. A negative PET scan excludes recurrence with a high certainty. Positive PET scan findings should be assessed with biopsy and follow up PET imaging if this is negative. It should be noted that physiological uptake of [^{18}F]fluorodeoxyglucose ([^{18}F]FDG) is observed due to vocal cord activity, so a 'silent protocol' should be employed.

2.6 Key Imaging Considerations

2.6.1 Tumour Volume

One of the critical factors in determining tumour-free survival and/or local control by radiation is tumour volume. For this reason, many imaging centres perform volumetric analyses of all laryngeal carcinomas. CT is the most common modality used to compute volumes. Supraglottic tumours measuring less than 6 ml and T3 glottic tumours measuring less than 3.5 ml have been demonstrated to have improved local control following radiotherapy and surgery [7]. Although tumour volume is closely associated with T stage and other findings such as cartilage invasion, it does appear to act as an independent predictor of survival.

2.6.2 Relationship of the Tumour to the Ventricular Complex

A key component of the imaging assessment is to define the three anatomical sites of supraglottis, glottis and subglottis. In order to define the tumour as supraglottic, glottic or subglottic, the radiologist must determine the level of the ventricular complex (comprising the true cord, false cord and the intervening ventricle). The superior aspect of the ventricular complex is defined by the superior margin of the arytenoid cartilages. The false cords are seen at this level running parallel and superior to the true cords. The inferior aspect of the ventricular complex is defined by the true cords. This is located radiologically by identifying a transition of paraglottic fat to soft tissue in the wall of the larynx. This soft tissue represents the thyroarytenoid muscle which stretches from the arytenoid cartilages posteriorly to the thyroid cartilage anteriorly.

Transglottic is a term used to describe tumours encroaching on both glottis and supraglottis with or without subglottic components and when the site of origin is unclear (these usually develop from glottic tumours).

Imaging identification of transglottic extension is a further indicator that primary radiotherapy may fail. Transglottic extension by supraglottic carcinoma will contraindicate a supraglottic laryngectomy, transglottic extension by glottic carcinoma with contraindicate vertical hemilaryngectomy, whilst extension to the subglottis excludes all voice-conserving partial laryngeal surgery. Coronal reformats or scanning is helpful in the assessment of such infiltration, particularly if no 'normal' axial section is seen between the tumour and the soft tissue of the thyroarytenoid muscle.

2.6.3 Involvement of the Submucosal Spaces

The fatty C-shaped pre-epiglottic space is bounded anteriorly by the thyroid cartilage and thyrohyoid membrane and posteriorly by the epiglottis and quadrangular membrane. The fat and connective tissue within the paraglottic space is confined by the thyroid cartilage and cricothyroid membrane anterolaterally, inferomedially by the conuselasticus, superomedially by the ventricular complex or vestibule and posteriorly by the pyriform sinus.

An understanding of the pre-epiglottic and paraglottic spaces allows the radiologist to predict and identify patterns of tumour spread which have a critical impact on therapeutic decisions.

Epiglottic carcinoma may spread directly into the pre-epiglottic space through dehiscences in the epiglottic cartilage.

Paraglottic space involvement may occur secondary to glottic and supraglottic carcinoma. Paraglottic spread is also a key pathway for spread of false cord and aryepiglottic fold tumours.

CT and MRI are 88–93% accurate in the assessment of tumour extension within these spaces [8].

Pre-epiglottic fat encroachment upstages supraglottic tumour to T3 and increases the possibility of cervical nodal involvement. Substantial involvement reduces the possibility of local control and preservation of laryngeal function by radiotherapy alone. Bulky pre-epiglottic disease with potential involvement of the hyoid bone will contraindicate supraglottic and supracricoid laryngectomies and may necessitate the removal of a cuff of tongue base.

Supraglottic and glottic carcinomas with paraglottic invasion with or without minor cartilage invasion are staged T3 by the UICC sixth edition, and they represent a high-risk group for recurrence post-radiotherapy [9]. A glottic tumour invading deeply to the paraglottic fat usually precludes local laser resection or cordectomy. A supraglottic carcinoma infiltrating the paraglottic space inferiorly to ventricular level will preclude a supraglottic laryngectomy. It should prompt the radiologist to assess for piriform sinus, pre-epiglottic and extralaryngeal extension, which will further influence treatment decisions.

2.6.4 Anterior and Posterior Extension

This is particularly important at the level of the glottis.

Extension of laryngeal carcinoma (usually from anterior glottic carcinoma) to the anterior commissure is significant in that it is frequently associated with thyroid cartilage invasion, particularly if there is involvement of the base of epiglottis. The cartilage is prone to invasion at this site because the internal perichondrium is deficient and the external perichondrium is thinner. Tumour may also extend from the anterior commissure to an extralaryngeal location caudal to the thyroid cartilage (via the cricothyroid membrane) and inferiorly to the subglottis. These findings would preclude partial laryngectomy and upstage the tumour. Extension of glottic carcinoma across the midline to involve greater than one-third of the contralateral vocal cord would also contraindicate a vertical hemilaryngectomy. CT is 75% accurate in predicting anterior commissure involvement [10].

Posterior extension of glottic tumour to the interarytenoid region is important since it will preclude supracricoid laryngectomies and may be a precursor to post-cricoid pharyngeal extension. Such extension of laryngeal carcinoma to the pharynx or upper oesophageal segment will necessitate an additional pharyngeal resection with its associated morbidity.

2.6.5 Laryngeal Cartilage Invasion

The presence of significant laryngeal cartilage invasion has been considered a negative indicator for conservative therapeutic strategies such as primary modality radiotherapy or partial laryngectomy; however, recent studies have shown that tumours with limited cartilage involvement may be cured with radiotherapy. The laryngeal cartilage may be evaluated with CT or MRI. CT signs of erosion and extralaryngeal tumour of the thyroid, cricoid and arytenoid cartilages together with sclerosis of the cricoid and arytenoid cartilages result in a sensitivity of 64–72% and specificity of 86–94% for cartilage involvement [10]. Sclerosis is the most sensitive criterion, but this often corresponds to reactive inflammation, particularly with respect to the thyroid cartilage. MRI criteria for cartilage involvement by tumour are high signal on fat-suppressed T2-w images and/or enhancement on post-gadolinium fat-suppressed T1-w images in the cartilage adjacent to the tumour or the presence of extralaryngeal tumour.

MRI has a tendency to overestimate cartilage involvement by tumour since it may be indistinguishable from that due to peritumoural inflammation. These changes are most commonly seen in the thyroid cartilage so specificity is lowest at this location. New criteria of moderately high T2-w signal and moderate enhancement as compared to the marked signal changes and gadolinium enhancement with inflammation have been proposed to overcome this problem.

2.6.6 Nodal or Systemic Metastases and Synchronous Tumour

CT diagnosis of malignant lymph nodal involvement is primarily based on morphological assessment. Important factors are size criteria, loss of reniform shape (resulting in rounded nodes) and necrosis (central low attenuation and no enhancement on post contrast scan). The cutoff sizes vary for different levels of neck nodes. For level I and II, it is greater than or equal to 1.5 cm; for retropharyngeal nodes, the cutoff is 0.8 cm; and for all other neck nodes, it is 1 cm.

The prognosis of the squamous cell cancer largely depends on the nodal involvement, and therefore, it is essential to evaluate the common draining lymph nodes. Bilateral nodal disease downgrades favourable prognosis further by 25% from unilateral disease. Lymph nodal metastasis is common with supraglottic carcinoma and usually involves levels 2–4 [11]. In glottic tumours the nodal metastasis is rare. In subglottic disease prelaryngeal or Delphian nodes are first involved.

The major limitation with CT scan is smaller lymph nodes may also be harbouring the metastatic disease. PET-CT scores over the conventional CT scanning in evaluation of these lymph nodes. Multiple studies have shown significant increase in identifying the nodal disease with the help of FDG-PET [12, 13].

The lungs followed by the mediastinum, bones and liver are the most common sites for systemic metastases. Approximately 15% of patients with supraglottic carcinoma and 3% of patients with glottic carcinoma will develop distant metastases within 2 years of diagnosis. Carcinoma of the larynx is also characterised by a high incidence of second primary tumours, particularly in the setting of supraglottic carcinoma. The likelihood of metastases is low in patients with early-stage disease, and routine workup is generally with a chest radiograph. A CT chest may be appropriate in patients with more advanced T staging or in those with paratracheal nodal disease. CT-PET may play a greater role in the future with regard to screening for distant metastases, particularly in patients with recurrent disease.

2.7 Supraglottic Carcinoma

Supraglottic cancer is entirely above laryngeal ventricle. It may arise in the epiglottis, aryepiglottic folds, false vocal cords, pre-epiglottic or paraglottic fat. Supraglottic cancers are usually larger than glottis tumours at the time of diagnosis and present with enlarged cervical lymph nodes because these are usually asymptomatic as compared with the tumours involving the vocal cords.

The tumours originating from aryepiglottic fold can involve the epiglottis anteriorly or paraglottic space laterally. The epiglottis lesions can invade the pre-epiglottic space anteriorly and pharyngeal wall laterally. The tongue base may also be involved if the lesion spreads along the glossoepiglottic fold. The false vocal cord or laryngeal ventricle lesions may also spread into the paraglottic space. The advanced tumours can directly destroy the thyroid cartilage, glottis or subglottis.

Coronal images are helpful for evaluating craniocaudal extension, whereas sagittal and axial images best evaluate the pre-epiglottic space. The inferior margin of supraglottic tumours to assess the invasion of the laryngeal ventricles, arytenoid cartilages or the anterior commissure of the larynx is essential because this rules out supraglottic laryngectomy as treatment option (Figs. 2.8 and 2.9).

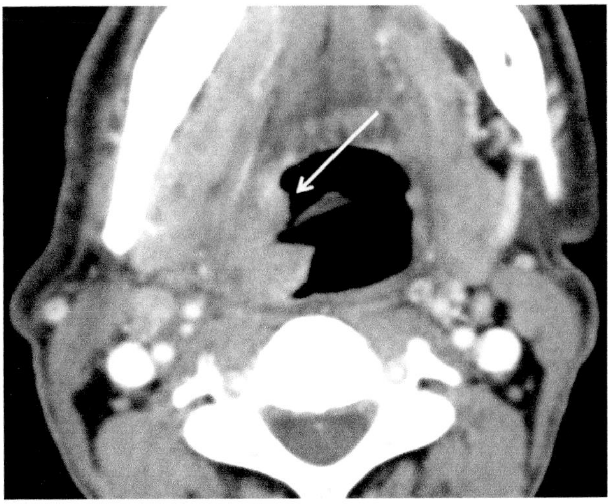

Fig. 2.8 Supraglottic squamous cell carcinoma: axial contrast CT image shows lobulated enhancing mass filling the right vallecula and extending in pre-epiglottic space

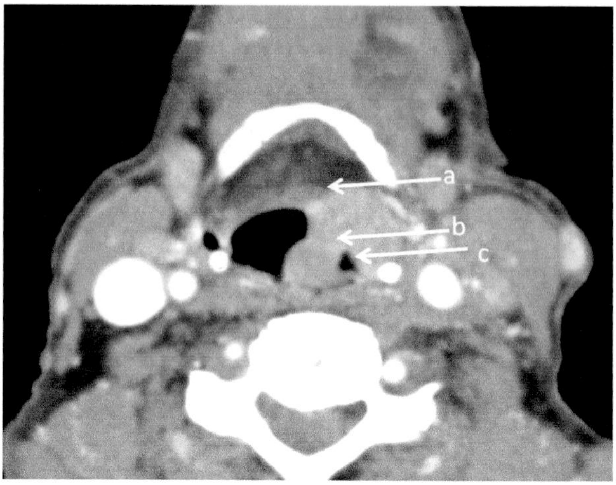

Fig. 2.9 Supraglottic squamous cell carcinoma: axial contrast CT image shows enhancing mass of the left aryepiglottic fold mass invading pre-epiglottic (*a*) and left paraglottic space (*b*) and narrowing of left pyriform sinus (*c*)

2.8 Glottic SCC

Glottis has poor lymphatic drainage and therefore nodal disease is uncommon. More so, patients with glottic disease present early with hoarseness of voice. Small-sized lesions might be difficult to detect on imaging. Early diagnosis is essential as T1 tumours carry a favourable prognosis with survival rates exceeding 90% [14].

The anterior commissure involvement is identified as soft tissue thickening greater than 1 mm. These tumours have tendency to spread to the contralateral cord. PET-CT also plays a pivotal role in diagnosis of opposite cord involvement. FDG uptake in opposite cord is highly suspicious of malignant spread. Anteriorly the thyroid cartilage, superiorly the paraglottic space and inferiorly the subglottis may be involved through the anterior commisure. Posterior commisure involvement may lead to invasion of arytenoid cartilage, cricoid cartilage or cricoarytenoid cartilage.

Coronal images are very helpful in evaluating the extension of tumour and determining whether there is transglottic spread 0 (cranial extension through the laryngeal ventricles) and/or subglottic extension. Such extensions denote T2 staging. Paraglottic and periglottic space invasion denote T3 staging. Tumours with hemilarynx fixation also denote T3 staging. Subglottic extension necessitates total laryngectomy (Fig. 2.10).

2.9 Subglottic SCC

Patients with subglottic cancer usually present with large masses and invasive disease because these tumours are clinically silent for long time. The nodal spread is uncommon, but the local invasion and surrounding soft tissue involvement results in poor prognosis.

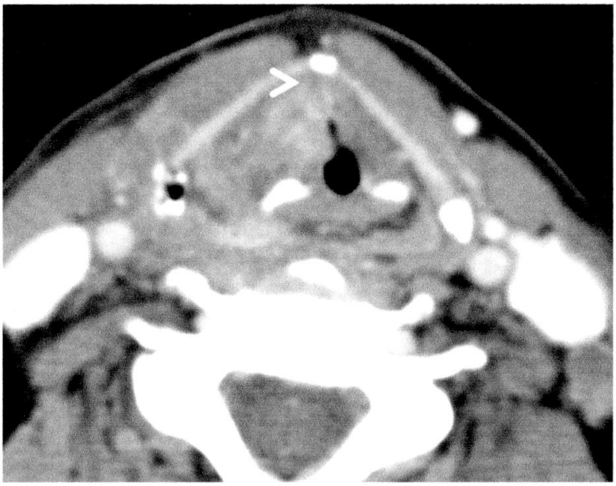

Fig. 2.10 Glottic SCC: axial CECT image shows a glottis mass involving right true vocal cord involving anterior commisure (arrow head)

Coronal images aid in evaluating craniocaudal extension and involvement of the true vocal cords. Since cricoid cartilage invasion upstages the primary tumour, close attention to its contour and density/signal is imperative.

The subglottic lesions may spread to true cords and supraglottis due to superior extension and the tracheal involvement by inferior extension, anteriorly through the cricothyroid membrane, the thyroid gland or posteriorly the cricoid cartilage and oesophagus.

Due to close apposition of the mucosa with the cricoid cartilage, any tissue seen in the airways should be graded as tumour invasion.

2.10 Post Treatment Imaging

Residual disease detection and early recurrence are main aims of imaging follow-up. It is crucial to differentiate the postsurgical anatomical distortion and residual disease. Also, the nodal involvement needs assessment. Direct laryngoscopy, although the reference standard for diagnosing the recurrent/residual disease, being invasive is not a preferred technique in follow-up cases. Also the nodal disease cannot be assessed with laryngoscopy. Especially in asymptomatic patients undergoing routine surveillance, a noninvasive technique is preferable.

Local recurrence is substantially high in patients with laryngeal carcinoma. The poor prognosis associated with these tumours is usually due to local recurrence. The accurate detection of the recurrent disease is cornerstone of imaging. This is because the local anatomy is usually distorted owing to tissue fibrosis, inflammatory changes and postsurgical clips creating streak artefacts in the region.

Out of CT, MRI, PET and PET-CT/MR, the FDG-PET-CT has been proven to be superior modality in detection of recurrent/residual disease in almost all head and neck cancers. This is due to ability of PET-CT to identify the lymph nodes below the morphological cutoff and supplementing differentiation of radiotherapy changes from recurrence. It is usually recommended that the FDG-PET-CT be advised after 2–3 months of radiotherapy and 4–8 weeks after chemotherapy to allow inflammatory changes to subside [15].

As the lungs are the most common sites of metastatic disease, for the evaluation of low-stage laryngeal malignancy, chest radiograph are sufficient. For higher-stage disease, CECT is necessary; for other suspicious regions, PET-CT is necessary.

2.11 Conclusion

Cross-sectional imaging is essential in imaging laryngeal malignancy. It provides accurate assessment of the locoregional extent of disease and thus planning the operative roadmap of the treatment and prognostication of outcome. PET-CT/MRI are the cornerstone to evaluate the recurrent/residual disease and metastatic disease.

References

1. Issa MR, Samuels SE, Bellile E, Shalabi FL, Eisbruch A, Wolf G. Tumor volumes and prognosis in laryngeal cancer. Cancers. 2015;7(4):2236–61.
2. Sulica L. Laryngoscopy, stroboscopy and other tools for the evaluation of voice disorders. Otolaryngol Clin North Am. 2013;46(1):21–30.
3. Loevner LA, Yousem DM, Montone KT, Weber R, Chalian AA, Weinstein GS. Can radiologists accurately predict PES invasion with MR imaging? AJR Am J Roentgenol. 1997;169:1681–7.
4. Zbaren P, Becker M, Läng H. Pretherapeutic staging of laryngeal carcinoma: clinical findings, CT and MRI with histopathology. Cancer. 1996;77:1263–73.
5. Becker M, Burkhardt K, Dulguerov P, Allal A. Imaging of the larynx and the hypopharynx. Eur J Radiol. 2008;66:460–79.
6. Caddy GR, Chen RY. Current clinical applications of endoscopic ultrasound. ANZ J Surg. 2007;77:101–11.
7. Connor S. Laryngeal cancer: how does the radiologist help? Cancer Imaging. 2007;7(1):93–103.
8. Wu J-H, et al. Comparison of CT and MRI in diagnosis of laryngeal carcinoma with anterior vocal commissure involvement. Sci Rep. 2016;6:30353. *PMC*. Web. 10 May 2018.
9. American Joint Committee on Cancer. Cancer staging handbook. 6th ed. New York: Springer; 2002.
10. Joshi VM, Wadhwa V, Mukherji SK. Imaging in laryngeal cancers. Indian J Radiol Imaging. 2012;22(3):209–26.
11. Sheahan P. Management of advanced laryngeal cancer. Rambam Maimonides Med J. 2014;5(2):e0015.
12. Curtin HD. The larynx. In: Som PM, Curtin HD, editors. Head and neck imaging. 4 th ed. St Louis: Mosby; 2003. p. 1595–699.
13. Mukherji SK, Bradford CR. Controversies: is there a role for positron-emission tomographic CT in the initial staging of head and neck squamous cell carcinoma? AJNR Am J Neuroradiol. 2006;27(2):243–5.
14. Zhang S-Y, et al. Retrospective analysis of prognostic factors in 205 patients with laryngeal squamous cell carcinoma who underwent surgical treatment. PLoS One. 2013;8(4):e60157.
15. Chu MM, Kositwattanarerk A, Lee DJ, Makkar JS, Genden EM, Kao J, et al. FDG PET with contrast enhanced CT: a critical imaging tool for laryngeal carcinoma. Radiographics. 2010;30:1353–72.

Diagnosis, Assessment and Staging of Carcinoma of the Larynx

3

Sudhir Bahadur and Junaid Malik

3.1 Introduction

Detailed assessment and staging of carcinoma of the larynx is mandatory as this will impact the treatment protocol. Decision-making is often complex and demanding. It is useful to remember that in most patients, the disease is resectable and treatable but not all are curable.

It is important that all patients are worked up in detail with clinical, radiological and endoscopic work-up and are biopsy proven. The inputs thus arrived at are discussed in the combined tumour clinic consisting of a surgeon, a radiation oncologist and a medical oncologist. The first step to decide is whether the treatment planned for the patient is curative or palliative. A patient with obvious unresectable disease or even with advanced but resectable disease with poor general condition may be treated with palliative intent.

However, if the decision is to treat the patient with curative effort, then the next question will be how? For early and intermediate stage, it is usually possible to offer treatment strategies which offer both cure and organ preservation. In advanced disease, though, curative treatment often involves a total laryngectomy with its sufficient morbidity and disability. Either way the decision is communicated to the patient in a simple manner which he can understand well. Also, the implications of treatment including the morbidity and likely cure rates should be explained.

S. Bahadur (✉)
Department of Otolaryngology and Head-Neck Surgery, Formerly at All India Institute of Medical Sciences, New Delhi, India

J. Malik
Department of Otolaryngology and Head-Neck Surgery, Hamdard Institute of Medical Sciences and Research, Jamia Hamdard, New Delhi, India

S. Bahadur et al. (eds.), *Carcinoma of the Larynx and Hypopharynx*,
https://doi.org/10.1007/978-981-13-3110-7_3

3.2 Clinical Evaluation

3.2.1 Age

In younger patients long-term curative effort and quality of life are both extremely important. Also, professional status of the patient is taken into account while planning treatment. Elderly patients may have, on the other hand, significant co-morbidities which may impact the prognosis [1]. These are also less likely to be suitably rehabilitated. Besides, patients above 70 years of age are usually not good candidates for chemoradiation treatment.

3.2.2 Related History

The clinical symptoms include features of primary tumour, metastatic disease and general effects of malignant process. History taking is no different in a cancer patient than with other medical or surgical conditions.

Usually the chief symptom of carcinoma of the larynx is hoarseness. It is persistent and may progressively become worse with increasing size of the tumour and may also result in stridor—stridor may also be a feature of bulky supraglottic tumours overhanging the laryngeal inlet. Aspiration of liquids may be another symptom with fixity of the hemilarynx. Both the stridor and aspiration are indicators of laryngeal dysfunction and are predictors of poor response to larynx preservation techniques with chemoradiation.

A majority of supraglottic tumours present with cervical node metastasis, and thus a neck mass may be a presenting symptom. Other features may include progressive difficulty in swallowing, weight loss and otalgia. However, dysphagia is associated more often with hypopharyngeal cancers.

3.2.3 Personal History (Risk Factors)

It is important to note the association of risk factors such as tobacco and alcohol consumption. It is useful to quantify the amount of tobacco and alcohol used daily and note the duration for which these have been consumed.

Similarly, it is important to note the presence of associated co-morbidity like diabetes and ischaemic heart disease which are likely to impact the prognosis as well as the recovery phase following surgery. Besides, conditions which are likely to affect the anaesthesia or surgery such as bleeding disorders or the use of anticoagulants and aspirin, etc. should be recorded.

History of the previous treatment should be noted in detail including the prior radiotherapy or surgery. Lastly, taking the psychosocial history is important.

Table 3.1 Eastern Cooperative Oncology Group (ECOG scale)

Grade	description
0	Fully active. Able to carry out all pre-disease activities without restriction (Karnofsky 90–100)
1	Restricted in physical strenuous activity, but ambulatory and able to carry out work of a light or sedentary nature (Karnofsky 70–80)
2	Ambulatory and capable of self-care but unable to carry out any work activities up and about 50% of waking hours (Karnofsky 50–60)
3	Capable of only limited self-care, confined to bed or chair 50% or more of waking hours (Karnofsky 30–40)
4	Completely disabled. Cannot carry out self-care (totally confined to bed or chair (Karnofsky 10–20)

3.2.4 General Physical Examination

It is always useful to note the general condition of the patient by using one of the methods of measuring performance status such as the Eastern Cooperative Oncology Group (ECOG) or the Karnofsky status (Table 3.1) [2]. These parameters can guide the treatment strategy, e.g. a patient with poor Karnofsky's scale may not be a good candidate for curative treatment with radical surgery and/or chemoradiation.

Systemic examination should include assessment of the chest and abdomen.

3.2.5 Examination of the Neck

Careful examination of the neck is essential to note any evidence of laryngeal enlargement (widening), presence or absence of post-cricoid crepitus and presence of neck node metastasis. The laryngeal enlargement suggests advanced disease (T_4), probably because of thyroid cartilage involvement. Similarly, the absence of post-cricoid crepitus may indicate post-cricoid tumour.

It is well known that the presence of clinically palpable neck node metastasis lowers the prognosis significantly, and it is therefore essential to assess the neck (N stage). The neck should be examined standing behind the patient, one side at a time, palpating systematically the different levels of nodes (levels I–V). The examination of the neck may be more difficult in fat patients or in those who have received previous radiotherapy or surgery.

3.2.6 Clinical Examination of the Larynx

In patients presenting with hoarseness or difficulty in swallowing, careful examination of the larynx is essential. An indirect laryngoscopy is usually carried out in the outpatient clinic (Figs. 3.1 and 3.2).

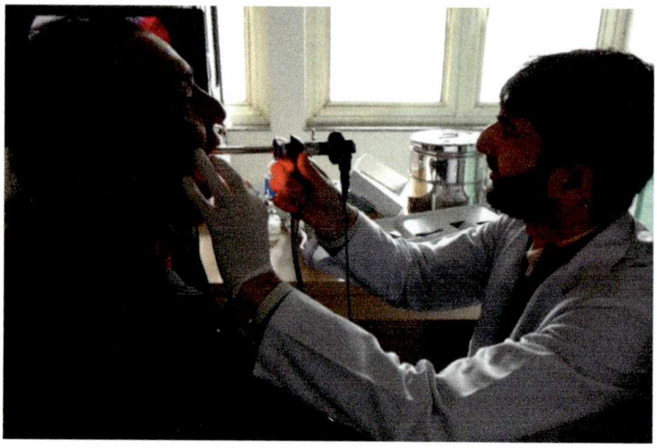

Fig. 3.1 Endoscopic examination with 90° rigid telescope

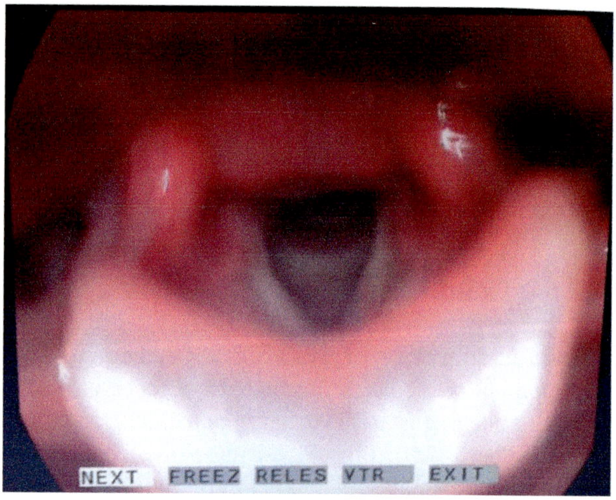

Fig. 3.2 Telescopic view of the larynx

The precise location of the lesion, its extension to the adjacent subsites, vocal cord mobility and stage of disease (T stage) are carefully noted and mapped with the help of a diagram. Indirect laryngoscopy has some limitations including the perceptional errors, learning curve and skills [3, 4]. However, indirect laryngoscopy is usually complemented by the use of 70° or 90° telescopes and/or flexible fibre-optic nasolaryngoscopy.

Endoscopic assessment either with a rigid or flexible laryngoscope has supplanted the mirrors due to better optical resolution and higher sensitivity [5, 6]. The rigid Hopkins rod system uses 70°- or 90°-angled lenses and allows an excellent view of the larynx through a transoral approach. The advantage of flexible fibre-optic laryngoscope is better visualization of base of the tongue, pyriform fossa and the larynx. Assessment of vocal cord mobility is categorized as mobile, impaired mobility or fixed.

Flexible endoscopes are expensive and relatively fragile instruments. They require care, maintenance and regular cleaning. Likewise, documentation and sterilization are important aspects. Disposable sheaths have been introduced to reduce the necessity of formal sterilization between the procedures. These have been shown to be effective in acting as a barrier to infection and protect the tips from damage and preserve the image quality [7–9].

Hopkins telescope should be used in order to comprehensively examine the laryngeal subsites. This can be coupled to video camera system to allow accurate recording of the primary tumour. The lesion can also be digitally recorded and reproduced later once the telescope is linked to the camera. The system thus helps the tumour clinic discussion in arriving at decision-making for treatment protocol.

Videostroboscopy, though not essential, may have a role in assessment of early lesions before planning partial laryngectomy. Another advantage of this instrument is that intra-laryngeal detail can be recorded and the subtle changes in vocal cord mobility can be appreciated better.

3.3 Clinical TNM Staging

It is important that following complete clinical evaluation, the disease should be staged according to TNM classification, describing the primary tumour, nodal metastasis (N stage) and any obvious evidence of distant metastasis. The clinical evaluation shall be later complemented by doing the radiological and endoscopic work-up.

3.3.1 Radiology

All patients should have an X-ray of the chest carried out to exclude evidence of distant metastasis and any other pulmonary pathology. If need be, it may be worthwhile ordering for CT of the chest. A plain soft tissue lateral neck may show increased distance between the cervical spine and the trachea suggesting the possibility of a post-cricoid tumour and Ba swallow may show a filling defect.

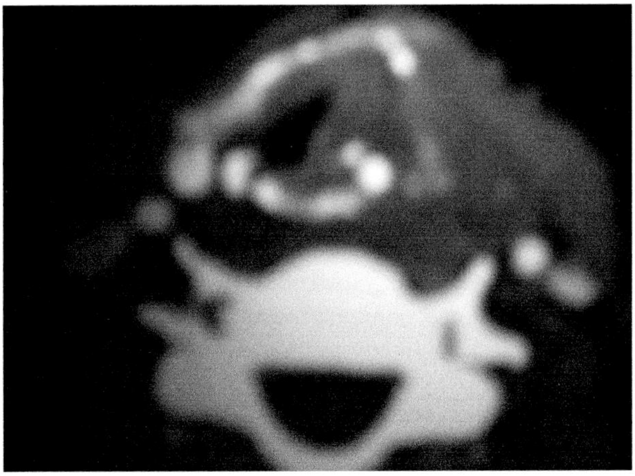

Fig. 3.3 CT of the larynx showing cartilage destruction

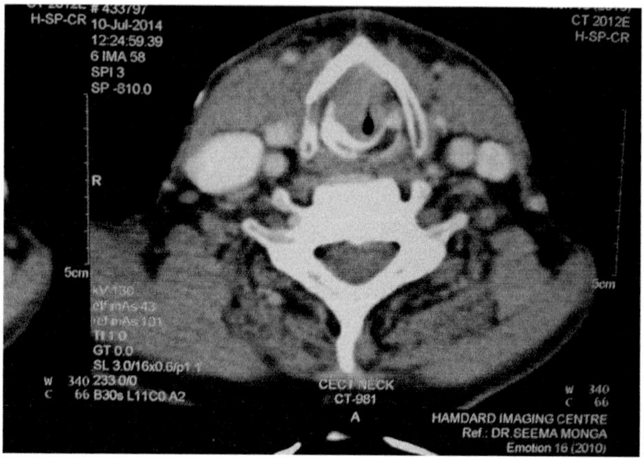

Fig. 3.4 CT scan of the larynx showing T_3 transglottic lesion

In order to further assess the primary neoplasm in the larynx or in the hypopharynx, it is important to carry out CECT of the neck. It helps to note the tumour extent and staging and helps in planning the treatment protocol. If cartilage invasion is seen on the CT scan (Fig. 3.3), it will be obviously better to consider such a patient for surgery than for organ preservation protocol using chemoradiation. The imaging techniques are extremely useful not only for advanced disease but also in assessment of early disease status in the paraglottic and pre-epiglottic spaces, anterior commissure and subglottic involvement (Fig. 3.4).

Whether CT scan should be done or the MRI, it is a subject of debate, but both are complementary to each other. MRI may also be valuable in patients of poor renal functions when intravenous contrast cannot be administered.

3.4 Direct Laryngoscopy (Microlaryngoscopy)

Once the lesion is identified in the larynx, it is mandatory to assess and stage the disease and to take biopsy, under general anaesthesia. However, it is important to assess the patient's fitness for anaesthesia beforehand by carrying out chest X-ray, electrocardiograms (ECG), full blood count, liver function tests, blood urea and sugar tests.

If on clinical examination of the larynx, the patient is found to have advanced disease causing obstruction to the airway, it may be brought to the notice of the anaesthetist for the possibility of performing the tracheostomy beforehand.

The microlaryngoscopy requires proper-size cuffed endotracheal tube for anaesthesia; proper instrumentation including the different size of rigid endoscopes and operating microscope. However, if transoral laser microsurgery is planned, specifically designed non-combustible non-reflective laser tubes are used. These have indicator dyes incorporated into the cuff to identify if it is damaged, in order to reduce the risk of airway fire hazard [10–14]. Direct laryngoscopy using a Jackson or Negus laryngoscope can help in assessment of the extent of tumour and to obtain a biopsy by lifting the larynx off the posterior pharyngeal wall mucosa.

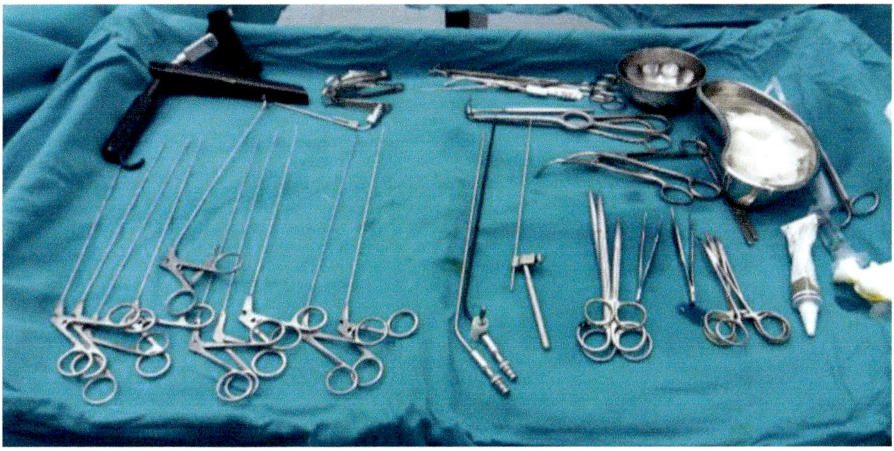

Fig. 3.5 Trolley of microlaryngeal instruments

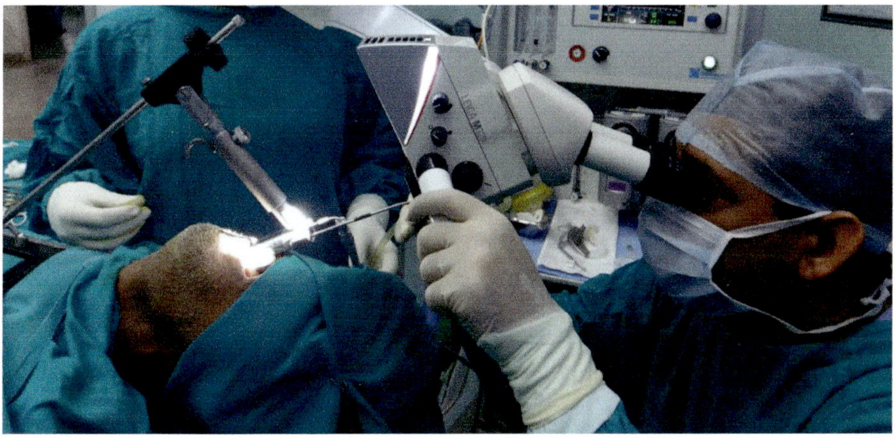

Fig. 3.6 Microlaryngoscopic procedure in progress

Microlaryngoscopy performed under general anaesthesia using a suspension laryngoscope is the standard procedure for diagnosis and endoscopic treatment for early laryngeal cancer and its precursor lesions (Figs. 3.5, 3.6, 3.7 and 3.8). However, it alone may not always assess epithelial dysplasias and carcinoma with precise delineation.

The primary tumour should be carefully assessed with regards to precise location, extension into adjacent structures and subsites and staging noted. All the three subsites of the larynx, i.e. supraglottis, glottis and subglottis, are examined. The ventricle, anterior commissure, laryngeal surface of epiglottis and false cord are sometimes difficult to assess for disease extension. Similarly, assessment of surrounding structures like pyriform fossa, post-cricoid region, postpharyngeal wall

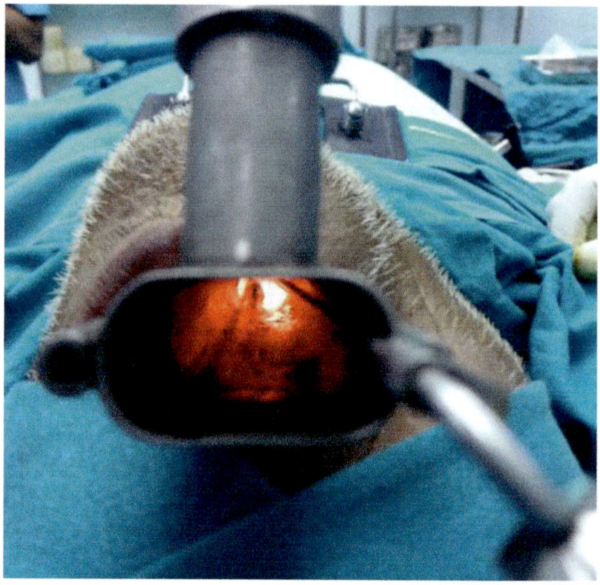

Fig. 3.7 Use of suspension laryngoscope

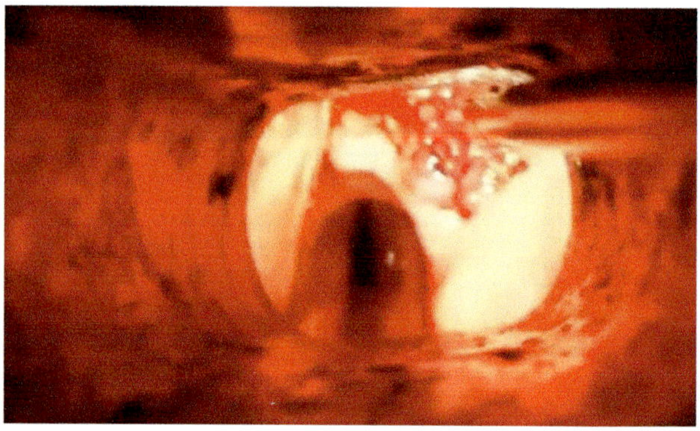

Fig. 3.8 Microlaryngoscopic view of the larynx

and base of the tongue should be undertaken. Vocal cord mobility and patency of the airway should be recorded, and a diagram may also be drawn. Similarly, photo-documentation is also useful.

3.4.1 Staging of Laryngeal Cancer

The basic premise of tumour staging is that disease progression takes place with expansion and invasion into the adjacent structures by the primary neoplasm (T). This is followed by the spread of disease into the regional lymph nodes (N) and further spread beyond the nodes to the distant metastatic sites (M).

The tumour staging is designed to mention the extent of disease and prognosis. Besides it is extremely useful in treatment planning and comparison of results following therapy either at the same centre or between different centres. Two principal staging systems of the AJCC and the UICC have in recent years come closer to each other and for practical purposes have become identical. Clinical classification (CTNM) is the pretreatment staging based on clinical evaluation, radiological assessment and endoscopy (and biopsy).

An important factor to determine the treatment planning in carcinoma of the larynx is accurate tumour staging prior to therapy. The limitations of clinical and endoscopic assessment are well known [15–17]. These two result in low staging accuracy [18] (57.5%). The anterior commissure and subglottic region can be difficult to assess because of bulky tumours. Besides, tumour extension into the pre-epiglottic space and paraglottic space, cartilaginous skeleton and extra-laryngeal structures cannot be evaluated by clinical examination or endoscopy.

Since the 1970s computed tomography (CT scan) has become an important adjunct to pre-therapy assessment of carcinoma of the larynx [18–20]. However, CT of the larynx has limitations, particularly in assessing cartilage invasion, due to irregular mix of calcified, ossified and non-calcified cartilage [21–23].

Magnetic resonance imaging (MRI) has proved to be a better method for evaluation of tumour stage. It is suggested that MRI is more suitable than CT in predicting the cartilage involvement by the tumour [24–26]. MRI is more sensitive but less specific than CT in detecting cartilage invasion. The combination of clinical/endoscopic evaluation and an additional examination, either CT or MR imaging, has significantly improved staging accuracy (80% vs 87%) [17, 18]. Few studies have even compared MRI findings with the histology of whole organ studies [22–25]. There are no statistical differences noted between CT and MRI in detecting cartilage invasion; the high false-positive rate of MRI may sometimes result in overtreatment in the form of total laryngectomy [17].

However, gross extra-laryngeal spread combined with extensive cartilage penetration and destruction is reasonable criteria for considering primary laryngectomy, particularly if pretreatment aspiration is already present [26].

It is also known that pathologically proven extra-laryngeal spread without thyroid cartilage penetration can occur in a significant number of cases underlying the importance of extra-laryngeal spread by alternate routes.

3.4.2 The Neck Nodal Metastasis (N Staging)

Detection of cervical lymph node metastasis is an important prognostic factor in patients with head and neck cancer as it is associated with the risk of distant metastasis [27]. Nodal size, shape, presence of central necrosis and possible extracapsular spread of disease are considered important parameters for detecting metastatic neck disease on MRI. It has been shown that minimal axial diameter of 7 mm for level II and 6 mm for all other levels should be considered significant lymphadenopathy [28]. However, the current morphologic parameters permit the detection of large node with central necrosis or extracepsular spread on the MRI, but it is not considered reliable for detecting micrometastasis in the neck nodes.

The lymph nodes mass over 3 cm are usually not single nodes but are confluent nodes or tumour in the soft tissues. The lymph nodes are grouped into seven levels. The pattern of lymphatic drainage varies for different anatomic sites. When primary tumour is located in the larynx and hypopharynx, the lymphatic drainage occurs usually into nodes at levels II, III and IV. However, lower level of lymph node involvement, increasing size of the node, number of nodes involved and extracapsular spread of disease indicate adverse prognostic significance.

There is some doubt about the reliability of clinical evaluation of the neck nodes particularly in patients with thick neck tissues or previously irradiated neck and whether the palpable nodes always harbour the metastatic foci. However, in large majority of patients, there is consistency between clinical positivity and final histopathology.

3.4.3 Pathological Staging (PTNM)

This is the most accurate staging regarding excised primary tumour and neck dissection status which would guide the postoperative adjuvant treatment.

3.4.4 Distant Metastasis (M) Staging

It is important to exclude presence of distant metastases before contemplating curative treatment for a patient. The presence or absence of distant metastases is indicated by M_1 or M_0, respectively. Incidence of distant metastases is lower in carcinoma of the larynx, accounting for nearly 7% of all patients with negative neck and 50% in patients with three positive nodes [27]. However, whenever it occurs it is usually in the lungs, liver, bones and brain and occasionally in the form of cutaneous nodules.

3.5 Recent Update in Early Diagnosis

There is increasing realization that diagnosis of laryngeal cancer is often delayed until the disease is far advanced. Often the early changes are not appreciated and diagnosed. There is evidence in recent literature to suggest that contact endoscopy, fluorescence endoscopy and endoscopy using high-frequency ultrasound can complement the microlaryngoscopic findings to diagnose the different stages of dysplasia, carcinoma in situ and early cancers of the larynx.

3.5.1 Contact Endoscopy and MLS

The new technique allows for microscopic assessment of epithelial cells in vivo and in situ. The process involves staining the epithelium with methylene blue or Lugol's iodine. A modified Hopkins rod telescope is applied against the mucosa of the larynx at magnification of ×60 and ×150, and cytological characteristics of cells, nuclei and cytoplasm can be appreciated [29, 30]. Premalignant changes such as dysplasia may also be noted. Preliminary studies show good correlation between cytological changes occurring in the epithelium from normal to disease and final histopathology.

3.6 Fluorescence Endoscopy

Fluorescence endoscopy has been found to be effective in the diagnosis of early laryngeal cancer and its precursor lesions. In this respect non-induced, i.e. autofluorescence endoscopy (AFE), and induced fluorescence endoscopy (IFE) show promising new imaging techniques [31]. Both AFE and IFE can be equally applied to the primary detection of these lesions showing better evaluation of the horizontal extension. Overall AFE is more useful, whereas IFE is more suited for assessment of recurrent disease. However, fluorescence endoscopy should be combined with white light illumination.

Both AFE and IFE can be useful to guided biopsy and surgical resection. Besides, it is also useful as follow-up of precancerous lesions and assessment for any recurrences.

In AFE, healthy laryngeal mucosa and benign lesions present a green colour. Precancerous lesion from severe dysplasia upwards displays red-violet colour (marked loss of autofluorescence). The ulcerated tumours may lead to yellow-orange colour.

Arens et al. [32] examined patients in different stages of laryngeal dysplasia, carcinoma in situ and laryngeal cancer by means of imaging techniques during microlaryngoscopy (autofluorescence endoscopy) or contact endoscopy high-frequency ultrasound, and results were compared to histology. In autofluorescence endoscopy, laryngeal mucosa was illuminated using blue-filtered light (380–460 nm) to obtain autofluorescence of optical demarcation of the lesion.

Precancerous and cancerous lesions show a red to violet fluorescence outlined against the light-green autofluorescence of the normal. The endoscopic high-frequency ultrasound examination is performed after flooding the larynx with 0.9% saline. The ultrasound catheters with frequencies between 10 and 20 MH_3 are inserted in the laryngeal lumen and moved in a standardized pattern. This is able to measure the vertical extension of laryngeal carcinoma bigger than 3 mm [30]. These authors concluded that *autofluorescence contact endoscopy* and *endoscopy high-frequency ultrasound* are promising new imaging techniques which supplement microlaryngoscopy. Autofluorescence along with contact endoscopy are suitable to differentiate dysplasia, carcinoma in situ and microinvasive lesion and at the same time can evaluate tumour margins. Ultrasound improves the assessment of tumour infiltration into the depth. These imaging techniques enable the surgeon to perform a more accurate diagnostic work-up.

Similar views were observed by Zargi et al. [33] who showed autofluorescence can be useful complement to microlaryngoscopy for detecting early lesions of larynx.

3.6.1 Narrow-Band Imaging

The value of laryngoscopy using narrow-band imaging (NBI) system in the diagnosis of precancerous and cancerous lesions of the larynx has been highlighted by several authors. Watanabe et al. [34] studied patients who underwent laryngoscopy with NBI system to determine whether the lesions were malignant before biopsy. The diagnostic criteria of malignancy by NBI view were the presence of demarcated brown spots in the lesion. Sensitivity and specificity for the diagnosis of malignancy by means of NBI view compared with histopathology were 91.3% sensitivity and 91.6% for specificity.

3.7 Author's Comments

Careful history taking in a patient suspected to have lesion in the larynx is important. Detailed assessment of the primary neoplasm as well as the neck node status both clinically and radiologically is extremely important to stage the disease (TNM) and plan the treatment. Besides, several other factors concerning the tumour location, its extension and those concerning the patient (age, general condition, co-morbidity, preference, etc.) and physician (availability of facilities and expertise) need to be considered. A variety of Hopkins telescopes and flexible fibre-optic endoscopes are available and should be used to supplement indirect laryngoscopy findings. Similarly, the recent literature highlights the usefulness of contact endoscopy, fluorescence endoscopy and endoscopy using high-frequency ultrasound findings to diagnose various stages of dysplasia, carcinoma in situ and early cancers of the larynx.

Index of suspicion for diagnosis and patient selection for specific treatment protocol are two key areas in successful management of carcinoma of the larynx. Radiology (CT scan/MRI) can help a great deal in staging and selecting a patient for either organ preservation protocol or surgical ablation.

3.8 Follow-Up

It is extremely important to follow up all the treated cases of carcinoma of the larynx and hypopharynx in the combined tumour clinic. First follow-up meeting with the patient may be 2 weeks after his discharge from the hospital after surgery. But the subsequent visits should be at monthly intervals in the first year, at two monthly interval in the second year and at three monthly interval in the third year, and later he may be seen after every 6 months. Following are the reasons why regular follow-up should be maintained.

(a) To initiate postoperative adjuvant treatment of radiotherapy or chemoradiotherapy in some patients based on final histopathology suggesting adverse prognostic factors.
(b) To monitor and reassure the disease-free status of the patients and to educate them regularly about the importance of stopping tobacco intake.
(c) Rehabilitation: Regular follow-up following treatment gives an opportunity to rehabilitate the patient with regard to speech and swallowing. If the patient is trying to learn oesophageal speech, he would require help from a professional speech therapist. In the meantime he also requires assurance that he may be able to go back to his job.

    If tracheoesophageal prosthesis has been performed at the time of surgery, the patient has to be educated about the maintenance and care of the prosthesis. Similarly, if the latter needs to be changed because of leakage of fluids or fungal infection, the otolaryngologist can suggest accordingly.
(d) Quality of life: To diagnose treatable morbidity like dental decay and hypothyroidism which would improve the quality of life of the patients.
(e) Research Tool: The follow-up clinic and the records also serve as a teaching guide for the residents of different subspecialities. Besides, patient data can be stored and used later for research purposes.
(f) Regular follow-up also ensures early detection of any local or regional or systemic recurrence of disease and some of which can still be salvaged with potential cure.

3.9 Role of Radiology (Follow-Up)

It is important to have an X-ray of the chest carried out at least once a year or even earlier if need be. Similarly, CT scan or preferably MRI may be asked for if clinical features suggest the possibility of residual or recurrent disease either at the primary or regional site or both. In post-irradiated cases it is more difficult to assess the disease status clinically, and MRI is more useful in such situations. Role of PET scan or diffusion-weighted MRI in monitoring the follow-up cases is increasingly receiving more attention in situations where deep invasive cancer is accompanied by laryngeal oedema [35]. Diffusion-weighted magnetic resonance imaging (DW-MRI) has been introduced recently and appears to be more specific than FDG PET in detection of residual or recurrent tumour after initial treatment with radiotherapy or chemoradiotherapy [36] (Table 3.2).

Table 3.2 TNM classification of laryngeal cancer

Larynx	
	Primary tumour (T)
T_x	Primary tumour cannot be assessed
T_o	No evidence of primary tumour
T_{is}	Carcinoma in situ
Supraglottis	
T_1	Tumour limited to one subsite of supraglottis with normal vocal cord mobility
T_2	Tumour invades mucosa of more than one adjacent subsite of supraglottis or region outside the supraglottis (e.g. mucosa of base of the tongue, vallecula or medial wall of pyriform fossa) without fixation of the larynx
T_3	Tumour limited to larynx with vocal cord fixation and/or invades any of the following: post-cricoid area, pre-epiglottic space, paraglottic space and/or inner cortex of thyroid cartilage
T_{4a}	Moderately advanced local disease. Tumour invades through thyroid cartilage and/or invades tissues beyond the larynx (e.g. trachea, soft tissues of neck including muscles of the tongue, strap muscles, thyroid or oesophagus)
T_{4b}	Very advanced local disease. Tumour invades prevertebral space, encases carotid artery or invades mediastinal structures
Glottis	
T_1	Tumour limited to the vocal cords (may involve anterior or posterior commissure) with normal mobility
T_{1a}	Tumour limited to one vocal cord
T_{1b}	Tumour involves both vocal cords
T_2	Tumour extends to supraglottis and/or subglottis and/or with impaired vocal cord mobility
T_3	Tumour limited to the larynx with vocal cord fixation and/or invasion of paraglottic space and/or inner cortex of the thyroid cartilage
T_{4a}	Moderately advanced local disease. Tumour invades through outer cortex of the thyroid cartilage and/or invades tissues beyond the larynx (e.g. trachea, soft tissues of the neck including deep extrinsic muscles of the tongue, strap muscles, oesophagus thyroid)
T_{4b}	Very advanced local disease. Tumour invades prevertebral space, encases carotid artery or invades mediastinal structures
Hypopharynx	
T_1	Tumour limited to one subsite of hypopharynx and/or 2 cm or less in greatest dimension
T_2	Tumour invades more than one subsite of hypopharynx or an adjacent site or measures more than 2 cm but not more than 4 cm in greatest dimension without fixation of hemi larynx
T_3	Tumour more than 4 cm in greatest dimension or with fixation of hemi larynx or extension to oesophagus
T_{4a}	Moderately advanced local disease. Tumour invades thyroid/cricoids cartilage/thyroid bone, thyroid gland or central compartment of soft tissue (includes prelaryngeal strap muscles and subcutaneous fat)
T_{4b}	Very advanced local disease. Tumour invades prevertebral fascia, encases carotid artery or involves mediastinal structures
Reginal lymph nodes (N)	
N_x	Regional lymph nodes cannot be assessed
N_o	No regional lymph node metastasis

Table 3.2 (continued)

N_1	Metastasis in a single ipsilateral lymph node 3 cm or less in greatest dimension
N_{2a}	Metastasis in a single ipsilateral lymph node more than 3 cm but not more than 6 cm in greatest dimension
N_{2b}	Metastasis in multiple ipsilateral lymph nodes, none more than 6 cm in greatest dimension
N_{2c}	Metastasis in bilateral or contralateral lymph nodes, none more than 6 cm in greatest dimension
N_3	Metastasis in a lymph node, more than 6 cm in greatest dimension
Distant metastasis (M)	
M_O	No distant metastasis (no pathologic M_O)
M_1	Distant metastasis

References

1. Roland N. Assessment and staging. In: Watkinson JC, Gilbert RW, editors. Stell Maran's. Text book of head & neck surgery and oncology. London: Hoddar Arnold; 2012: p. 38–56.
2. Karnofsky DA, Abeman WH, Craver LF, Burchenail JH. The use of nitrogen mustards in palliative treatment of carcinoma. Cancer. 1948;1:634–56.
3. Goldman JL, Roffman JD. Indirect laryngoscopy. Laryngoscope. 1975;85:530–3.
4. Calhoun KH, Steinberg CM, Quinn FB, Clarke WD. Teaching indirect mirror laryngoscopy. Ototaryngol Head Neck Surg. 1989;100:80–2.
5. Shao J, Stern J, Wang JM, Henson D, et al. Clinical evaluation of 70° and 90° laryngeal telescopes. Arch Otolaryngol Head Neck Surg. 2002;128:941–4.
6. Barker M, Dort JC. Laryngeal examination. A comparison of mirror examination with a rigid lens system. J Otolaryngol. 1991;20:100–3.
7. Yanagisawa E, Yanagisawa K. Stroboscopic video-laryngoscopy: a comparison of fibroscopic and telescopic documentation. Ann Otol Rhinol Laryngol. 1993;102:255–65.
8. Baker KH, Chaput MP, Clavet CR, et al. Evaluation of endoscopic sheaths as viral barriers. Laryngoscope. 1999;109:636–9.
9. Sibermann HD. Non-inflatable sterile sheath for introduction of flexible nasopharyngolaryngoscope. Ann Otol Rhinol Laryngol. 2001;110:385–7.
10. Altissimi G, Gallucci L, Prattichizzo L, et al. Laryngeal microscopy under general anesthesia using a small bore endotracheal tubes: blood gas analysis. Laryngoscope. 1994;104:325–8.
11. Edelist G, Alberth PW. Anesthesia for Co_2 laser surgery of the larynx. J Otolaryngol. 1982;11:107–10.
12. Shaker MH, Konechigeri HN, Andrews AH. Anaesthetic management for carbon dioxide laser surgery of the larynx. Laryngoscope. 1976;86:857–61.
13. Hawkins JB, Joseph MM. Avoiding a wrapped endotracheal tube in laser laryngeal surgery. Experiences with apnoeic anesthesia and metal laser flex endotracheal tubes. Laryngoscope. 1990;10:1283–7.
14. Williams SR, Van Hasselt CA, Aun CS, et al. Tubeless anesthetic technique for optimal carbon dioxide lease surgery of the larynx. Am J Otolaryngol. 1993;14:271–4.
15. Pillsbury HRC, Kirchner JA. Clinical versus histopathology staging in laryngeal cancer. Arch Otolaryngol. 1979;105:157–9.
16. Sulfaro S, Barzan L, Qurein F, et al. T staging of laryngopharyngeal carcinoma. Arch Otolaryngol. 1989;15:613–20.
17. Zbaren P, Becker M, Lang H. Staging of laryngeal cancer: endoscopy, computed tomography and magnetic resonance versus histopathlogy. Eur Arch Otorhinolaryngol. 1997;254(Suppl. 1):S117–22.

18. Zbaren P, Becker M, Lang H. Pre-therapeutic staging of laryngeal carcinoma clinical findings, computed tomography and magnetic resonance imaging compared with histopathology. Cancer. 1996;70:1263–70.
19. Archer CR, Yeager VL. Computed tomography of laryngeal cancer with histopathological co-relation. Laryngoscope. 1982;92:1173–80.
20. Horowitz BL, Woodson GE, Bryan RN. CT of laryngeal tumours. Radiol Clin North Am. 1984;22:265–79.
21. Archer CR, Yeager VL, Herbold DR. Computed tomography vs histology of laryngeal cancer: their value in predicting laryngeal cartilage invasion. Laryngoscope. 1983;93:140–7.
22. Beckar M, Zbaren P, Lang H, et al. Neoplastic invasion of the laryngeal cartilage: comparision of MRI and CT with histopathologic co-relation. Radiology. 1995;194:661–9.
23. Casteligns JA, Golding RP, Van SC, et al. MR findings of cartilage invasion by laryngeal cancer: value in predicting outcome of radiation therapy. Radiology. 1990;174:669–73.
24. Curtin HD. Importance of imaging demonstration of neoplastic invasion of laryngeal cartilage. Radiology. 1995;194:643–4.
25. Wortham DG, Hoover LA, Lufkin RB. Magnetic resonance imaging of the larynx: a co-relation with histologic sections. Arch Otolaryngol Head Neck Surg. 1986;94:123–33.
26. Beitler JJ, Muller S, Grist WJ, et al. Prognostic accuracy of computed tomography findings for patients with laryngeal cancer undergoing laryngectomy. J Clin Oncol. 2010;28:2318–22.
27. Leemans CR, Tiwari R, Nauta JJ, Van der Waal I, Snow GB. Regional lymph node involvement and its significance in development of distant metastasis in the head and neck carcinoma. Cancer. 1993;71:452–6.
28. Van de Brekal M, Castelings J, Snow G. The size of lymph nodes in the neck on sonograms as radiology criteria for metastasis: how reliable is it. Am J Neuro radiol. 1998;19:695–700.
29. Andrea M, Dias O, Sanbos A. Contact endoscopy during micro-laryngeal surgery. A new technique for endoscopic examination of the larynx. Ann Otol Rhinol Laryngol. 1995;104:333–7.
30. Wardrop PJ, Sim S, McLaren K. Contact endoscopy of the larynx, a quantitative study. J Laryngol Otol. 2000;114:437–40.
31. Kraft M, Betz CM, Leumig A. Value of fluorescence endoscopy for early diagnosis of laryngeal cancer and its precursor lesions. Head Neck. 2011;33:941–8.
32. Arens C, Dreyert T, Glanz H, Malzahn K. Indirect auto-fluorescence laryngoscopy in the diagnosis of laryngeal cancer and its precursor lesions. Eur Arch Otorrhinolaryngol. 2004;261:71–6.
33. Zargi M, Fajdiga J, Smid J. Auto-fluorescence imaging in diagnosis of laryngeal cancer. Eur Arch Otorhinolaryngol. 2000;257:17–23.
34. Watanabe A, Taniguchi M, Tsujie H. The value of narrow band imaging for early detection of laryngeal cancer. Eur Arch Otorhinolaryngol. 2009;266:1017–23.
35. Banko B, Dukic V, Milovanovic J, et al. Diagnostic significance of magnetic resonance imaging in preoperative evaluation of patients with laryngeal tumour. Eur Arch Otolaryngol. 2011;268:1617–23.
36. Dechen W, Vogal T, Zbaeran P, et al. Diffusion - weighted MR imaging including bi-exponential fitting for the detection of recurrent or residual tumour afte (chemo) radiotherapy for laryngeal and hypopharygeal cancers. Eur Radiol. 2013;23:562–9.

Metastatic Neck Disease

4

Tapaswani Pradhan and Sudhir Bahadur

4.1 Introduction

An important prognostic factor in carcinoma of the larynx and hypopharynx, as indeed in other sites of the head and neck, is the presence or absence of metastatic neck disease. The factors influencing the nodal metastasis include the different subsites in the region as well as the stage of primary neoplasm (T status). Most tumours may have different biological behaviour based on the presence of neck metastasis.

There are several controversies regarding the management guidelines for the metastatic disease in the neck. There are several questions that need to be addressed. The basic questions include how to treat the primary tumours with clinically negative (No) necks and those with clinically positive (N+) necks. Secondly, what should be the extent of neck dissection? Besides, role of radiotherapy or chemo-radiation has to be assessed particularly in the background of organ preservation. Also, what are the current guidelines for salvage surgery for residual/recurrent disease in the neck?

4.2 Clinical Significance

The presence of nodal metastasis in the neck indicates the primary tumour can metastasize locally and manifest itself at distant sites. This process shows a host response which allows the development of metastasis at both local level and in

T. Pradhan (✉)
Department of Surgical Oncology, BLK Super Speciality Hospital, Delhi, India

S. Bahadur
Department of Otolaryngology and Head-Neck Surgery, Formerly at All India Institute of Medical Sciences, New Delhi, India

S. Bahadur et al. (eds.), *Carcinoma of the Larynx and Hypopharynx*,
https://doi.org/10.1007/978-981-13-3110-7_4

distant organs [1]. Thus, lymph node metastasis indicates an aggressive tumour behaviour which in some cases has already spread to distant sites by lymphaticovenous channels or by haematological routes. This explains why the presence of lymph node metastasis indicates a poor prognosis as compared to patients without neck metastasis (No).

4.3 Lymphatic Drainage of the Larynx

The lymphatic drainage of the larynx is separated into the upper and lower systems based on the embryological origins, and the division occurs at the level of vocal cords.

The supraglottic structures drain through vessels which move along the superior laryngeal vessels via the thyrohyoid membrane to reach the upper deep cervical lymph nodes (levels II and III) with a tendency of bilateral nodal drainage [1]. The lower system drains into the deep cervical lymph nodes (levels III and IV) through vessels which pass through cricothyroid membrane and also into the pre-laryngeal, pretracheal or paratracheal nodes (level VI) and later enter the deep cervical lymph nodes. The vocal cords are relatively avascular, and they have sparse lymphatic drainage.

An incidence of neck metastasis in 34% cases of supraglottic carcinoma regardless of T stage and bilateral nodal metastasis in 26% cases has been reported [1–3]. A significant number of patients with clinically negative (No) necks also contain microscopic metastatic neck disease [4].

Isolated involvement of paratracheal lymph nodes has been reported in carcinoma of the larynx and hypopharynx [5, 6]. But pretreatment assessment of these lymph nodes through radiology (CT, MRI and PET-CT) is difficult [7, 8].

4.4 Lymphatic Drainage of Hypopharynx

Level II, III and IV lymph nodes are most frequently involved in hypopharyngeal cancers [9]. Besides, the inferior portion of the hypopharynx and post-cricoid area drains into paratracheal, paraoesophageal and supraclavicular group of neck nodes. The posterior pharyngeal wall lesions also drain into retropharyngeal nodes.

Due to rich lymphatic drainage, hypopharyngeal cancers present with palpable neck metastasis in 50–75% cases [9, 10]. The pyriform fossa cancers show neck node involvement in 60–70% cases, whereas posterior pharyngeal wall and post-cricoid area show an incidence of 30% and 40%, respectively [11, 12]. A significant number of cases may present with large neck node metastasis (N_2 or N_3 disease) and often with bilateral neck disease. In patients with clinically negative necks, micrometastasis may be seen in ipsilateral neck in nearly 40% cases and bilaterally in 30% [12–15].

Risk factors influencing the neck metastasis have been highlighted in hypopharyngeal cancers [16, 17]. These include tumour size, thyroid cartilage invasion, recurrent laryngeal nerve involvement and extralaryngeal soft tissue involvement. It has been seen that tumours larger than 4 cm show an incidence of 85% of neck node involvement as opposed to 50% nodal metastasis observed when the lesion is less than 4 cm, indicating that T stage generally co-relates with 'N' stage.

4.5 Neck Dissection

Traditionally, all positive neck nodes have been addressed with radical neck dissection because this has been the standard of care for nodal metastasis in the neck since the pioneering work of Crile in 1906. The operation has over the years provided reasonable chance of disease control at regional level. The radical neck dissection was subsequently popularised by Hayes Martin (1951) from Memorial Hospital, New York, who also wrote extensively on the subject [1].

A decade later in 1963, the Argentinian Suarez first introduced the systematic approach to functional neck dissection (FND) by demonstrating lymph nodes to be within well-defined fascial compartments. Later Suarez and Bocca (1964) published a detailed article outlining the principles of functional neck dissection while sparing the important structures and yet achieving the same oncologic outcome as the radical neck dissection [1, 18]. The latter is now advised for advanced metastatic neck disease (N_2/N_3 disease). As a result of new information on lymph drainage pathways, further modifications were developed in the 1960s such as modified radical neck dissection (MRND) and selective neck dissection (SND). There has also been a better understanding of the topographical distribution of lymph node metastasis with different primary sites. This has allowed confirmation of the role of selective neck dissection (e.g. clearance of levels II, III and IV) in carcinoma of the larynx and hypopharynx.

4.6 Neck Dissection After Chemo-radiation

It is known that radiotherapy/chemo-radiation tends to sterilise the subclinical disease in the neck in most situations, and therefore prophylactic neck dissection is not required in N_0 neck. However, in the early phase of organ preservation protocol, N-positive neck despite showing a good response to radiotherapy was subsequently planned for a neck dissection. This concept was developed by MD Anderson Cancer Center in the era where radiation alone coupled with neck dissection for advanced neck disease showed good control rates [16, 19]. It is known that nodes do not completely respond to radiation. However, in the recent years with improved radiological assessment, most surgeons have been able to streamline patients to be considered for neck dissection. Patients with small neck disease (N_1) with a complete response to the treatment are not considered for surgery any longer. The bulky nodes ($\geq N_{2a}$), at pretreatment, still remain a controversial issue with regard to planned neck dissection post-treatment. Most surgeons would prefer to perform surgery because of unreliable follow-up. However, upfront neck dissection in these groups may be considered over treatment in the era of chemo-radiation. Additionally if neck dissection is performed before and the primary lesion fail to show complete response to chemo-radiation, additional salvage surgery for the primary may be required.

Recent review by Ferlito et al. [20] has been clearly able to defy the need for planned neck dissection in complete responders. The review article which has a compilation of 24 retrospective studies, with a heterogenous treatment strategy group, did not show any benefit of planned neck dissection, and the regional failure rate were reported between 0 and 16%. PET-CT performed at the 12th week post-treatment had been used as the main radiological investigation for the assessment of the neck in all the cases. Similar views on the reduced need for planned neck dissection have been mentioned by Goguen et al. [21] where they found a correlation between histological positivity and nodal stage post-treatment. According to the study, complete response was seen in 40–70% of advanced neck disease. However, in a series by Stenson et al. [22], viable tumour cells increased from 12% for N_{2b} to 20% for N_{2c} to 30% for N_3 necks post-treatment (chemo-radiotherapy). Other studies have reported a complete response of 42–50% for N_3 neck [23, 24]. Clearly, the need to perform neck dissection is restricted to patients with residual neck disease. The extent of neck dissection in the salvage situation for years was always a comprehensive neck dissection and is probably still valid in Indian context. With time, a trend is being seen towards selective and superselective neck dissection. A study carried out by Dhiwakar et al. [24] stated that 88% of the residual neck diseases were located at levels II and III and the regional failure following the procedure was 6%. The feasibility of superselective neck dissection has now been studied by Robbins et al. [25]. The study had 177 patients treated with concomitant radiation and intraarterial cisplatin; 82% of the patients had disease confined to one nodal level only. The collected data on superselective neck dissection have been based on the fact that concurrent chemo-radiation would sterilise the occult metastases in various levels of the neck. Hence the residual disease could be addressed through superselective neck dissection.

In summary, planned neck dissection in a treated neck with negative radiology may not be necessary and is required only in N_2 and N_3 disease particularly where PET-CT is positive (also in N_1 disease with positive PET-CT following radiation).

4.7 Levels of Lymph Nodes

A description of regional cervical lymph nodes has been established with regard to their levels of location by the Memorial Sloan Kettering Cancer Center [18] (Fig. 4.1).

4.7.1 Level I Submental Group

The lymph nodes between the anterior belly of digastric muscle and hyoid bone. The submandibular group—lymph nodes in the triangular area between anterior and posterior belly or digastric muscle and the inferior border of the mandible. The lymph nodes adjacent to the submandibular salivary gland and facial artery are included in this group (Fig. 4.2).

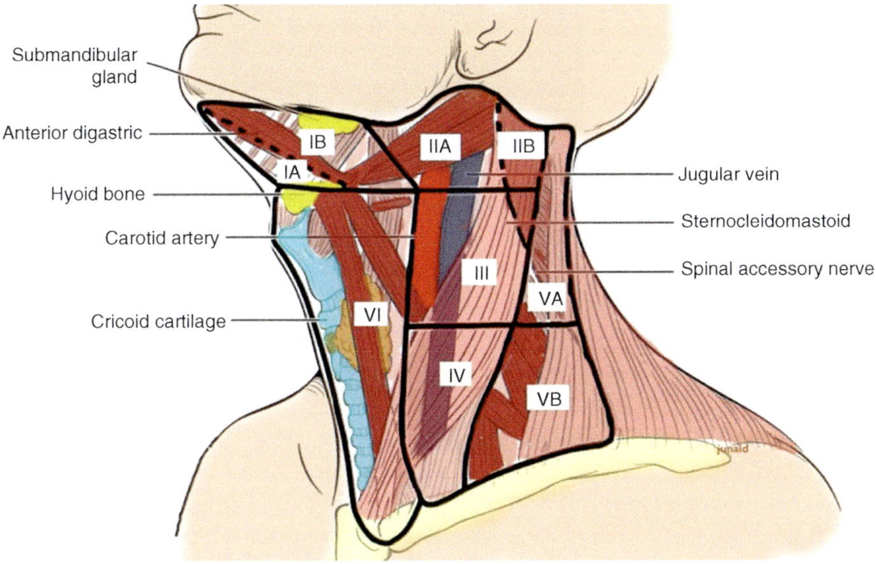

Fig. 4.1 Levels of lymph nodes in the neck

Fig. 4.2 Transglottic carcinoma with pyriform fossa involvement. Surgery included a radical neck dissection for palpable nodal metastasis

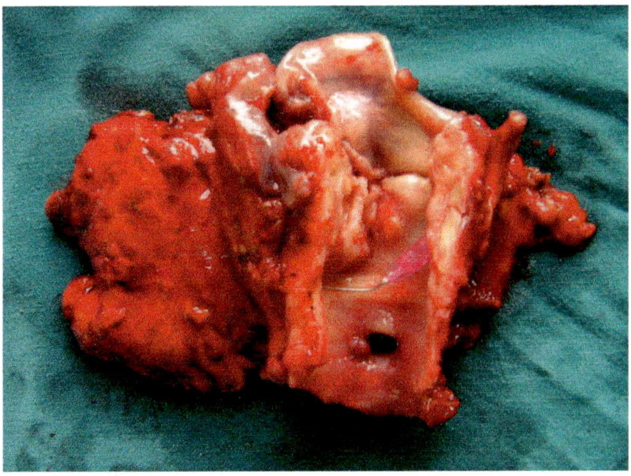

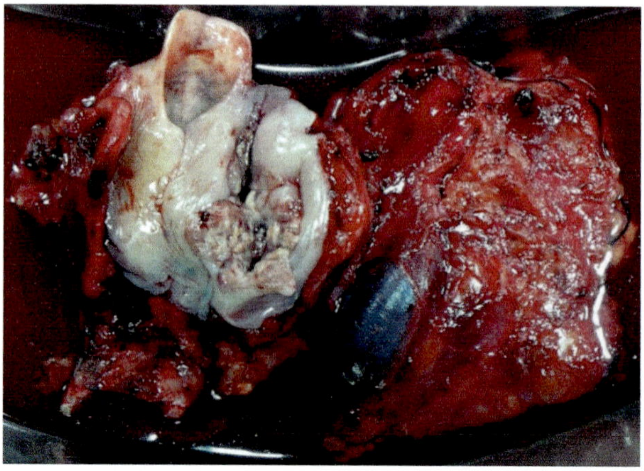

Fig. 4.3 Pyriform fossa cancer. Surgical specimen included a total laryngectomy and partial pharyngectomy with radical neck dissection for nodal disease

4.7.2 Level II Upper Jugular Group

Lymph nodes around the upper portion of the internal jugular vein and upper part of the spinal accessory nerve to the bifurcation of carotid artery (jugulodigastric group)

4.7.3 Level III Mid-jugular Group

Lymph nodes around mid-third of the internal jugular vein from inferior border of level II up to the omohyoid muscle (inferior border of cricoid cartilage)

4.7.4 Level IV Lower Jugular Group

Lymph nodes around the lower third of internal jugular vein up to the clavicle

4.7.5 Level V Post-triangle Group

Lymph nodes around the lower portion of the spinal accessory nerve and along the transverse vessels

4.7.6 Level VI Central Compartment Group

Lymph nodes in the pre-laryngeal, pretracheal (Delphian), paratracheal and tracheo-oesophageal groove

4.7.7 Level VII Superior Mediastinum Group

Lymph nodes in the anterior superior mediastinum and tracheo-oesophageal groove extending from the suprasternal notch to the innominate artery

N Staging of lymph node metastasis from squamous cell carcinoma of the head and neck except nasopharynx (AJCC/UICC)

N_x Regional lymph nodes cannot be assessed

N_0 No regional lymph node metastasis

N_1 Metastasis in a single ipsilateral lymph node, <3 cm in greatest dimension

N_{2a} Metastasis in a single ipsilateral lymph node >3 cm but <6 cm in greatest dimension

N_{2b} Metastasis in multiple ipsilateral lymph nodes none greater than >6 cm

N_{2c} Metastases in bilateral or contralateral lymph nodes, none greater than 6 cm in greatest dimension

N_3 Metastasis in a lymph node >6 cm in greatest dimension

Prognostic nodal features

- Site, size number
- Lower levels
- Extracapsular spread
- Morphology
- Bilateral and contralateral node

4.8 Nodal Factors Affecting the Prognosis

It is well realised that the presence of cervical lymph node metastasis adversely affects the prognosis. The nodal features influencing the prognosis include the size, the number, the level/levels and the bilateral neck disease. Thus involvement of level IV nodal disease carries much worse prognosis than involvement of level II. Similarly, other factors adversely impacting prognosis are perivascular and perineural infiltration. However, the factor which has received most attention in recent years is the presence of extracapsular spread (ECS) of disease impacting the prognosis [18]. There is enough evidence in the literature that the presence of ECS decreases the survival rates by nearly half compared to the patients whose disease was confined to the nodes [26–28]. Another meta-analysis concluded that ECS adversely affected 5-year survival [29]. It has been shown that ECS adversely affected survival in laryngeal cancer by increasing the risk of metastases nine times [30].

There is general agreement in literature that the standard treatment if ECS is detected following surgery is to additionally give postoperative radiotherapy or chemo-radiation [26, 31]. Currently, level I evidence in literature suggests that adjuvant chemo-radiation should be given in the postoperative period in the presence of extracapsular spread (ECS) of disease [32]. Lefebvre et al. [33], in a large study of

1330 patients, showed that irrespective of T staging, ECS or three or more positive nodes or positive level IV nodes increased the risk of regional failures twofold and increased the risk of distant metastasis three times.

4.9 Classification of Neck Dissection

The classification of neck dissection was carried out to include increasing variation in the types of neck dissection performed and to bring about uniformity in the nomenclature. The American Academy of Otolaryngology-Head and Neck Surgery jointly with the American Society of Head and Neck Surgery produced a standardised classification in 1991 [18]. Further update was produced in 2002 to refine the description of modified radical neck dissection and selective neck dissection. Classification of neck dissection identifies four categories.

(a) Comprehensive neck dissection
- Radical neck dissection—It involves excision of lymph nodes in levels I–V and three non-lymphatic structures including the sternocleidomastoid muscle, the internal jugular vein and the accessory nerve.
- Modified radical neck dissection—It involves the removal of lymph nodes in levels I to V but preserves one of the three non-lymphatic structures which are sacrificed in RND. The structure that is preserved should be specifically named, e.g. spinal accessory nerve and internal jugular vein.
- Extended radical neck dissection—Excision of more structures besides those removed in RND, e.g. level VII lymph node, hypoglossal nerve skin of the neck and carotid artery of the structures removed, should be identified.

(b) Selective neck dissection—Specific lymph node group draining the particular primary lesion are excised while preserving the remaining lymphatic and non-lymphatic structures, e.g. excision of level II–IV lymph nodes in patients with carcinoma of the larynx and hypopharynx.

Selective neck dissection (for clinically negative (No) necks)—The surgical procedures that selectively excise lymph node groups at specific levels in No neck which are at risk to contain micrometastasis [34] include:
- Supraomohyoid neck dissection (SOND)—This procedure includes dissection of lymph nodes at levels I, II and III (for primary tumours of the oral cavity). An extended SOND is advised for primary tumour located in the lateral border of the tongue.
- Jugular neck dissection (anterolateral neck dissection)—This surgical procedure includes dissection of level II, III and IV lymph nodes (for primary tumours of the larynx and hypopharynx).
- Central compartment neck dissection—This procedure includes dissection of lymph nodes at level VI in the central compartment (for thyroid cancer).

- Posterolateral neck dissection—This operation comprises of dissection of lymph nodes in the suboccipital triangle, posterior triangle of the neck, level V and deep jugular chain of lymph nodes at levels II, III and IV (for melanomas and squamous carcinoma of posterior scalp).

Surgical technique of Jugular (anterolateral) neck dissection—The surgical procedure is usually performed along with resection of primary tumour located in the larynx or hypopharynx. The operation may be performed on the ipsilateral side if lesions are strictly confined to one side or bilaterally if the lesion crosses the midline of the laryngopharyngeal area. The surgery may be performed through the same incision (usually Sorenson's or horizontal incision across the middle of neck) used for excision of primary neoplasm.

Skin flaps are elevated in the usual manner exposing the sternocleidomastoid muscle in its entire length. The internal jugular nodes (levels II, III and IV) that lie anteriorly, laterally and posteriorly to the vein are excised in a monobloc manner. The main surgical procedure begins by incising the fascia along with anterior border of the sternocleidomastoid muscle which is then grasped with haemostats to retract the muscle and continue the dissection on the medical surface of the muscle.

Once the careful dissection reaches the posterior border of the undersurface of the muscle, the internal jugular chain of lymph nodes from jugulodigastric area to supraclavicular region is exposed.

Surgical dissection is usually started at the upper end clearing the lymph nodes that are posterior to the spinal accessory nerve on the medial aspect of the muscle, and further dissection permits delivery of these lymph nodes beneath the nerve. The lymph nodes lie over the splenius capitis muscle and levator scapulae muscle in the floor of the posterior triangle. The dissection is carried forwards to join the jugulodigastric lymph nodes exposing the sensory roots and the lateral border of internal jugular vein. The dissection is continued to keep these lymph nodes in continuity with jugular lymph nodes in its entire length and completely exposing the vein, clearing the accessory chain of lymph nodes and exposing the cervical roots.

Further the dissection is continued anterolateral to the internal jugular vein clearing off all the lymph nodes from the jugular foramen superiorly to the supraclavicular region.

There is no need to dissect the lymph nodes in level I, and hence the submandibular gland can be preserved. However, pharyngeal branches draining into the internal jugular vein and the common facial vein have to be ligated and divided to complete the dissection of upper lymph nodes. Similarly, the hypoglossal nerve, the descendens hypoglossi and branches of superior thyroid artery are identified and preserved. The carotid artery remains under vision while excising the specimen.

The specimen is carefully marked with regard to the levels of lymph nodes before sending it to the pathologist. It is a monobloc resection and may be combined with laryngectomy or laryngopharyngectomy specimen (Fig. 4.3 to Fig. 4.12).

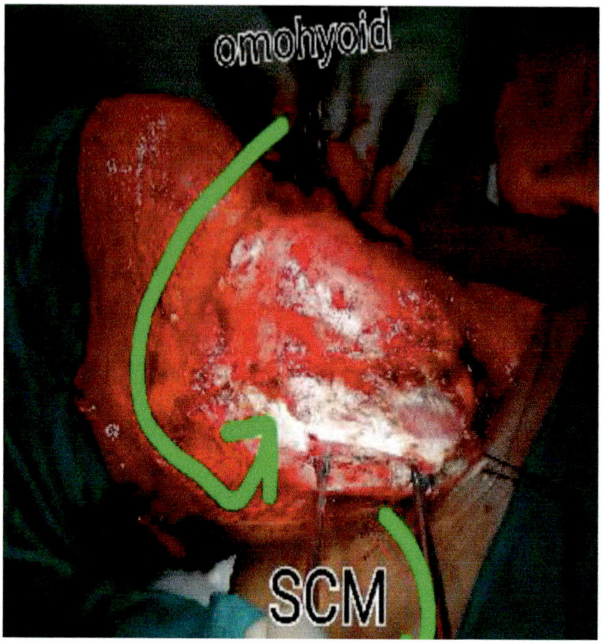

Fig. 4.4 Steps of selective neck dissection (Skin flaps elevated and carotid sheath exposed)

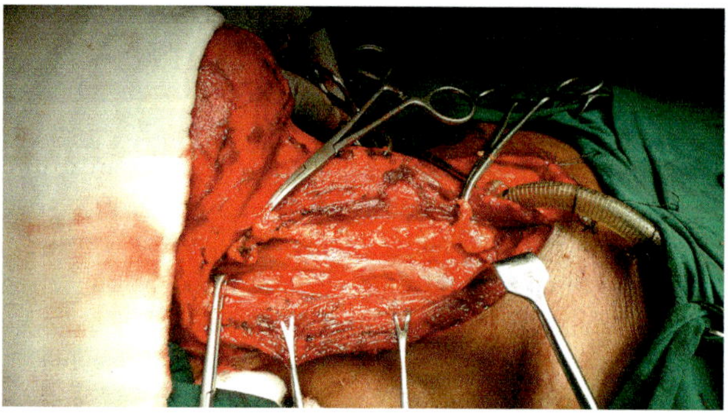

Fig. 4.5 Steps of selective neck dissection (clearance of level II, III and IV lymph nodes)

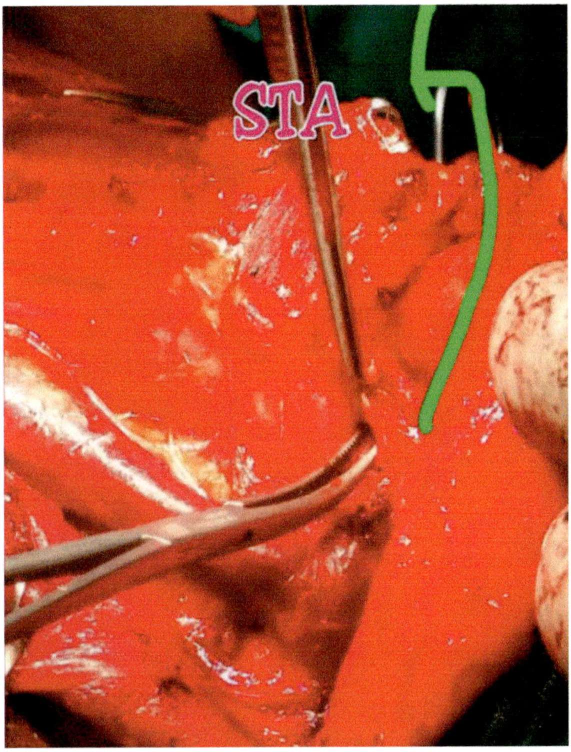

Fig. 4.6 Steps of selective neck dissection (Visualization of internal jugular vein and superior thyroid artery)

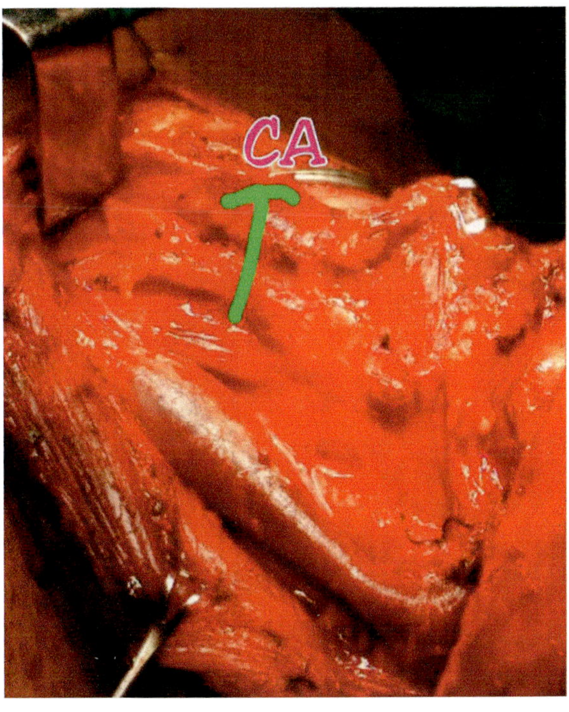

Fig. 4.7 Steps of selective neck dissection (Exposure of carotid artery)

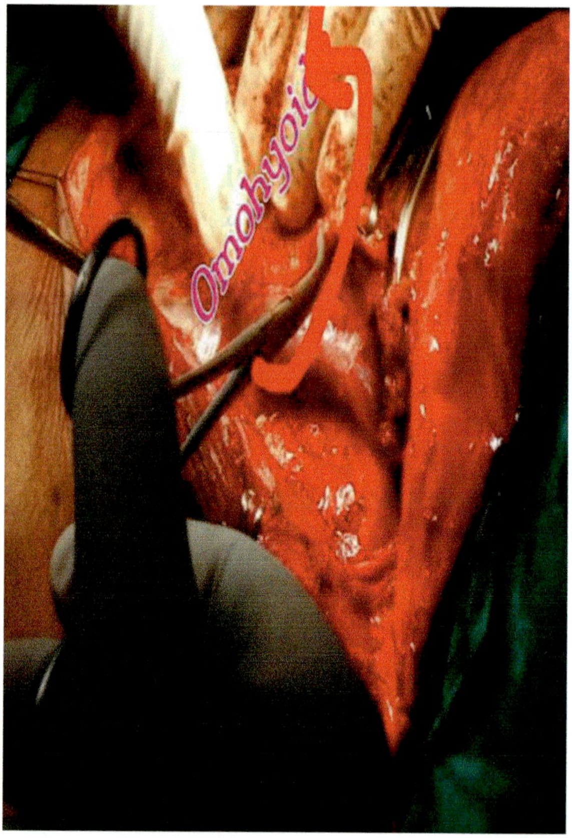

Fig. 4.8 Steps of selective neck dissection (clearance of level II, III and IV lymph nodes)

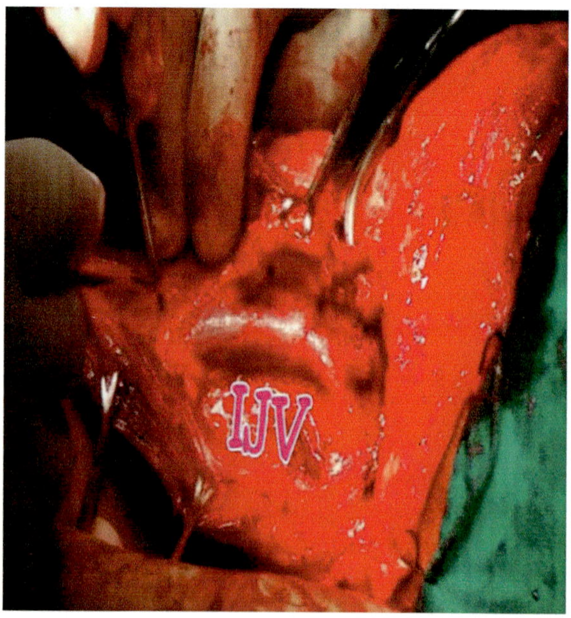

Fig. 4.9 Steps of selective neck dissection (clearance of level II, III and IV lymph nodes)

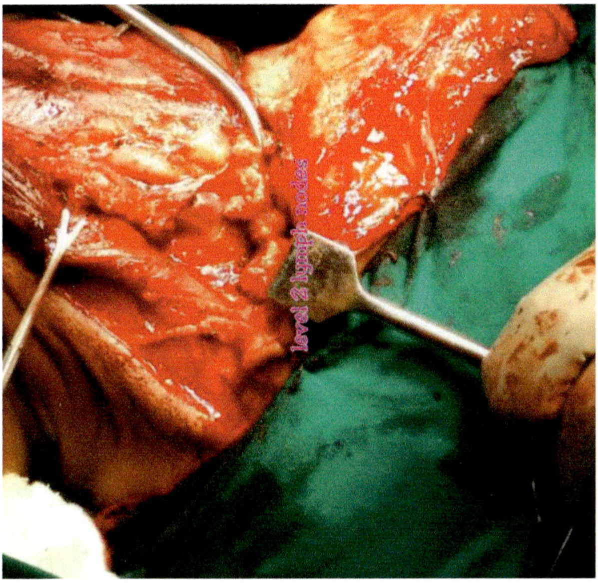

Fig. 4.10 Steps of selective neck dissection (clearance of level II, III and IV lymph nodes)

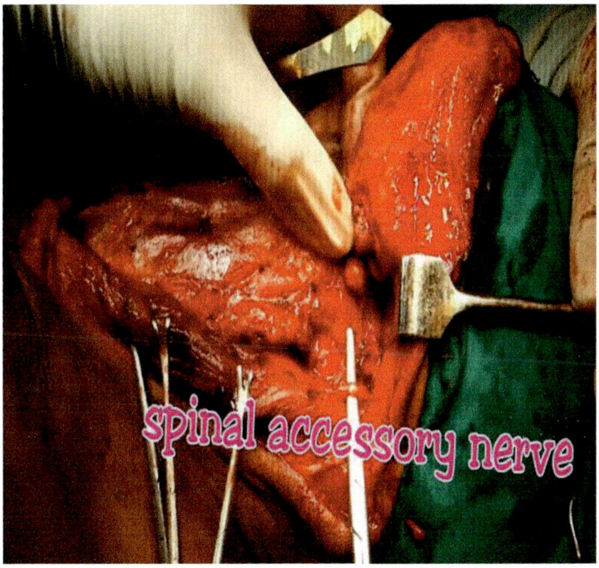

Fig. 4.11 Steps of selective neck dissection (exposure of spinal accessory nerve)

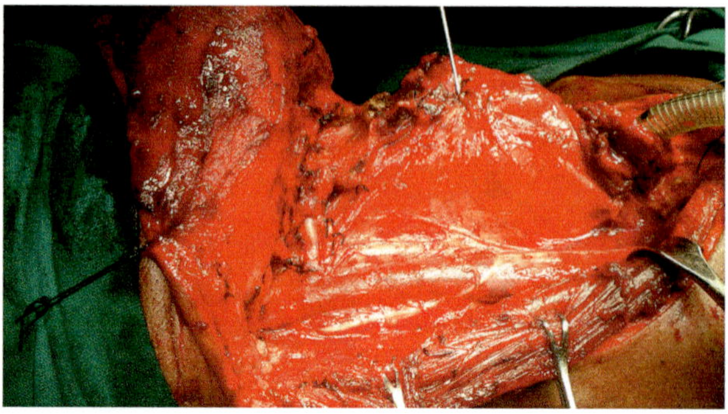

Fig. 4.12 Steps of selective neck dissection (visualization of posterior triangle structures)

4.9.1 Classic Radical Neck Dissection (RND)

The radical neck dissection has been the mainstay of surgery for palpable nodal metastasis in the neck for more than a century since Crile established the principles of neck dissection in 1906. This surgical procedure comprehensively excises the lymph nodes from levels I, II, III, IV and V but also includes sacrifice of the sternocleidomastoid muscle, spinal accessory nerve, internal jugular vein and submandibular salivary gland. It is realised that radical neck dissection carries a certain morbidity, and therefore, many surgeons prefer to carry out modified neck dissection without compromising on oncologic principles and reserve it for more advanced metastatic disease (N_3) or in recurrent disease following radiation failures [35] (Figs. 4.13, 4.14, and 4.15).

A variety of incisions are described for carrying out radical neck dissection, and most surgeons prefer using a modified ‘Conley’ (trifurcate T-shaped) incision when primary tumour is located in the oral cavity. However, since the primary tumour is located in the larynx or hypopharynx and exposure can be obtained by (Sorenson) incision, the same exposure can easily include the radical neck dissection.

The dissection begins by raising the skin flaps in the subplatysmal plane using first the scalpel and later the electrocautery. Similarly the skin hooks also help in raising the flaps by aiding in retraction. Anterior flap is raised in the middle of the neck reaching the hyoid bone. The posterior skin flap is raised till the anterior border of trapezius is reached, exposing the muscle from mastoid process superiorly to the clavicle inferiorly. However, platysma is not present in the posterior skin flap right up to the trapezius muscle.

The dissection may begin along the anterior border of trapezius, moving forwards into the posterior triangle, or may start with division of the lower attachment of sternocleidomastoid muscle close to the clavicle and pursue the infero-lateral neck dissection. The latter approach is usually preferred by a majority of surgeons [1, 36].

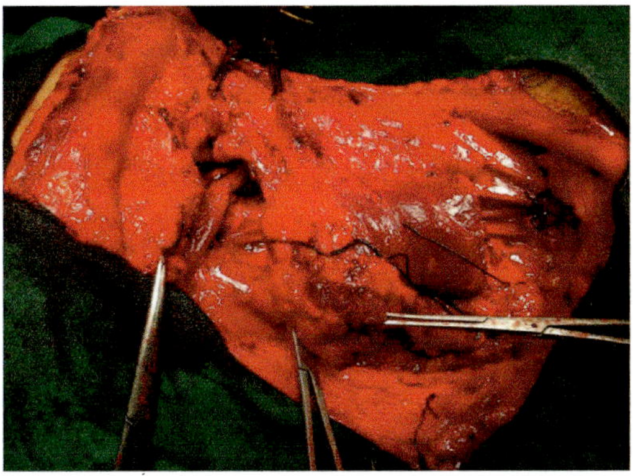

Fig. 4.13 Division of sternocleidomastoid muscle (lower end) ligature and division of internal jugular vein—part of infero-lateral dissection

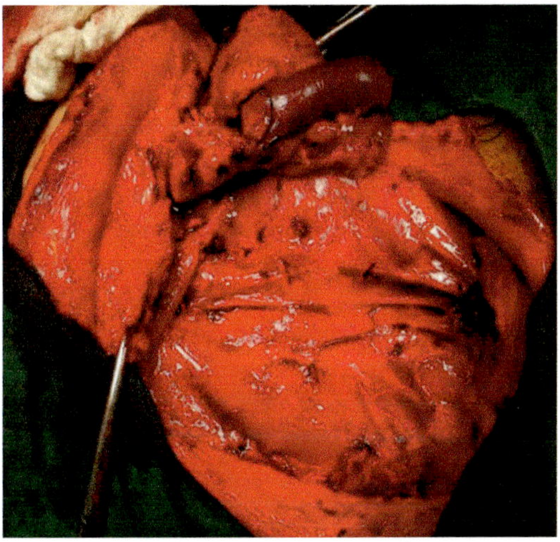

Fig. 4.14 Specimen has been pushed forwards towards the larynx exposing carotid artery vagus nerve and the posterior triangle

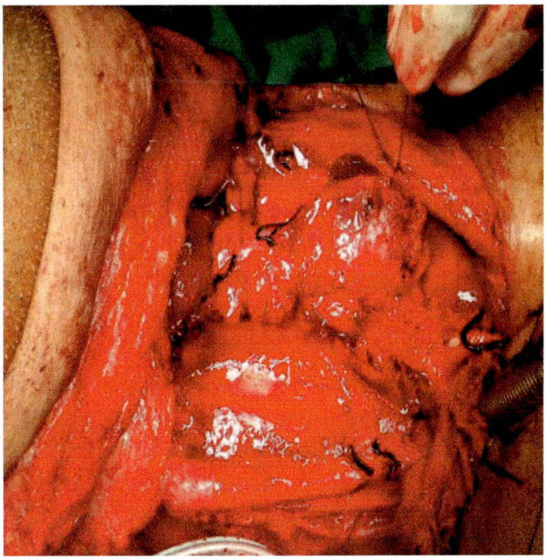

Fig. 4.15 Visualization of the tracheal and carotid structures after dissection

(a) The lower end of internal jugular vein

There is some debate whether the lower end or the upper end of the internal jugular vein should be tied first: Ligation of the lower end prevents the spread of possible tumour emboli into the blood stream, but this step also results in distension of the vein above the ligature making the dissection somewhat more difficult.

Usually the dissection proceeds infero-laterally along the upper border of the clavicle from suprasternal notch to the trapezius muscle. The supraclavicular nerve and vessels such as external jugular vein are divided, and division of sternal and clavicular fibres of sternocleidomastoid muscle is completed before attempting to expose, ligate and divide the internal jugular vein. The vein is encompassed in the carotid sheath which includes the artery, internal jugular vein, vagus nerve and branches of ansa cervicalis.

The carotid sheath is initially opened for several centimetres to have adequate exposure for ligation. It is important to separate out the vagus nerve which lies in the posterior relationship of the vein between the latter and the common carotid artery. The lower end of the vein is usually ligated with three sutures of 1-0 silk or 0/0 Vicryl. An additional transfixation suture may be applied at the lower end. It is also useful to check for any injury to the thoracic duct if doing the left-sided neck dissection: the former may enter the vein on its posterior and medial surface about 1–2 cm above the clavicle.

The internal jugular vein can easily be injured during dissection and manipulation, producing serious bleeding. Therefore, it is important to remain calm and composed and try and stop the bleeding by applying pressure and then identify the injured vessel and apply the arterial clamps before ligating the vessel. However, if the vein is torn, it is useful to place the patient in Trendelenburg position before clamping or ligating the vein because the main danger is not the blood loss but the risk of air embolism.

However, after the internal jugular vein has been ligated and divided, the dissection proceeds laterally towards the posterior triangle after having secured the carotid artery, vagus nerve and sympathetic chain. The scalene group of lymph nodes are included in the dissection and so also the fibro-fatty tissue and the nodes covering the roof of posterior triangle.

(b) Junction of clavicle and anterior border of trapezius

The dissection then proceeds in the posterior triangle exposing the deep fascia lining the muscles of the floor (scalene group, levator scapulae). Phrenic nerve and brachial plexus can be seen shining behind the deep fascia, and these structures are preserved. The fatty tissues in supraclavicular region are divided exposing the inferior belly of omohyoid muscle which is similarly divided and retracted superiorly.

The transverse cervical vessels are found medial to the omohyoid as these run laterally across the floor of the posterior triangle. They are usually ligated. There are small branches particularly from the vein across the anterior border of trapezius. These need to be tied as they can produce bleeding during the dissection of posterior triangle.

The neck dissection is carried forwards superiorly and anteriorly at the level of prevertebral fascia overlying the scalene muscles. Further exposure to structures lying directly beneath the prevertebral fascia, the phrenic nerve and the brachial plexus is obtained. The phrenic nerve descends from lateral to medial border of scalene anterior muscle. The bipolar cautery should be used in case bleeding occurs in this part of dissection.

The dissection continues superiorly along the anterior border of trapezius to the mastoid process where the trapezius and sternocleidomastoid muscle meet. The dissection is still carried on the prevertebral fascia on the floor of posterior triangle, over the splenius capitis and levator scapulae muscles, cranially. The accessory nerve should be identified before dissection of posterior triangle, running in the roof of posterior triangle.

The accessory innervates the trapezius muscle after exiting from its trajectory through the sternocleidomastoid muscle approximately at junction of upper third and lower two-thirds or 1 cm above Erb's point (where greater auricular nerve emerges) from posterior border of the sternocleidomastoid muscle. The nerve may also be identified as it enters the anterior border of trapezius, a few centimetres above the clavicle.

The dissected tissues are retracted forwards after dividing the branches of cervical plexus (C2, C3 and C4) which emerge posterolateral to the carotid artery and internal jugular vein; the latter is dissected with the specimen. The dissection continues from the mastoid process forwards after dividing the upper end of sternocleidomastoid muscle and tail of parotid gland and retracted caudally and exposing the posterior belly of digastric muscle which is an important landmark.

(c) The upper end of the internal jugular vein

The posterior belly of digastric muscle is cleared of fibro-fatty tissue, and using a Langenbeck retractor, the muscle can be retracted superiorly to expose the internal jugular vein and the accessory nerve; the latter descends along the vein from the jugular foramen and crosses the jugular vein, as it joins the sternocleidomastoid muscle at the level of upper and middle third of the muscle. The dissection is continued across the jugular vein, and it is useful to again identify the vagus and hypoglossal nerves. The hypoglossal nerve crosses the carotid bifurcation and the lingual and occipital arteries. Dissection close to the carotid bifurcation may produce bradycardia, and changes in blood pressure because of the stimulation of carotid sinus and application of cotton wool soaked in xylocaine may help in avoiding it.

It is important to ligate the branches entering the upper end of the internal jugular vein usually on the antero-medial surface. The main internal jugular vein once exposed adequately is ligated with 1-0 silk or Vicryl 0/0 and is also transfixed and divided, and the surgical specimen is mobilised both from cranial and caudal direction.

(d) The submandibular triangle

The contents of submandibular triangle include lymph nodes (level I) fatty tissue and the gland itself. Dissection in this area generally begins in the midline by dividing the fatty tissue covering the anterior belly of digastric muscle (fatty tissue of the submental triangle is included); the fascia enclosing the submandibular gland is incised in the middle and the upper layer containing the marginal mandibular nerve. Another landmark for the latter is where it crosses the facial vein. The facial vessels are carefully dissected, ligated and divided separately; the lymph nodes along the vessels are included in the surgical specimen.

The submandibular gland is retracted downwards exposing the floor of submandibular triangle including the lingual and hypoglossal nerve in the deeper plane formed by genioglossus and hyoglossus muscle. The submandibular ganglion attached to the lingual nerve is divided, permitting the nerve to retract upwards and dissecting the remaining connective tissue inferiorly.

The submandibular duct is divided and ligated as it emerges from the anterior border of mylohyoid muscle. The tissues are retracted infero-laterally to expose the facial artery again as it curves the posterior belly of digastric muscle. The artery is ligated and divided. It may be preserved if microvascular anastomosis is to be carried out for raising the free flap.

4.9.2 Modified Radical Neck Dissection

(a) Sparing of the accessory nerve

It is useful to localise the nerve at the early stage of neck dissection, during the raising of the posterior skin flaps because the nerve runs at the superficial level. There are several methods to identify the nerve.

The accessory nerve emerges from its trajectory through the sternocleidomastoid muscle, roughly at the junction of its upper third and lower two-thirds (about 1 cm about Erb's point). The nerve then runs in a caudo-lateral direction to reach the anterior border of trapezius, a few centimetres above the clavicle.

Another important place to locate the nerve is in its cranial part as it enters the neck with the internal jugular vein crossing it from medial to lateral aspect to innervate the sternocleidomastoid muscle where transverse process of the atlas serves as a useful landmark. The nerve can be dissected through the muscle, cutting its branch supplying the muscle after lifting the latter. The accessory nerve is subsequently dissected through the roof of posterior triangle to enter the trapezius.

(b) Preservation of internal jugular vein

It requires careful dissection on the surface of internal jugular vein in its entire length in the neck. The sternocleidomastoid muscle is divided first if it is to be sacrificed just above the clavicle. Dissection is carried out across the clavicle from trapezius to suprasternal notch. The supraclavicular nerves and the external jugular vein are divided. The carotid sheath is opened and the internal jugular vein is exposed. One has to be careful while dissecting on the surface of the vein. The dissection in the posterior triangle is similar to the one carried out in radical neck dissection. The upper part of the internal jugular vein is exposed after retracting the posterior belly of digastrics superiorly. Small tributaries draining into the vein are first tied and divided. Dissection is completed across the surface of internal jugular vein.

(c) Preservation of the sternocleidomastoid muscle
The dissection begins at anterior border of sternocleidomastoid muscle and is carried forwards on the medial surface of the muscle and simultaneously causing sufficient retraction on the muscle. However, the exposure may be difficult to obtain, and some surgeons prefer to divide the muscle at its caudal end, retracting it superiorly and completing the neck dissection. The muscle can be resutured into the place at the end of surgery.

4.10 Authors' Comments

Presence of cervical lymph node metastasis adversely affects the prognosis in carcinoma of the larynx and hypopharynx. It is also true there is high incidence of lymph node involvement in supraglottic and transglottic cancers as well as in most of hypopharyngeal lesions. The nodal features affecting the prognosis to varying degree include the size, location, number, the level/levels and whether the patient has bilateral neck disease. However, the most important feature adversely impacting the prognosis remains the extracapsular spread (ECS) of disease, detected on histology. It is known that a significant number of patients with clinically negative (No) neck have micrometastasis in the lymph nodes.

It is, therefore, important that No neck must be electively treated either by radiation/ chemo-radiation or by surgery (selective neck dissection) to address level II, III and IV lymph nodes as a part of treatment of primary neoplasm, except in early glottis lesions.

Traditionally, the nodal metastasis has been treated with radical or modified radical neck dissection along with laryngectomy. Usually, postoperative radiotherapy is recommended if the nodes are found to be histologically positive. In case the extracapsular spread of disease is detected following surgery, there is enough evidence available in literature that these cases should instead receive chemo-radiation.

There is a major dilemma in the treatment of neck in patients with advanced disease who are selected to be treated with chemo-radiation as a part of organ preservation. It is generally recommended that FDG PET done 3 months after treatment may be useful to select patients for neck dissection (if nodes have clinically disappeared after chemo-radiation). However, if such imaging facilities are not available, the nodal metastasis (N_2 and N_3) should be treated with neck dissection irrespective of the clinical status of the neck particularly in Indian set-up where reliable follow-up cannot be easily maintained. However, patients with N_1 disease may be observed if the node disappears after chemo-radiation.

Diagnosis of residual or recurrent disease whether in the neck node or at primary site or both is always difficult. Similarly, salvage surgery carries considerable morbidity and lower cure rates. Thus, proper case selection and regular follow-up are essential in the management of metastatic neck disease.

References

1. Paleri V, Watkinson JC. Metastatic neck disease. In: Watkinson JC, Gilbert RW, editors. Stell and Maran's textbook of head and neck surgery and oncology. London: Hoddar Arnold; 2011. 2012: p. 661–89.
2. Byers RM, Wolf PF, Ballantyne AJ. Rationale for elective modified neck dissection. Head Neck Surg. 1988;10:160–7.
3. Kowalski LP, Medina JE. Nodal metastasis : predictive factors. Management of the neck in head and neck cancer. Otolaryngol Clin North Am. 1998;31(5):803–14.
4. Canadela FC, Kothari K, Shah JP. Patterns of cervical nodal Metastasis from squamous carcinoma of the oropharynx and hypopharynx. Head Neck. 1990;12:197–203.
5. Plaat RE, de Bree R, Kuik DJ, et al. Prognostic importance of paratracheal lymph node metastases. Laryngoscrope. 2005;115:894–8.
6. Timon CV, Toner M, Conlon BJ. Paratracheal lymph node involvement in advanced cancer of the larynx, hypopharynx, and cervical esophagus. Laryngoscope. 2003;113:1595–9.
7. Kim JW, Roh JL, Kim JS, et al. Evaluation of 18F-FDG PET-CT and CT/MRI with histopathologic correlation in patient undergoing central compartment neck dissection for squamous cell carcinoma of the larynx, hypopharynx and oesophagus. Oral Oncol. 2013;49:449–53.
8. Peters TT, Castelinjns JA, Ljumanovic R, Witte BI, Leemans CR, De Bree R. Diagnostic value of CT and MRI in the detection of paratracheal lymph nodes metastasis. Oral Oncol. 2012;48:450–5.
9. Carpenter RJ, DeSanto LW. Cancer of the hypopharynx. Surg Clin North Am. 1977;57:723–35.
10. El Badawi SA, Goepfert H, Herson J, Oswald MJ. Squamous cell carcinoma of the pyriform sinus. Laryngoscope. 1982;92:357–64.
11. Stell PM. Cancer of the hypopharynx. J R Coll Surg Edinb. 1973;18:20–30.
12. Kraus DH, Pfister DG, Harrison LB, et al. Salvage laryngectomy for unsuccessful larynx preservation therapy. Ann Otol Rhinol Laryngol. 1995;104:936–41.
13. Davidson J, Briant D, Gullane P, Keane T, Rawlinson E. The role of surgery following radiotherapy failure. A prospective study. Arch Otolaryngol Head Neck Surg. 1994;120:269–76.
14. Buckley JG, Maclennan K. Cervical node metastases in laryngeal and hypopharyngeal cancer: a prospective analysis of prevalence and distribution. Head Neck. 2000;22:380–5.
15. Candela FC, Kothari K, Shah JP. Patterns of cervical node metastases from squamous cell carcinoma of the oropharynx and hypopharynx. Head Neck. 1990;12:197–203.
16. Peters LJ, Goepfert H, Ang KK, et al. Evaluation of the dose for post-operative radiation therapy of head and neck cancer: first report of a prospective randomised trial. Int J Radiat Oncol Biol Phys. 1993;26:3–11.
17. Newkirk KA, Cullen KJ, Harter KW, Picken CA, Sessions RB, Davidson BJ. Planned neck dissection for advanced primary head and neck malignancy treated with organ preservation therapy: disease control and survival outcomes. Head Neck. 2001;23:73–9.
18. Lecmans R, Eerenstein S, Paleri V. In: Watkins JC, Gilbert RW, editors. Neck dissection in Stell & Maran's textbook of Head and Neck Surgery and Oncology. London: Hodder Arnold; 2012. p. 699–713.
19. Barkley HT Jr, Fletcher GH, Jesse RH, Linberg RD. Management of cervical lymph node metastases in squamous cell carcinoma of the tonsillar fossa, base of tongue, supraglottic larynx, and Hypopharynx. Am J Surg. 1972;24:762–7.
20. Ferlito A, Corry J, Silver CE, Shaha AR, Robbins KT, Rinaldo A. Planned neck dissection for patients with complete response to chemoradiotherapy: a concept approaching obsolescence. Head Neck. 2010;32:235–61.
21. Goguen LA, Posner MR, Tishler RB, Wirth LJ, Norris CM, Annino DJ, et al. Examining the need for neck dissection in the era of chemoradiation therapy for advanced head and neck cancer. Arch Otolaryngol Head Neck Surg. 2006;132:526–31.
22. Stenson KM, Huo D, Blair E, Cohen EE, Argiris A, Haraf DJ, et al. Planned post-chemoradiation neck dissection : significance of radiation dose. Laryngoscope. 2006;116:33–6.

23. McHam SA, Adelstein DJ, Rybicki LA, Lavertu P, Esclamado RM, Wood BG, et al. Who merits a neck dissection after definitive chemoradiotherapy for N2-N3 squamous cell head and neck cancer. Head Neck. 2003;25:791–8.
24. Dhiwakar M, Robbins KT, Vieira F, Rao K, Malone J. Selective neck dissection as an early salvage intervention for clinically persistent nodal disease following chemoradiation. Head Neck. 2012;34:188–93.
25. Robbins KT, Shannon K, Vieira F. Superselective neck dissection after chemoradiation : Feasibility based on clinical and pathological comparisons. Arch Otolaryngol Head Neck Surg. 2007;133:486–9.
26. Bahadur S. Radical neck dissection. Indian J Otolaryngol Head Neck Surg. 1986;38:141–4.
27. Collins SL. Controversies in management of cancer of the neck in Thawley SE, Panje WR. In: Bataskis JG, Lindberg RD, editors. Comprehensive management of head and neck tumours. Philadelphia: WB Saunders; 1999. p. 1479–563.
28. Johnson JT, Barnes EL, Myers EN, et al. The extracapsular spread of tumour in cervical node metastasis. Arch Otolaryngol. 1981;107:725–9.
29. Ferlito A, Rinaldo A, Devaney KO, et al. Prognostic significance of microscopic and microscopic of extracapsular spread from metastatic tumour in the cervical lymph nodes. Oral Oncol. 2002;38:747–51.
30. Dunne AA, Muller HH, Elsiele DW, et al. Meta-analysis of prognostic significance of perinodal spread in head and neck squamous cell carcinoma patients. Eur J Cancer. 2006;42:1863–8.
31. Oosterkamp S, de Jong JM, Van den Ende PL, et al. Predictive value of lymph node metastasis and extracapsular extension for the risk of distant metastasis in laryngeal carcinoma. Laryngocope. 2006;116:2067–70.
32. Bahadur S, Kumar S, Tandon DA, et al. Combined therapy in advanced head and neck cancer. J Laryngol Otol. 1992;106:243–9.
33. Berner K, Cooper JS, Pajak TF, et al. Defining risk levels in locally advanced head and neck cancers: a comparative analysis of concurrent post-operative radiation plus chemo therapy trials of the EORTC (22931) and RTOG (9501). Head Neck. 2005;L27:843–50.
34. Gupta S, Bahadur S, Mathur M, Thakar A. Lateral neck dissection in cancers of the larynx and hypopharynx with No neck. Indian J Otolaryngol Head Neck Surg. 2000;52:253–6.
35. Lefebvre JL. Oral cavity, pharynx and larynx cancer Prognostic factors in cancer. New York: Weiley Lisa; 2001.
36. Shah J. Cervical lymph nodes. In: Shah JP, Patal S, editors. Head and neck surgery and oncology. 4th ed. Maryland Heights: Mosby; 2012: p. 353–94.

Guidelines in Management of Early Laryngeal Cancers (T_1 and T_2)

5

Sudhir Bahadur and Alok Thakar

5.1 Introduction

The aim of treatment in early cancers of the larynx is to obtain high cure rates and preserve all laryngeal functions, i.e. voice, airway and aspiration-free swallowing. Since the cure rates with different treatment modalities such as radiotherapy, endoscopic laser and open partial laryngectomy do not differ significantly, therapeutic decisions are influenced by factors such as voice quality, patient's choice, availability to treatment expertise and cost-effectiveness of treatment. However, during the last decade, the paradigm for treatment of early laryngeal cancer has shifted away from open partial laryngectomy as initial treatment to either radiotherapy or to TOLS (trans-oral laser surgery). The role of open partial laryngectomy has been mostly relegated to salvage setting following radiation failures.

Once the patient has been worked up in detail clinically, radiologically and staged (TNM) and biopsied, the case is then discussed in the multidisciplinary tumour board. It is important to have the CT/MRI images to properly stage and plan the treatment. Treatment decision is influenced by tumour factors (site, stage, behaviour, nodal metastasis), patient factors (age, co-morbidity, Karnofsky scale, pulmonary reserve and preference) and physician factors (treatment facilities and expertise available).

It is important to remember that for early cancers of the larynx, a single modality of treatment should be employed, and, therefore, choice should be carefully made based upon above factors.

S. Bahadur (✉)
Department of Otolaryngology and Head-Neck Surgery, Formerly at All India Institute of Medical Sciences, New Delhi, India

A. Thakar
Department of Otolaryngology and Head-Neck Surgery, All India Institute of Medical Sciences, New Delhi, India
e-mail: drathakar.orlhns@aiims.edu

S. Bahadur et al. (eds.), *Carcinoma of the Larynx and Hypopharynx*,
https://doi.org/10.1007/978-981-13-3110-7_5

5.2 Glottic Cancer

Treatment options for early glottic (T_1 and T_2) cancer include radiation therapy, trans-oral laser surgery and open partial laryngectomy. The choice is based on 'T' stage, the site within glottis region, cord mobility, anterior commissure involvement, age and occupation of the patient and availability of laser.

5.2.1 Carcinoma In Situ

Trans-oral endoscopic CO_2 laser surgery (TOLS) is the optimum way of treating carcinoma in situ. If the facilities for CO_2 laser are not available, trans-oral microlaryngoscopy and stripping of the vocal card are advisable. Regular follow-up and complete avoidance of smoking are essential. Besides, radiotherapy should not be used when there is no invasive cancer.

5.2.2 T_1 Glottic Cancer

All the three treatment modalities of treatment, i.e. narrow field radiation therapy or open partial laryngectomy or tans-oral CO_2 laser surgery (TOLS), normally provide excellent results. However, the quality of voice with radiotherapy is probably superior to that following surgery. Therefore, radiation therapy may be considered treatment of choice particularly if patient's profession demands good quality of voice. Several authors have reported excellent results of more than 90% 5 years cure rates in T_1 glottic lesions [1–4]. These authors also believe that functional results are better with radiation therapy.

However, advantage with trans-oral endoscopic laser surgery lies in its simplicity, short hospital stay and excellent outcome, and cure rates are approximately 90% [5–8]. The voice quality is good, though marginally inferior to the one following radiotherapy.

Trans-oral laser surgery further has the advantage of offering precise and tailored excisions for different categories of tumours. Further details of this technique are available in another chapter on the subject. Laser excisions for glottic lesions are classified as per the European Laryngological Classification and are listed in Table 5.1.

Table 5.1 CA glottis-endoscopic cordectomy

Type I	Subepithelial cordectomy
Type II	Subligamental cordectomy
Type III	Transmuscular cordectomy
Type IV	Total or complete cordectomy
Type V	Extended cordectomy encompassing
Type Va	Contralateral fold/anterior commissure
Type Vb	Arytenoids
Type Vc	Ventricular fold
Type Vd	Subglottis

ELS European Laryngological Society Classification

Table 5.2 Summary of recommended treatments for early laryngeal cancers

Glottic cancer
• Carcinoma—in situ
(a) Trans-oral endoscopic laser surgery
(b) MLS and stripping of vocal cord
• T_1 glottic cancer
(a) Mid-cordal lesion
– TOLS
– Radiotherapy
(b) Anterior commissure involvement
– Radiotherapy
– TOLS
– Fronto-lateral hemilaryngectomy
• T_2 glottic cancer
(a) T_2a (freely mobile cord)
– TOLS
– Radiotherapy
– Open partial laryngectomy
(b) T_2b (impaired vocal cord mobility)
– Open partial laryngectomy
– TOLS
– Radiotherapy
Supraglottic cancer (T_1/T_2)
Treatment decision is based upon location of tumour, pre-epiglottic space involvement, pulmonary status, age of patient and status of nodal disease N0/N+
• Marginal zone
(a) TOLS
(b) Radiotherapy
• Infrahyoid epiglottis
(a) Supraglottic laryngectomy
(b) Radiotherapy (if pulmonary reserve is poor)
• Suprahyoid epiglottis
(a) Radiotherapy
(b) TOLS

Voice results following laser resections depend to a large extent on the extent of resection undertaken. Minimal resections such as Type I and Type II cordectomy have minimal effects on the voice, while Type IV cordectomy (total cordectomy) and Type Va cordectomy (anterior commissure excision) often lead to initial complete aphonia. Typically voice results following laser surgery improve over time.

Similar good results are available with open partial laryngectomy, which are comparable to radiotherapy and laser cordectomy, though temporary tracheotomy is required for open partial laryngectomy and voice quality is usually somewhat inferior to one following endoscopic CO_2 laser excision [9].

5.2.3 Anterior Commissure Lesion or Vocal Fold Lesion Extending to the Anterior Commissure

Lesions of anterior commissure present complex issues in management. These lesions have a propensity for superior and inferior extension along the anterior commissure ligament and also for thyroid cartilage invasion as the inner perichondrium of this cartilage is known to be anatomically deficient at the anterior commissure. All such cases require careful endoscopic evaluation by flexible or rigid video-endoscopy for superior/inferior extension and also thin section contrast-enhanced CT evaluation for thyroid cartilage erosion.

In general some compromise in oncologic results has been noted with both radiation therapy [10–12] and trans-oral laser surgery [13, 14]. Partial laryngectomy was advocated in the past as it also covered for the risk of occult cartilage involvement [11, 12], but with improving radiology, this risk is now minimized (though not excluded). With current radiology, cartilage involvement at the anterior commissure is now more easily identified. Such candidates with anterior commissure thyroid cartilage involvement but with mobile cords are best treated by partial laryngectomy but no longer classified as early cancer as they are upstaged to T3/T4.

For the anterior commissure tumour with no cartilage involvement, current improvements in radiation techniques have also enabled better cure rates than was the case earlier. Mendenhall in a review of 450 patients of early cancer treated with radiotherapy did not find any difference in results even when anterior commissure was involved [10].

Trans-oral laser surgery is noted to be as effective but should be carried out by experienced surgeons since the procedure is technically more demanding. Loco-regional failures of 21–30% have been reported in patients with anterior commissure involvement [13, 14], as opposed to 5% recurrence rate in case anterior commissure is not involved [14]. Also, voice results can be initially very disappointing as both vocal cords lose their anterior attachment as so lose tension, but this tends to improve once the healing and scarification again lead to a tensioning of the vocal fold.

5.2.4 T_2 Glottic Cancer

T_2 glottic tumours include two subcategories which may behave differently. T_{2a} lesions are cancers with surface extension beyond the glottis (i.e. tumour extension onto supraglottis or subglottis). T_{2b} lesions are cancers wherein the vocal cord mobility is impaired (but not fixed) because of tumour infiltration. It is suggested that overall T_2 glottic tumours treated with surgery produce better results than with radiation therapy. Wang [15] has shown local control rates of 86% in T_{2a} lesions and 63% in T_{2b} lesions when these were primarily treated with radiotherapy. Similar results have been reported by other authors [9, 16], who advocate radiation therapy for treatment of T_{2a} lesions but prefer treating T_{2b} lesions (impaired vocal cord mobility) with vertical partial laryngectomy or supracricoid laryngectomy with cricohyoidoepiglottopexy. Alternatively, if facilities exist, these lesions can be effectively treated by trans-oral endoscopic CO_2 laser surgery [7, 8].

5.2.5 Supraglottic Cancer (T_1 and T_2)

Supraglottic cancers have a relatively high propensity for metastasis to the neck nodes. The rate of occult neck metastasis in the otherwise N_0 neck exceeds 20%, and all such patients therefore merit elective neck treatment. Cure rates are relatively poorer in comparison to glottis disease primarily because of disease involvement of the neck.

In case of supraglottic cancer with mobile vocal cords and minimal neck disease (N_0/N_1), the important parameters for decision-making include the site of disease, pulmonary status of the patient, and presence or absence of pre-epiglottic space involvement.

Lesions located in the infrahyoid epiglottis are more prone to involve the pre-epiglottic space, and horizontal supraglottic laryngectomy gives superior cure rates than radiation therapy [17, 18]. Therefore in younger patients with good pulmonary status, surgery is the preferred option. However, in case of poor pulmonary reserve, open partial laryngectomy may produce severe aspiration and considerable morbidity, and therefore such patients are better treated with radiation therapy, particularly if imaging studies do not show any pre-epiglottic space involvement, and reserving total laryngectomy for surgical salvage. However if CT/MRI shows definite pre-epiglottic space involvement, surgery comprising of near-total or total laryngectomy may be a preferred option. Suprahyoid lesions of the epiglottis on the other hand respond well to radiation therapy, partly because these are exophytic and do not involve the pre-epiglottic space, and the neck is included in the radiation field.

However, if early supraglottic cancers (T_1 and T_2) are accompanied by bulky nodal disease (N_2/N_3), supraglottic laryngectomy with an appropriate neck dissection is recommended. These patients will need postoperative radiotherapy, if the neck nodes are found to be histologically positive. In cases of bilateral neck disease, it is to safer to perform a functional neck dissection on the side of less bulky disease and a radical neck dissection on the side of more extensive disease.

5.3 TOLS for Supraglottic Cancer

If complete resection can be achieved, the oncologic results of TOLS are comparable to those of open supraglottic laryngectomy with the advantage that functional results are superior in terms of early restoration of swallowing and avoidance of tracheostomy. Besides, low incidence of pharyngocutaneous fistula formation and shorter hospital stay are other advantages [19, 20]. Management of the neck remains of paramount importance as survival of supraglottic cancer patients depends more on status of cervical metastasis than on the primary tumour [20].

Various authors have reported excellent results treating supraglottic tumours with trans-oral endoscopic laser (TOLS). Steiner [5] and Ambrosch et al. [20] have mentioned 5-year local control rates of 100% for T_1 and 89% for T_2 supraglottic tumours. Three-year disease-free and overall survival in T_2 lesions were 83 and 76%, respectively. Similar good results have been reported elsewhere [21–23]. In the USA prior to availability of laser surgery, supraglottic laryngectomy had been the favoured modality of treatment because of high rate of laryngeal preservation [21, 24].

The availability of the da Vinci Robot has led to a trend from trans-oral laser supraglottic laryngectomy to the trans-oral robotic supraglottic laryngectomy. The robot offers the advantages of enabling an en bloc excision in a shorter surgical time. Anatomical restrictions of space and access may however restrict its use, and it is not appropriate for all patients.

5.4 Radiation Therapy

There have been a very few reports of results of radiotherapy in treatment of supraglottic cancer. Mendenhall [25, 26] reported a cause-specific survival of 100% for T_1 and 83% for T_2 supraglottic lesions.

The local control and preservation of laryngeal function by radiotherapy are related to tumour volume [27, 28]. On univariate analysis in the latter study, local control rates were 92.6% and 73.6% for small and bulky tumours ($P = 0.03$) and 89.6% and 75.9% for patients without and with anterior commissure involvement, respectively ($P = 0.01$). On multivariate analysis, tumour bulk was the only significant factor that affected local control ($P = 0.007$).

In supraglottic cancers, local control rate is influenced by pre-epiglottic space involvement which in turn is reflected by tumour volume. Studies have demonstrated that supraglottic tumours staged T_1–T_3 with tumour volumes less than 6cc as determined by computed tomography achieved 83% local control, whereas if tumour volume was greater than 6cc, local control rate was achieved in 46% of patients ($P = 0.038$). This difference was independent of both T stage and primary site [27, 28].

5.5 Partial Laryngectomy

Open partial laryngectomy has been an important tool in treatment of early laryngeal cancer for almost a country. It provides excellent results in suitably selected patients with laryngeal preservation. However, in recent years, with advances in radiation techniques and trans-oral endoscopic laser surgery, open partial laryngectomy is rarely employed as the initial treatment of early-stage cancer. Partial laryngectomy is now mostly used for salvage surgery for radiotherapy failed cases. Nevertheless, the surgeons should be familiar with the surgical technique and post-operative care.

5.6 Vertical Partial Laryngectomy

The vertical partial laryngectomy has been so named because the endolarynx is opened by a vertical incision through the thyroid cartilage near the anterior commissure. A variety of vertical partial laryngectomies have been described. The most common are laryngofissure and cordectomy, vertical hemilaryngectomy, frontolateral hemilaryngectomy, extended vertical hemilaryngectomy, and the epiglottic laryngoplasty [29]. There have been excellent articles on techniques of fronto-lateral hemilaryngectomy. The basic feature of all the procedures is vertical transection of the thyroid cartilage and resection of the glottis extended into the paraglottic space. The vertical partial laryngectomy is indicated for T_1 and T_2 glottic lesions. However, in patients with vocal card fixation because of invasion of cricoarytenoid joint, a hemilaryngectomy should not be considered [30]. The survival rates at 5 years with this technique have been more than 90% [31, 32]. Another study reported local control in T_1 lesions was 91% but decreased to 74% (with anterior commissure involvement) and further dropped to 69% in T_2 lesions [33]. However, rates of local control and survival at 5 years were significantly lower for T_3 lesions [12, 34]. It is apparent that vertical partial laryngectomy is a useful procedure in selected cases. However, cases that are suitable for open partial laryngectomy can be still better managed with trans-oral endoscopic laser surgery, which provides similar rates of local control, better voice quality and swallowing function and lower complication rates [35].

5.7 Supraglottic Laryngectomy

The surgical technique for supraglottic tumours was initially described by Som [17] and Alonso [36]. The surgery involves resection of epiglottic, the bands, the aryepiglottic folds, hyoid bone, superior portion of thyroid cartilage and contents of preepiglottic space. Usually supraglottic laryngectomy is performed sparing both arytenoids, both true vocal cords and the tongue base. The resection can be extended to include one arytenoid, part of base of the tongue or the pyriform sinus. However, the rehabilitation process following surgery and depending upon extent of resection and age of the patient and pulmonary reserve is often very long and complicated.

Normally, the indications for supraglottic laryngectomy include T_1 and T_2 lesions, but it may be performed in select T_3 and T_4 lesions involving the preepiglottic space or one of the arytenoids, the pyriform sinus or minimally the base of the tongue, but patients selected for supraglottic laryngectomy need to have adequate pulmonary function. The overall survival at 5 years is almost comparable to that obtained with total laryngectomy for similar lesions, ranging for 67–90%. The survival rate is approximately 85% for stage I and II, 75% for stage III and over 55–70% for stage IV tumours [37–41]. Overall, laryngeal preservation rate and functional results are good and in over 85% cases. Thus, overall supraglottic laryngectomy is a good surgical technique in selected cases of small and advanced tumours; still, it has been replaced by trans-oral endoscopic laser surgery which provides better functional advantage [28].

5.8 Supracricoid Partial Laryngectomy

The surgical technique for SCL was initially described by Majer and Reider [42] and later by Laccoureye [43]. Two forms are described depending upon involvement of epiglottis, the cricohyoidopexy and cricohyoidoepiglottopexy (CHEP). The surgery involves resecting the vocal folds, the aryepiglottic folds, the epiglottis, the thyroid cartilage, contents of pre-epiglottic and paraglottic spaces and also the part of subglottis corresponding to upper surface of the cricoid cartilage. The resection may include one arytenoid but preserve the hyoid bone. The SCL may also be used as a salvage surgery following RT/concurrent chemoradiotherapy. Nakayama et al. [44] in their review of 73 patients treated by SCL-CHEP reported larynx preservation rates and overall survival rates to be 92% and 85%, respectively. The oncologic and functional outcomes were satisfactory and did not vary between irradiated and nonirradiated patients. It has been suggested that in selected cases, SCL could be an alternative to total laryngectomy [45]. After SCL, intensive rehabilitation over weeks is needed until speech and swallowing are restored, and 80%–90% patients are expected to recover swallowing function within first year [44, 46–48].

5.9 Authors' Comments

The main objective of treatment in early cancers of the larynx is to achieve high cure rates in oncologic terms and to preserve the larynx and its functions. Ideally, a single modality of treatment should be employed, and therefore, choice of treatment should be carefully made based on tumour factors (site, stage, tumour extension, cord mobility, nodal metastasis), patient factors (co-morbidity, pulmonary reserve and preference) and physician factors (facilities and expertise available).

It is also realized that cure rates with different treatment strategies such as radiotherapy, endoscopic laser surgery and open partial laryngectomy may not significantly differ. Therefore, decision-making also takes into account factors such as voice quality, morbidity of the treatment and its cost-effectiveness. Decisions need to be individualized for individual patients. Particularly difficult are treatment decisions between radiation therapy and trans-oral laser surgery in the T_1/T_{2a} cancers. The pros and cons of each are summarized in Table 5.3.

Table 5.3 Pros and cons of radiation treatment and trans-oral laser surgery for early laryngeal cancers

Radiation treatment	Trans-oral laser surgery
7 weeks treatment duration	Single surgical treatment—often day care
Better preservation of anatomy	Avoids overtreatment (tailored Rx as per disease extent)
Functional voice results better initially	Functional voice results equivalent after healing
	Avoids long-term radiation morbidity
Option of radiation Rx limited for subsequent recurrence/2nd primary (10%)	All treatment options including radiation Rx/laser surgery/conventional surgery preserved for subsequent recurrence/2nd Primary (10%)
Recurrence may need total laryngectomy	Overall laryngeal preservation rates possibly better [49]

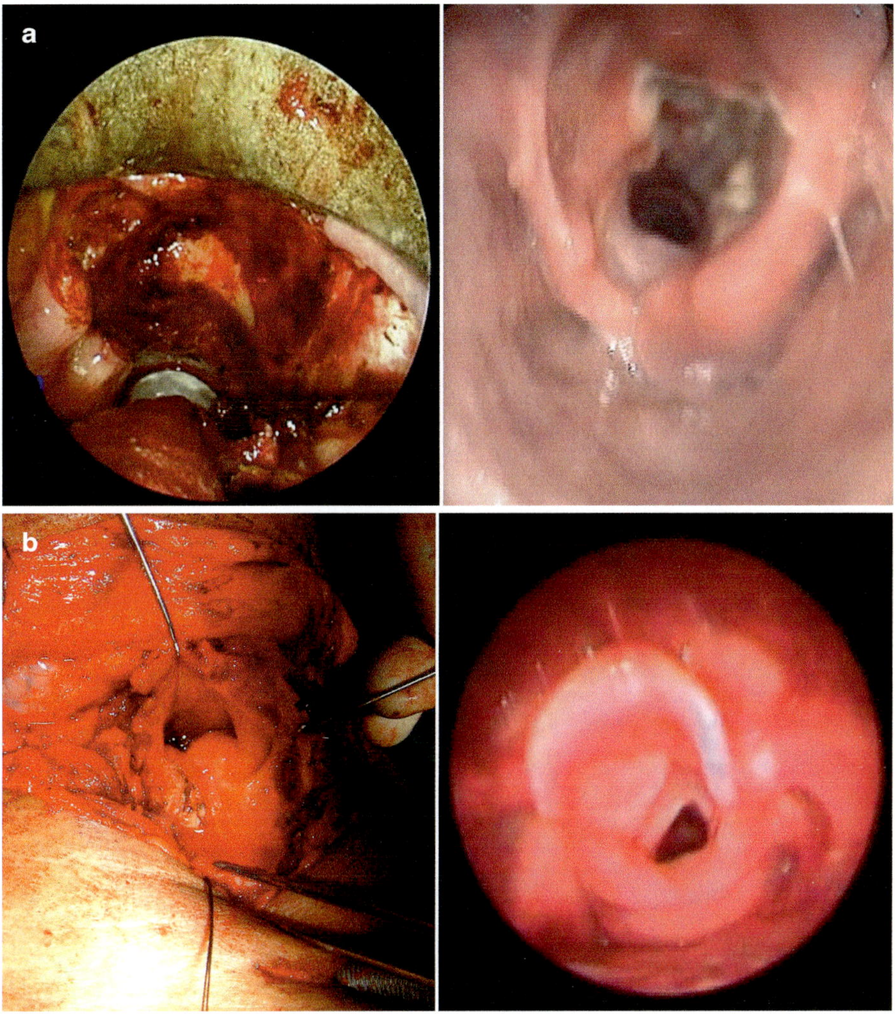

Fig. 5.1 Surgical pictures and postsurgical laryngoscopy of (**a**) trans-oral laser resection of Rt Type IV cordectomy + anterior commissure resection. Transected edges of Lt vocal fold and ventricular fold noted; (**b**) right vertical partial laryngectomy, fibrotic Rt. neo-cord and absence of ventricular fold noted in the postsurgical laryngoscopy; (**c**) horizontal partial laryngectomy and (**d**) supracricoid laryngectomy with cricohyoidoepiglottopexy, postsurgical laryngoscopy demonstrating only remnant of epiglottis and bilateral arytenoids and absence of bilateral ventricular and vocal folds

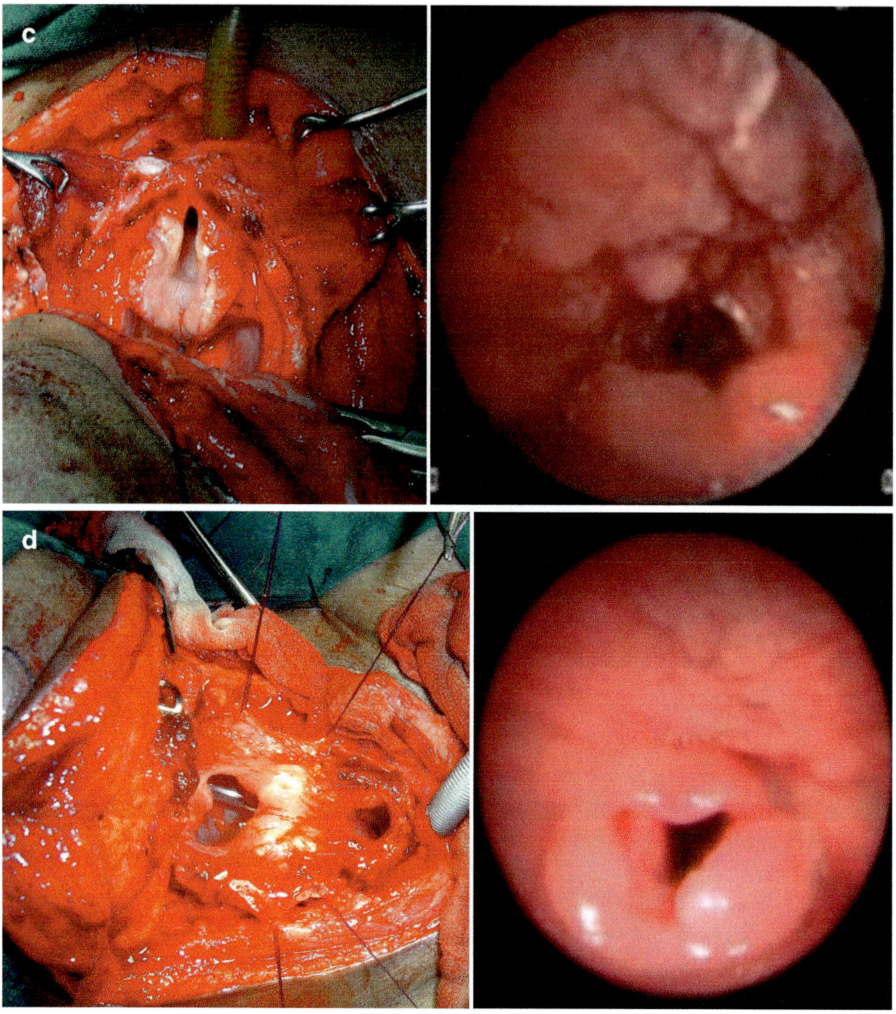

Fig. 5.1 (continued)

T_1 glottic tumours (mid-cordal lesions) can be treated equally well with either of three modalities. However, if facilities for laser are available, it should be preferred because of good oncologic outcome, short hospital stay and little morbidity. Radiotherapy is an excellent alternative if laser is not available. It produces high cure rates with good quality of voice. Open partial laryngectomy is still useful in the salvage setting in cases of radiation failure. The glottis lesions with involvement of anterior commissure present complex problem. Treatment with endoscopic laser, if considered, should be carried out by experienced surgeons because of higher local recurrence rate reported. Most of good radiotherapy centres still report excellent cure rates in this situation with recurrence rates only marginally different than when anterior commissure is not involved.

T_2 glottic lesion as shown by paraglottic space involvement (seen on the CT scan) respond better to surgery (open partial laryngectomy or TOLS) as compared to radiotherapy, particularly in cases where vocal cord mobility is impaired or minimal subglottic extension is noted. Still, radiotherapy produces good overall outcome and excellent voice quality in T_2 glottic lesions.

Important parameters for decision-making for treatment of supraglottic cancers (T_1 and T_2) include the precise location of tumour, pre-epiglottic space involvement and pulmonary status. Lesions of infrahyoid epiglottis (prone to involve the pre-epiglottic space) respond better to horizontal partial laryngectomy than to radiation therapy. Therefore in younger patients with good pulmonary reserve, surgery is the preferred option. Patients with poor chest condition may be treated with radiotherapy while reserving salvage total laryngectomy for failures. Suprahyoid lesions of the epiglottis respond well to radiotherapy.

References

1. Mendenhall WM, Parsons JT, Stringer SP, et al. T_1 and T_2 vocal cord carcinoma. A basis for comparing the results of radiotherapy and surgery. Head Neck Surg. 1988;10:373–7.
2. Tamura Y, Tanaka S, Asato R, Hirano S, et al. Therapeutic outcomes of laryngeal cancer at Kyoto university Hospital for 10 years. Acta Otolaryngol Suppl. 2007;557:62–5.
3. Mohanti BK, Tandon DA, Bahadur S, Rath GK, Tanwar RK, Lal P, Biswal BM. Results of definitive radiotherapy in T_1 and T_2 glottic carcinoma: Institute of Rotary Cancer Hospital experience. Australas Radiol. 1996;40:287–90.
4. Dinshaw KA, Sharma V. Radiation therapy in early glottic carcinoma: significance of prognostic factors and dose fractionation. Indian J Cancer. 1990;27:143–53.
5. Steiner W. Results of curative laser micro-surgery of the laryngeal carcinomas. Am J Otolaryngol. 1993;14:116–21.
6. Eckel HE, Thumfart WF. Laser Surgery for treatment of larynx carcinoma: indications, techniques and preliminary results. Annals Otol Rhimol Laryngol. 1992;101:113–8.
7. Pradhan SA, Pai PS, Neeli SI, D'Cruz AK. Trans oral laser surgery for early glottic cancer. Arch Otolaryngol Head Neck Surg. 2003;129:623–5.
8. Steiner W, Ambroch P. Endoscopic laser surgery of the upper aerodigestive tract. Stuttgart: Thieme; 2000. p. 56–60.
9. Pradhan S. Voice conservation surgery for laryngeal and hypopharyngeal cancer. Mumbai: Lloyds; 2006.
10. Mendenhall WM, Amdur RJ, Morris CG, Hinerman RW. $T_1 - T_2$ N_0 squamous cell carcinoma of the glottic larynx treated with radiation therapy. J Clin Oncol. 2001;19:4029–36.
11. Laccourrey O, Weinstein G, Brasun D, et al. Vertical partial laryngectomy. A critical analysis of local recurrence. Ann Otol Rhinol Laryngol. 1991;100:68–71.
12. Kessler DJ, Trap TK, Calcaterra TC. Treatment of T_3 glottic carcinoma with vertical partial laryngectomy. Arch of Otolaryngology. 1987;113:1196–9.
13. Chone CT, Yonchera E, Marthtins JE, et al. Importance of anterior commissure in recurrence of early glottic cancer after laser endoscopic resection. Arch, Otolargyngol Head and Neck Surg. 2007;133:882–7.
14. Steiner W, Ambrosch P, Rodal RM, Kron M. Impact of anterior commissure involvement on local control of early glottic carcinoma treated by laser microresections. Laryngoscope. 2004;114:1485–91.

15. Wang CC. Treatment of glottic carcinoma by megavoltage radiation therapy and results. Am J Roentgenol Rad Ther Med. 1974;120:157.
16. Harwood A. Cancer of the larynx. The Toronto experience. J Otolaryngol. 1982;11:1–21.
17. Som M. Conservation Surgery for carcinoma of the supraglottis. J Laryngol Otol. 1970;84:655–78.
18. Robbins KT, Davidson W, Petars LT, Geopfart H. Conservations Surgery for T_2 and T_3 carcinoma of the supraglottic larynx. Arch Otolaryngol Head Neck Surg. 1988;114:421–6.
19. Rodrigo JP, Suraez C, Silver CE, et al. Trans oral laser surgery for supraglottic cancer. Head Neck. 2008;30:658–66.
20. Ambrosch P, Kron M, Steiner W. Carbon dioxide laser microsurgery for early supraglottic carcinoma. Ann Otol Rhinol Laryngol. 1998;107:680–8.
21. Zeitels SM, Koufman JA, Davis RK, Voughn CW. Endoscopic treatment in supraglottic and hypopharynx cancer. Laryngoscope. 1994;104:71-78.
22. Grant DG, Salassa JR, Hinni ML, et al. Trans oral microsurgery for carcinoma of supraglottic larynx. Ototlaryngology Head and Neck Surgery. 2007;136:900–6.
23. Cabanillhas R, Rodrigo JL, Llorante JL, Suarez C. Oncologic outcomes of trans oral laser surgery of supraglottic carcinoma compared with transcervical approach. Head Neck. 2008;30:750–5.
24. Sessions DG, Lenox J, Spector GJ. Supraglottic laryngeal cancer: analysis of treatment results. Laryngoscope. 2005;115:1402–10.
25. Mendenhall WM, Parsons JT, Strigner SP, et al. Carcinoma of the Supraglottic larynx for comparing results of radiotherapy and surgery. Head Neck. 1990;12:204–9.
26. Mendenhall WM, Mancuso AA, Hinerman RW, et al. Multidisciplinary management of laryngeal carcinoma. Int J Radiat Oncol Biol Phys. 2007;69(Suppl):12–4.
27. Reddy SL, Hong RL, Nagda S, Emami B. Effect of tumour bulk on local control and survival of patients with T_1 glottic cancer: a 30 year experience. Inj J Radiat Oncol Biol Phys. 2007;69:1389–94.
28. Freeman DE, Mancuso AA, Parsons JT, Mendenhall WM, Million RR. Irradiation alone for supraglottic larynx carcinoma: can CT findings predict treatment results? Int J Radiat Oncol Biol Phys. 1990;19:485–90.
29. Weinstein GS, Lacourrey O, Brasano D, Laccourrey W. Organ preservation for laryngeal cancer. San Diego, CA: Singular Publishing Group; 2000.
30. Rodrigo JP, Suarez C, Silver CE. Transoral laser surgery for supraglottic cancer. Head Neck. 2008;30:658–66.
31. Johnson JT, Hao S, Myers ENF, Wegner RI. Outcome of open partial laryngectomy for glottic carcinoma. Ann Otol Rhinol Laryngol. 1993;102:752–5.
32. Thomas JV, Oslen KD, Neal HB, et al. Early glottic carcinoma treated with open partial laryngeal procedures. Arch Otolaryngeal Head Neck Surg. 1994;120:264–8.
33. Burmund KT, Gutierrez-Fonsea R, Gracia D, et al. Frontolateral vertical partial laryngectomy without tracheostomy for invasive squamous cell carcinoma of the true vocal cord: a 25 year experience. Ann Otol Rhinol Laryngol. 2005;114:314–22.
34. Biller HF, Lawson W. Partial laryngectomy for vocal cord cancer with marked limitation or fixation of the vocal cord. Laryngoscope. 1986;96:61–4.
35. Keratzanis AD, Pyhogios G, Waldjaher F, et al. Comparison among different available surgical approaches in T_1 glottic cancer. Laryngoscope. 2009;119:1704–8.
36. Alonso CM, Jackson CL. Conservation of function in surgery of cancer of the larynx. Bases technique and results. Trans Am Acad Opthalmol Otolaryngol. 1952;56:722.
37. Sevilla MA, Ridrigo JP, Llorente JL, et al. Supraglottic laryngectomy – analysis of 267 cases. Eur acrh Otolaryngology. 2008;265:11–6.
38. Scola B, Fernandez Vega M, Martinez T. Management of cancer of supraglottis. Otolaryngol Head Neck Surg. 2001;124:194–8.
39. Herranz J, Martinez Vidal J, Martinej Moran A. Supraglottic laryngectomy. Still ongoing. Acta Otolarygol Esp. 2006;57:235–41.

40. Robbins KT, Davidson N, Peters LT, Goepfert H. Conservation surgery for T_2 and T_3 carcinoma of supraglottic larynx. Arch Otolaryngol. 1998;114:421–6.
41. Suarez E, Rodrigo JP, Herranz J, et al. Supraglottic laryngectomy with or without post operative radiotherapy. Annals Otol Rhinol Larygol. 1995;104:358–63.
42. Major H, Rider A. Technique de laryngectomie permanent de conserva ta permeabilita repiratorira (ta crico-hyoidopexie). Ann Otolaryngol Chir Carvicofac. 1959;76:677–83.
43. Laccourrey O, Laccourreye L, Garcia D. Vertical partial laryngectomy versus supra cricoid partial laryngectomy for selected T_2N_0 carcinoma of true cord. Ann Otol Rhinol Laryngol. 2000;109:965–71.
44. Nakayama M, Laccourreye O, Hdsinger FC, et al. Functional organ preservation for laryngeal cancer: past, present and future. Jpn J Clin Oncol. 2012;42(3):155–60.
45. Silver CE. Laryngeal Cancer. In: Silver CE, editor. New York: Thieme Medical Publishers; 1991: p. 140–14.
46. Hartl DM, Fertilo A, Brasnu DF, et al. Evidence based review of treatment options for patients with glottic cancer. Head Neck. 2011;33:1638–48.
47. Castro A, Sanchez-Cuedrado I, Bernaldez R. Larynx function preservation following supracricoid partial laryngectomy. Head Neck. 2012;134:162–7.
48. Nando P, Laccourreye O, Weinstein GS, et al. Functional outcome and prognostic factors after supracricoid partial laryngectomy with cricohyoidopexy. Ann Otol Rhinol Laryngol. 1997;106:291–6.
49. Bron LP, Soldati D, Zouhair A, Ozsahin M, Brossard E, Monnier P, Pasche P. Treatment of early stage squamous-cell carcinoma of the glottic larynx: endoscopic surgery or cricohyoidoepiglottopexy versus radiotherapy. Head Neck. 2001;23:823–9.

Guidelines in the Management of Advanced Carcinoma of the Larynx

6

Sudhir Bahadur

6.1 Definition

The term advanced laryngeal cancer generally designates stage T_3 or T_4 disease according to UICC/AJCC staging. These may attain advanced stage by virtue of advanced T classification (T_3 or T_4), N classification (N_1–N_3) or M classification (M_1). However, it also allows early T classification (T_1, T_2) to be included in advanced lesions if they are associated with nodal metastasis.

Laryngeal cancers attain T_3 classification if they have vocal cord fixation, paraglottic space or pre-epiglottic space invasion, post-cricoid extension or minor thyroid cartilage erosion. T_4 classification is attained in tumours with cartilage destruction or extra-laryngeal invasion. Accurate staging of laryngeal cancers demands careful clinical, radiological and endoscopic assessment for standard treatment. Curative radiotherapy has been an accepted modality of treatment for early laryngeal cancer, and it provides excellent results both in terms of oncologic cure rates and organ preservations [1]. In small number of patients where disease persists or recurs, timely intervention with salvage surgery can boost the overall survival rates. However, results of radiotherapy alone in advanced lesions are less satisfactory, and more failed cases need salvage surgery [2, 3].

6.2 Introduction

Management of advanced carcinoma of the larynx is a complex issue. Often the diagnosis is delayed, such as in supraglottic cancers, which may have a few symptoms until the disease is far advanced with high incidence of lymph node

S. Bahadur (✉)
Department of Otolaryngology and Head-Neck Surgery, Formerly at All India Institute of Medical Sciences, New Delhi, India

S. Bahadur et al. (eds.), *Carcinoma of the Larynx and Hypopharynx*,
https://doi.org/10.1007/978-981-13-3110-7_6

involvement. Both the supraglottic and transglottic cancers usually carry aggressive tumour behaviour with guarded prognosis. However, glottic lesions tend to have better prognosis because of their early presentation and rare lymph node involvement.

Overall 40–80% of laryngeal carcinomas present with stage III or IV disease when first evaluated [4–6]. Most cases are associated with history of tobacco and alcohol intake, so treatment is often impacted by medical comorbidity and development of second primary cancers [7, 8].

Total laryngectomy with postoperative radiotherapy for advanced lesions is the gold standard treatment for advanced carcinoma. Unfortunately, total laryngectomy also results in permanent tracheostoma and loss of speech, which is why most patients are reluctant to undergo surgery fearing social isolation and loss and depression [9, 10]. Still, in terms of oncologic outcome and disease-free survival, surgery provides better results. Speech rehabilitation with oesophageal speech or tracheo-oesophageal prosthesis (TEP), however, helps in overcoming the handicap.

Results of open partial laryngectomy and laser microsurgery are well established and comparable to those of RT [11]. There has been increased interest in the use of combination or chemo-radiation since the early 1990s for laryngeal preservation in advanced disease. The combined treatment has focused on two aims: of increased survival and functional organ preservation. The strategies consist of induction chemotherapy as initially established in the Veterans Affairs Larynx preservations trial [12] and subsequently with concomitant chemo-radiotherapy as described by Radiation Therapy Oncology Group (RTOG)91-11 [13].

The primary end point in the latter study was overall survival and organ preservation (laryngectomy-free survival, LFS). Both induction chemotherapy and concurrent chemotherapy resulted in superior LFS as compared to radiation alone. However, concurrent chemo-radiotherapy was the superior approach to laryngeal preservation, though overall survival was not significantly different [13].

Despite the advantages of higher laryngeal preservation rate following chemo-radiotherapy, it is associated with significant toxicity and morbidity and even mortality. These patients require increased care in specialized centres and regular follow-up besides the increased cost of treatment. However, the most important parameter is the careful selection of patients for chemo-radiotherapy protocol.

6.3 Surgical Treatment of Metastatic Neck

Surgical treatment includes management of neck metastasis. The lymph node metastasis significantly and adversely affects the survival in patients with carcinoma of the larynx [14–16]. The management depends upon the stage and site of primary tumour and whether the neck is clinically negative or positive. It is well realized that there is high propensity of lymph node involvement in supraglottic and transglottic cancers, varying between 50% and 70% cases. Similarly, the rate of occult neck disease (PN+) even in clinically negative necks in these cancers is high except in glottic lesions, and when such is the case (PN+), it produces disease-free rates similar to those found in clinically positive nodes [15]. There is thus a case for doing elective neck dissection in supraglottic cancers [16, 17]. Besides, regional failure of 20% has been demonstrated on the contralateral side in supraglottic cancer, and these authors recommended bilateral neck dissection to impact the failure rate from 20% to 9%. However, there is also a suggestion that close observation with latter treatment reserved for subsequent neck metastasis is a valid form of treatment.

A radical neck dissection or a modified neck dissection is performed on the side of the lesion in patients with clinically positive neck, with resection of primary neoplasm.

6.4 Surgery for Primary Neoplasm

The ultimate aim of total laryngectomy with or without a neck dissection is to achieve maximum locoregional control. Tumour-free margins are confirmed by frozen section studies during surgery, and the pharynx is closed primarily as enough mucosa is available for repair. However, sometimes a patched pectoralis major myocutaneous flap may be useful if surgery is carried out in radiation failed cases.

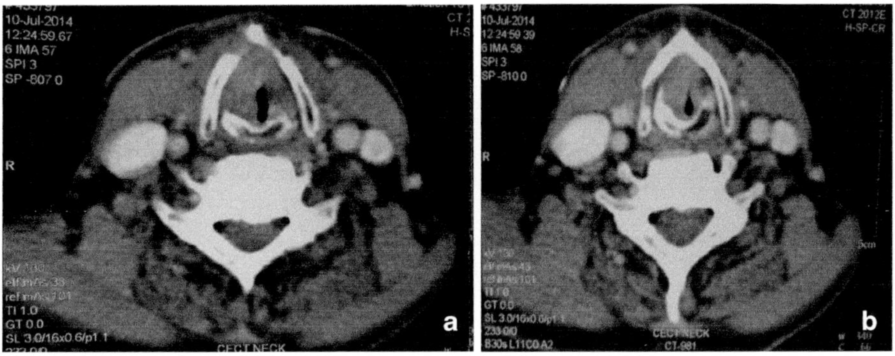

Fig. 6.1 (**a**, **b**) CT scans showing extensive laryngeal tumour (T_4 N_1) suggesting cartilage invasion. It would be better to treat such a case with total laryngectomy

Fig. 6.2 Advanced lesion showing obvious cartilage destruction. Will have guarded prognosis despite radical surgery and postoperative radiotherapy

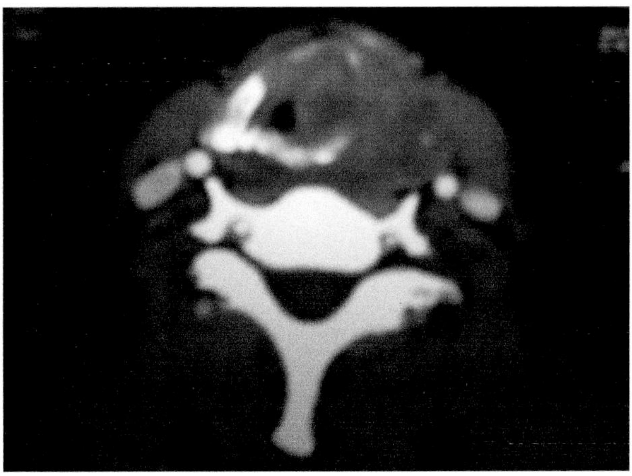

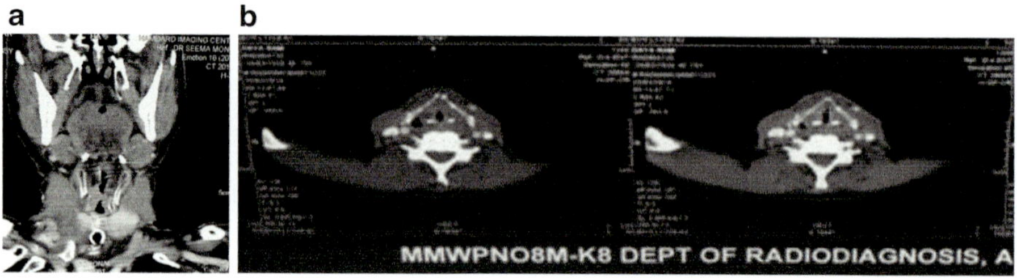

Fig. 6.3 (**a**, **b**) CT scans of T_3 glottic carcinoma may be considered for chemo-radiation protocol based on patient factors

Fig. 6.4 Total laryngectomy with radical neck dissection specimen for T_4 N, transglottic lesion

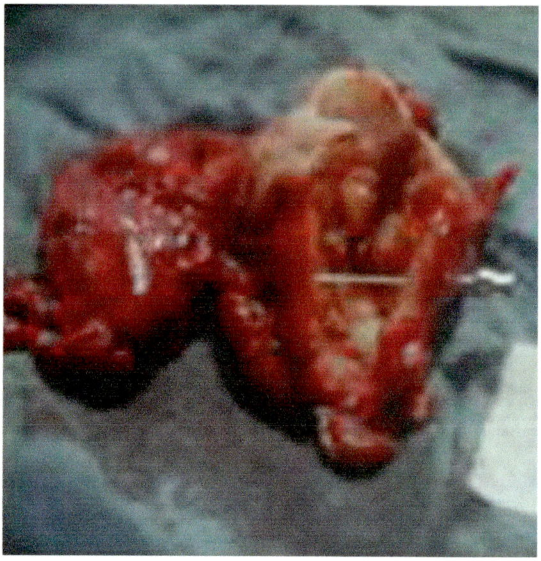

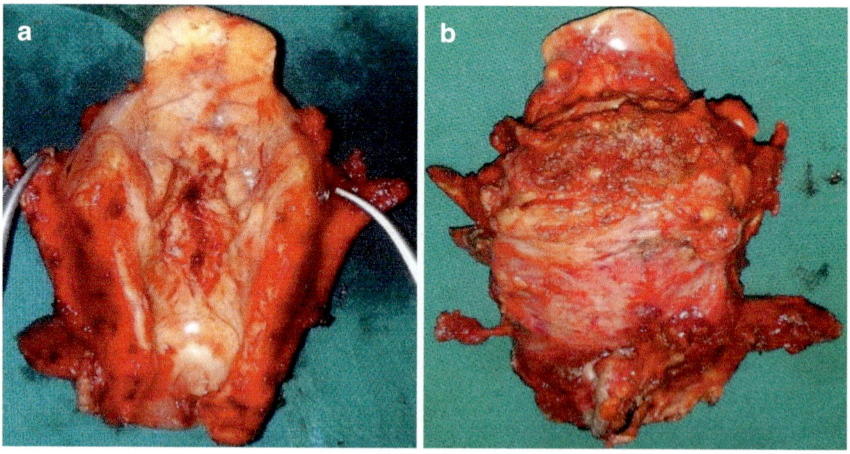

Fig. 6.5 (**a**, **b**) Laryngectomy specimen of advanced transglottic carcinoma. A cuff of soft tissue is included anteriorly in the specimen

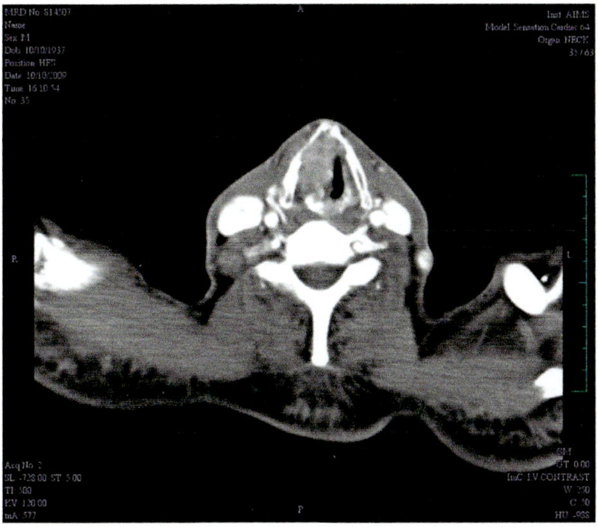

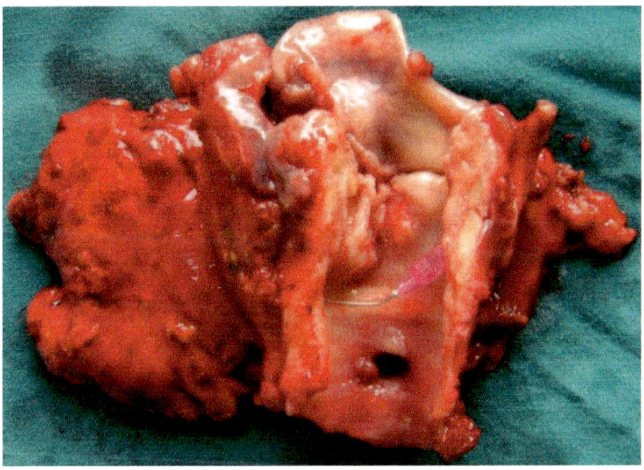

Fig. 6.6 Surgical specimen of T_4N_1 transglottic carcinoma with obvious involvement of pyriform fossa (prior tracheostomy site included in the specimen)

6.5 Selection of Patients for Surgery

There are several factors that have to be considered in the final decision-making for treatment.

6.5.1 Indications

1. Tumour Factors
   (a) Tumour stage and extent of invasion of thyroid cartilage/cricoid cartilage (T_4 disease) as seen on CT scan or MRI is an important indication for total laryngectomy (Figs. 6.1, 6.2, 6.3, 6.4 and 6.5). Patients with extensive tumours

have been shown to have worse disease control when treated by radiotherapy alone compared with surgery and postoperative radiotherapy [3]. If these patients were placed in organ preservation trials, they are more likely to need salvage laryngectomy. The patients with such advanced tumours (T_4 disease) have been excluded from participation in the trials [13].

(b) Total laryngectomy should also be considered in patients who have severe aspiration at the time of diagnosis. Similarly advanced nodal disease (N_2/N_3) may also be a pointer to consider surgery.

(c) Apart from the advanced T_4 lesions with cartilage invasion, primary total laryngectomy may also be considered in T_3transglottic carcinoma with fixed vocal cords. The latter lesions were not included in the larynx preservation trial [13]. It is possible that because of their tendency to involve the cartilage early and limited response to radiotherapy, these cases were not included in the study.

(d) Besides, there are situations where total laryngectomy may be an appropriate option for advanced laryngeal cancer. These include unreliable patients and those who are unlikely to come for regular follow-up or (1) who do not wish to undergo physically the ordeal of chemo-radiotherapy, (2) treatment centres that are located in areas where facilities for multimodality treatment are not available or (3) cost of treatment, which is a serious concern.

2. Patient Factors

The age of patient, Karnofsky Performance Status Scale and comorbidity may be important criteria to influence the choice of treatment. Patients above 70 years of age are usually not considered for chemotherapy. Similarly patients with poor results in the Karnofsky Performance Status Scale may receive palliative treatment instead of curative effort. Similarly cardiac illness may necessitate change of chemotherapy regimen or fractionated radiotherapy.

Besides patients' professional work, lifestyle and social support system may also influence treatment protocol. Teachers or lawyers may prefer to undergo organ preservation with chemo-radiation rather than opting for total laryngectomy. Likewise, many self-employed individuals may prefer to be treated with short procedure like endoscopic laser microsurgery rather than extensive and long chemo-radiation protocol.

3. Physician Factors

The expertise of the treating physician and centre is an important consideration for influencing the treatment decision, e.g. conservation surgery using trans-oral laser microsurgery should not be undertaken by an occasional surgeon.

Finally the patient's preference should be respected. If surgery is chosen for treatment protocol details and nature of surgery, its likely implications and morbidity must be explained to the patient.

Theodor Billroth performed the first total laryngectomy in 1873 and first hemilaryngectomy 5 years later in 1878 for the carcinoma of the larynx [18]. After the initial reports and results, that the surgery was safe and satisfactory, modern-wide field total laryngectomy came to be accepted as the treatment of choice for the advanced laryngeal cancer from the second half of the twentieth century.

6.5.2 Prognostic Factors and Postoperative Radiotherapy

Zhang et al. [19] observed that clinical stage, surgical resection margins and comorbidity were found to be independent factors affecting the prognosis of laryngeal cancer. The postoperative irradiation (radiation doses up to 60–66 Gy) improves the outcome of advanced squamous cell carcinoma, and in most institutions it has become the standard adjuvant treatment to ablative surgery in advanced lesions [20–23].

Whether radiotherapy should be administered pre- or postoperatively has been addressed [22], and these authors observed that locoregional control was significantly better for patients undergoing postoperative radiotherapy than for the ones receiving preoperative radiation. Eighteen percent of the former group and 31% of the latter group of patients failed locally at the end of 2 years, though overall survival was similar. After this period incidence of distant metastasis and second primary cancers become the predominant failure pattern. This shift in late failures tends to negate any advantage in absolute survival for patients receiving postoperative radiotherapy. Most authors report incidence of distant metastasis as between 4% and 13% [23, 24].

6.5.3 Survival Data

Yimaz et al. [25] similarly studied the pattern of failures in 236 patients who received radiotherapy following surgery and compared these with patients treated with surgery alone. The multivariate analysis revealed that locoregional recurrences were determined independently by tumour 'T' and pathological (pn) staging ($p < 0.05$).

The distant metastasis rates were significantly dependent upon N stage ($p < 0.05$), whereas multiple primary cancers were affected by age and radiation status.

Most authors have reported 5-year locoregional control rates of 70–74% in patients of advanced laryngeal cancers, treated with surgery and postoperative radiotherapy [24–27]. However, patients treated with surgery plus chemo-radiation were found to have better prognosis and disease-specific survival [27, 28]. Overall survival rates were 41.1% and 16.7% ($P < 0.001$). The presence of regional metastasis affected the prognosis, and disease-specific survival (DSS) rates were 66% for

N_0 and 46% for N_+ cases ($P = 0.002$). Similarly OS rates were 44.9% and 29.5%, respectively.

Megwaler and Sikora et al. [29] reviewed the survival outcomes in a population-based cohort study of 5394 patients with stage III and IV laryngeal carcinoma and reported patients who received surgical therapy as opposed to non-sugical therapy had 2- and 5-year disease-specific survival rates of 70% vs 64% and 55% vs 51%, respectively ($P < 0.001$).

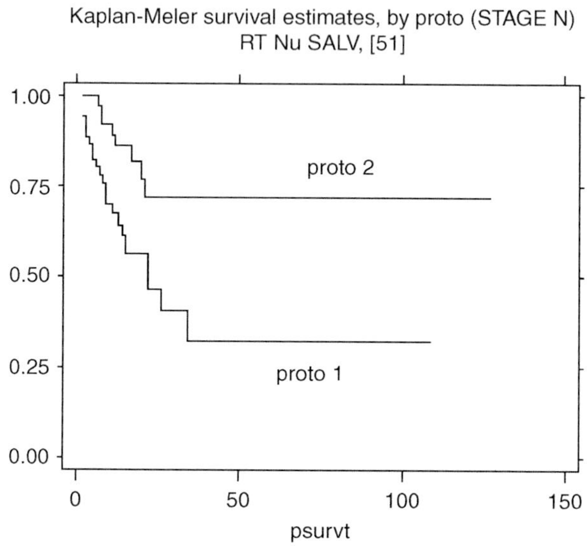

6.5.4 Postoperative Concurrent CT + RT

The poor prognostic factors that are predictors for recurrences include microscopically involved surgical margins, extracapsular spread of disease in positive lymph nodes, two or more positive lymph nodes, perineural infiltration and lymphovascular invasion. These patients have particularly high rates of recurrences (27–61%) and distant metastasis (18–21%) and have a 5-year survival rate of 27–34% (Cooper et al. [30]). This issue was addressed by two similar large-scale prospective randomized clinical trials designed by the European Organisation for Research and Treatment of Cancer (EORTC) and Radiation Therapy Oncology Group (RTOG) and was carried out in order to evaluate the role of concurrent chemo-radiotherapy on postoperative treatment of high-risk head and neck cancers [21, 30].

It was observed that in the presence of adverse prognostic factors, postoperative concurrent chemo-radiotherapy was found to be more effective as compared to postoperative radiotherapy alone in terms of locoregional control and survival [21]. The authors enrolled 439 patients in the study and found that 2-year rate of local and regional control was 82% in combined chemo-radiation group in postoperative setting compared to 72% in the radiotherapy group. However, the combined chemo-radiation group was associated with substantial increase in adverse effects.

6.5.5 Trans-oral Laser Microsurgery for Advanced Laryngeal Cancer

In recent years, different strategies have been reported with comparable outcomes while carrying out conservation or organ preservation surgery. These strategies have not made significant impact on the survival, though there is emphasis on achieving the functional results. Trans-oral laser microsurgery is a relatively new type of conservation surgery for advanced laryngeal cancer [31–32].

It uses the carbon dioxide laser via an endoscopic approach to the larynx. The procedure was initially used by Strong and Jacko for the treatment of early lesions of the larynx in the 1970s. However, the technique has been extended for advanced disease in recent years [11, 31, 33–35].

In TLM, the tumour is repeatedly divided and resected piece by piece, allowing the surgeon to microscopically map tumour depth and assess margins in multiple planes thus resulting in minimal loss of healthy tissue.

Besides fewer surgical complications, other advantages of TOLs include:

1. Avoidance of extensive reconstruction, therefore minimizing the morbidity of donor site
2. Avoiding the tracheostomy
3. Early postoperative swallowing
4. Option of salvage surgery in cases of local recurrences

Advantages of this method point to a more logical tumour resection and greater preservation of normal tissues' structure and function. Indications of neck dissection are determined by surgeon's preference, presence of positive nodes or risk of occult metastasis. The adjuvant radiotherapy is usually considered for the primary site and the neck based on tumour stage and characteristics, adverse prognostic factors including the neck node positivity and presence of extracapsular spread of disease.

Hinni et al. [32] observed the results of TLM in 117 patients with stage III and stage IV laryngeal cancers. The complications included bleeding in 5% and mortality in 3% of cases. The mean duration of hospital stay was 5.7 days. The actual 2-year laryngeal preservation rate was 92% with TLM, and locoregional disease control rates were 77% and 74% at 2 and 5 years, respectively. The disease-free survival rates were 68% and 58% at 2 and 5 years. However, 3% of patients were found to be tracheostomy dependent, and 7% of patients were feeding tube dependent following treatment. There was no significant difference in patients who received postoperative radiotherapy and those who did not.

Carnis et al. [36] reported 5-year organ preservation rate and local control rate of 80% and 67% in patients with T_{4a} laryngeal cancer treated with trans-oral laser microsurgery. These authors concluded that these results were comparable to total laryngectomy while being superior to primary chemo-radiotherapy.

6.5.6 Laryngeal Preservation with Chemo-radiation

It is well realized that results of curative radiotherapy are poor, despite its potential to preserve the larynx. Since the 1990s attempts have been made in the management of advanced disease with multimodality treatment aimed at laryngeal preservation. The continued development of new treatment protocols include new adjuvant and concurrent chemo-radiotherapy, advances in radiation techniques and targeted molecular therapy. These new advances have the potential to improve clinical outcomes, functional results and quality of life.

6.5.7 Induction of CT + RT

It was observed that chemotherapy response predicted the radiotherapy response and complete or partial response was a satisfactorily important factor regarding local control rates [37]. This concept was highlighted to select patients most likely to respond to radiotherapy in a large prospective study published in 1991 by the Department of Veterans Affairs Laryngeal Cancer Study Group (VALCSG) [12]. This study demonstrated the potential value of non-surgical therapy in achieving laryngeal preservation (64%) with survival rates comparable to total laryngectomy as the primary treatment. This landmark trial utilized three cycles of induction chemotherapy (cisplatin plus fluorouracil) followed by radiotherapy. This group was compared with surgery plus postoperative radiotherapy arm, and the 2-year survival rate was 68% in both groups. No significant difference in survival has been reported after more than 10 years of follow-up [37].

The ability to preserve the larynx in two-thirds of the patients without jeopardizing survival established the use of induction chemotherapy followed by radiotherapy as an alternative to laryngectomy for locally advanced laryngeal carcinoma.

The similarly designed European Organisation for Research and Treatment of Cancer (EORTC) larynx preservation study, which focused on patients with advanced carcinoma of the hypopharynx, further supported the principle of VA trial [38].

6.5.8 Concomitant Chemo-radiotherapy

Subsequent important randomized study conducted by the Radiation Therapy Oncology Group (RTOG) study 91-11 was undertaken in collaboration with the Head and Neck Intergroup and published in 2003 [13] to investigate three radiation-based treatment protocols:

(a) Induction cisplatin plus fluorouracil followed by radiotherapy if there was response to chemotherapy
(b) Radiotherapy with concurrent administration of cisplatin
(c) Radiation alone

The primary objective of the trial was to compare the rates of laryngeal preservation. The patients with poor partial response underwent total laryngectomy followed by adjuvant radiotherapy. A total of 547 were randomly assigned to one of the study groups. All patients had biopsy-proven, previously untreated stage III or IV squamous cell carcinoma of the glottic or supraglottic larynx (surgical treatment of which would require total laryngectomy). However, large-volume T_4 disease eroding the cartilage was not included in the study.

The dose of radiation was the same in all three study groups. The dose of radiation to the primary tumour and clinically positive nodes was 70 Gy, given in 35 fractions of 2 Gy each over a 7-week period.

Patients who had either a single node 3 cm or greater in diameter or multiple lymph node metastasis on initial preservation were required to undergo neck dissection 8 weeks after completion of radiotherapy. Total laryngectomy was performed in patients who had histologically proven persistent or recurrent carcinoma after completion of treatment or who had inadequate response after two courses of induction chemotherapy.

6.5.9 Preservations of the Larynx

The rate of laryngeal preservation at a median follow-up for 3.8 years was significantly higher among patients with radiotherapy and concurrent chemotherapy (145/172 patients, 84%) than among those receiving induction chemotherapy followed by radiotherapy (125 of 173 patients) (72%) ($P = 0.005$) or radiotherapy alone (116 of 173 patients) (67%) ($P < 0.001$). Laryngectomy-free survival rates for the composite end point at 2- and 5-year estimated rates for induction and chemotherapy (cisplatin plus fluorouracil) followed by radiotherapy group were 59% and 43%, respectively. However, for concurrent chemo-radiotherapy group, laryngectomy-free survival rates were 66% and 45%, and for those assigned for radiotherapy alone, these rates were 53% and 38%, respectively. There was a significant difference in laryngectomy-free survival when concurrent chemo-radiotherapy was compared with radiotherapy alone ($P = 0.001$) survival outcomes.

The median follow-up among surviving patients was 3.8 years. Two- and 5-year estimates of disease-free survivals were 52% and 38%, respectively, for induction chemotherapy plus radiotherapy, 61% and 36% for concurrent chemo-radiotherapy group and 44% and 27% for radiotherapy alone. However, another study showed better survival with surgery group [38].

Chemotherapy reduced the rate of distant metastasis at 2 years. The incidence of distant metastasis was 15% in patients receiving induction chemotherapy plus RT, 8% and 12% in patients treated with concurrent CT + RT, 16% and 22% in patients who were treated with radiotherapy alone.

Forastiere et al. [39] in 2013 published long-term results of RTOG 91-11 trial at a median follow-up of 10.8 years. Both the chemotherapy regimens significantly improved laryngectomy-free survival compared with RT alone. Concomitant cisplatin with radiotherapy significantly improved the larynx preservation rate over that of induction CT + RT as well as over RT done. Overall, survival did not differ significantly though deaths not attributed to laryngeal cancer or treatment were higher in concomitant CT + RT group (30.8% vs 20.8% with induction CT and 16.9 with RT alone). There have been reports of late toxicity in 39–45% cases with laryngopharyngeal primary site, older age and advanced T stage being predictors for worse prognosis [37, 38, 40, 41].

Induction chemotherapy predominantly improves systemic control, whereas concomitant chemo-radiation primarily improves the locoregional control [13]. However, it has been debated if induction chemotherapy helps in laryngeal preservation by helping in patient selection or whether it has any therapeutic effect [42]. It has been suggested that sequential administration of both induction chemotherapy and concurrent chemo-radiotherapy (or bio-radiotherapy with cetuximab) may result in still better survival results and laryngeal preservation [43, 44].

Another randomized phase II Tremplin trial was carried out by Lefebvre in 2013 [44] to check the above hypothesis by comparing TPF induction chemotherapy followed by concurrent chemo-radiotherapy TPF followed by cetuximab and radiotherapy. However, authors concluded, because of poor response or toxicity, one should either use induction or concurrent chemotherapy, but not both.

Posner et al. [45] carried out TAX 324, a large phase III trial of sequential therapy comparing induction chemotherapy with either TPF (docetaxel plus cisplatin and fluorouracil) or PF (cisplatin and fluorouracil) followed by carboplatin-based chemo-radiotherapy. The trial showed that TPF improves survival rate by 30% in patients with locally advanced head and neck cancer. The subgroup analysis of patients with carcinoma of the larynx and hypopharynx, analysed by the same authors in 2009, demonstrated that TPF improves the laryngectomy-free and overall survival and that there was absolute improvement of 20% at 3 years compared with PF. The authors concluded that results of their sub-analysis provide confirmatory evidence for results from GORTEC 2000-01 [46] trial, showing that TPF is superior to PF for organ preservation as well as for survival.

6.6 Toxic Effects

During induction chemotherapy and radiotherapy, toxicity was manifested primarily as neutropenia stomatitis and nausea or vomiting. The grade and frequency of toxic effects during induction chemotherapy plus radiotherapy and in radiotherapy alone group were nearly identical. In contrast, patients receiving radiotherapy with concurrent chemotherapy had severe toxic effects, e.g. neutropenia and nausea or vomiting and increased rates of severe radiation-related mucosa, pharyngeal and oesopharyngeal effects [13]. The authors indicated that total number of deaths were probably treatment related and occurred in 3%, 5% (concurrent CT + RT) and 3% (radiotherapy alone group).

Silver et al. [47] noted that chemotherapy-related systemic complications like neutropenia, pneumonia and pharyngeal strictures occur with significant incidence.

These authors also observed aspiration to be significantly worse in patients receiving chemo-radiation.

Even though advances have taken place in chemo-radiation strategy in laryngeal preservation in the treatment of laryngeal cancer, there is serious concern that preservation of anatomy does not necessarily result in the preservation of adequate function. Post-radiation xerostomia, fibrosis, oedema and mucositis could have a negative effect on both voice and swallowing functions. The addition of chemotherapy may precipitate the harm of radiotherapy. Forastiere et al. [13] observed speech and swallowing from patients who were disease-free and had an intact larynx and found no difference among three treatment groups with regard to speech at 12 months of follow-up. There was mild-to-moderate speech impairment equally in three groups in a small number of cases (approximately 10%). However, at 1 year, 23% of patients had dysphagia and required gastrostomy tube (PEG) insertion at some stage during treatment with chemo-radiotherapy [47]. The group was able to swallow only soft food or liquids, and 3% could not swallow at all; in contrast of patients in induction chemotherapy group and radiotherapy alone group, 9% were limited to soft food or liquids ($P = 0.004$) at 2 years, and there was no significant difference among the three groups with regard to difficulty in swallowing (nearly 15% in each).

However, difficulty in swallowing following chemo-radiation remains an important issue. Nearly 5–10% will require regular oesophageal dilatation or will be on gastrostomy (or PEG). Similarly a small number of cases will be on permanent tracheostomy. These issues impair the functional results and thus quality of life of patients and thus need to be discussed beforehand.

6.7 Conclusions

The management of advanced carcinoma of the larynx is a challenging issue. Since a majority of patients (nearly 80–85%) in India belong to this group which also contains a significant number of supraglottic and transglottic cancers, often with cervical lymphadenopathy, overall prognosis remains guarded in these cases. Final decision regarding the treatment for advanced laryngeal cancers is made in the multidisciplinary team meeting after reviewing the clinical details and radiology.

Total laryngectomy with neck dissection and postoperative radiotherapy has been the standard care for advanced lesions until recently. Unfortunately it is also associated with significant morbidity in terms of permanent stoma and loss of speech, though most patients can be suitably rehabilitated with either oesophageal speech or trachea oesophageal prosthesis or electronic larynx. However, in terms of oncologic outcome and survival, surgery is probably still the best option for T_4 lesions with obvious cartilage invasion or even for T_3 transglottic cancer or patients with advanced disease who do not wish to go through the long grind of chemo-radiation or patients who cannot come for regular follow-up.

6.8 Trans-oral Laser Microsurgery

TLM is a relatively new type of conservation surgery for advanced laryngeal cancer. Advocates of this method point to several advantages of this technique, including more logical tumour resection and greater preservation of normal tissues and function. There are very few complications, and the hospital stay and duration of treatment is short. Locoregional control rate is excellent [11, 33], and the laryngeal preservation of 5 years is technology dependent. However, it is not available in all centres and also requires considerable surgical experience, though it provides comparable organ and function preserving results compared to the chemo-radiation protocol without significant morbidity.

6.9 Laryngeal Preservation with Chemo-radiation

Since the 1990s there have been significant advances in the role of chemo-radiation in laryngeal preservation [12, 13, 31]. Initial studies highlighted the role of induction chemotherapy followed by radiotherapy in producing laryngeal preservation in significant number of patients and survival rate of nearly 68% (of 2 years) compared to group receiving surgery and postoperative radiotherapy.

Subsequent study by RTOG 91-11 published by Forastiere et al. [13] in 2003 showed that the overall survival and organ preservation (laryngectomy-free survival (LFS)) was superior to both induction and with concurrent chemotherapy and radiotherapy as compared to radiotherapy alone. However, concurrent chemotherapy was found to be superior in terms of laryngeal preservation although overall survival was not significantly affected. Further improvements in laryngeal preservation and survival rates have been reported by Postner et al. [44] in a large trial of sequential therapy comparing induction chemotherapy using either TPF (docetaxel plus cisplatin and fluorouracil) or PF (cisplatin and fluorouracil) followed by carboplatin-based chemo-radiotherapy. The authors concluded that TPF regime is superior to the PF regime for laryngeal preservation.

However, recommendations by panel headed by Lefebvre et al. [48] recommended that eligible patients for laryngeal preservation protocol should include T_2 or T_3 glottic, supraglottic or hypopharyngeal lesions not considered for partial laryngectomy. In consideration of *N* stage, there is an increased risk of distant metastasis in patients with N_2/N_3 disease. These authors demonstrated a reduction in distant metastasis in patients who received induction chemotherapy (13%) versus no chemotherapy (22% $P = 0.03$) prior to chemo-radiation.

The exclusion criteria recommended by Lefebvre et al. include laryngeal dysfunction, defined as pretreatment tracheostomy vocal cord fixation, tumour-related dysphagia requiring feeding tube or recurring pneumonia within the preceding 12 months. These authors also suggested excluding patients more than 70 years of age because it was realised that elderly patients did not benefit from addition of chemotherapy to radiotherapy [39].

Despite the advantages of higher laryngeal preservation rate with chemo-radiotherapy, it is associated with significant toxicity and morbidity and, therefore, should be practised in a centre where facilities of multimodality treatment are available and careful follow-up can be maintained. Besides, the need for salvage surgery can be carried out for patients with residual tumours. Important decision in patient selection for treatment protocol whether medical or surgical is mandatory.

However, observation by Chen and Halpern [49] and Hoffmen et al. [50] of the trend towards decreasing survival in laryngeal cancer should be kept in mind particularly because of popularity of non-surgical treatment.

6.10 Authors' Comments

Final decision regarding the treatment for advanced laryngeal cancer is made in the multidisciplinary cancer team meeting after reviewing the clinical details, radiological and endoscopic findings, based on patient factors (age, Karnofsky Performance Status Scale, profession and comorbidity, etc.), tumour factors (stage, tumour extension and location) and physician factors (facilities and expertize available). Once the treatment protocol has been decided, its implications and likely morbidity must be explained to the patient, and his preference should be noted.

Patients with extensive resectable tumours have been shown to have worse disease control when treated by radiotherapy alone as compared to similar tumours treated by surgery and postoperative radiotherapy. Current indications for surgery should include (1) advanced T_4 lesions with cartilage invasion, (2) patients with prior tracheostomy and aspiration problems, (3) patients who are unlikely to come for regular follow-ups or patients who do not wish to undergo ordeal of chemo-radiation or elderly patients above 70 years of age who are generally not considered medically fit for chemotherapy as a part of chemo-radiation for laryngeal preservation protocol, or (4) T_3transglottic tumours with fixed vocal cords or (5) in a centre where facilities for multimodal treatment are not available.

There has been serious research advances to achieve organ preservation both by trans-oral endoscopic laser resection and by radiation or chemo-radiation protocol. Larynx preservation in T_3 laryngeal lesions, when treated with curative radiotherapy, was possible in 37% patients at the end of 4 years [51], and though a significant number of residual, recurrent lesions could be salvaged with surgery, a few became unresectable with progression of disease. Overall, the results were inferior to the group that was treated with planned regimen of surgery and postoperative radiotherapy. These organ-preserving strategies have not made significant impact on the survival, though there is emphasis on achieving functional results. However, both the strategies require considerable facilities, cost and expertise in the treating centre. Besides the case of organ preservation with chemo-radiation protocol, extra effort is required to monitor these patients for additional toxicity and thus morbidity and extra mortality. However, morbidity as a result of chemo-radiation protocol is considerably less in patients treated with induction chemotherapy and radiation protocol (in responders) [52], though larynx preservation rate and long-term survival rate are also less as compared to concurrent chemo-radiation. Another factor to be seriously considered is the quality of organ preservation because it is known that preservation of anatomy does not result necessarily in the preservation of function. Difficulty in swallowing following chemo-radiation because of stricture formation remains an important issue, and nearly 5–10% of cases will be on gastrostomy tube or on PEG. Likewise, a small number of cases will be on permanent tracheostomy. These issues that impair the quality of life need to be told to the patient prior to the treatment.

Finally, patient selection is extremely important to decide in favour of chemo-radiation (organ preservation). The indications for such a strategy should include T_3 glottic and T_2/T_3 supraglottic cancers; the latter may be associated with neck node metastasis. The protocol may even be considered for extremely select T_4 lesions (without cartilage involvement). However, it is important to consider the patients' general fitness, his commitment and willingness to complete the protocol and preparedness to come for regular follow-up. Local conditions should be taken into account along with the cost of treatment. The possibility of managing a residual or recurrent neoplasm following chemo-radiation in nearly one-third to one-half of the patients should always be kept in mind and is part of the protocol. It is known that diagnosis in such cases is difficult both by clinical and radiological means. Subsequently, morbidity will be higher, and final outcome following salvage surgery may be lower in advanced tumours. And some cases may even become unresectable with the progression of disease. These points should be carefully considered right in the beginning before deciding in favour of either primary surgery followed by postoperative radiotherapy or organ preservation protocol with chemo-radiation. However, advanced unresectable lesions or even resectable lesions with extremely poor general condition may be treated with palliative radiotherapy [53].

6.11 Surgery for Advanced Resectable Cancer

The main surgical procedures considered for advanced resectable lesions are near total laryngectomy (NTL) and total laryngectomy. Whereas it is possible to treat select T_3 laryngeal cancer with partial laryngectomy, most of these are treated with concurrent chemo-radiation protocol. Similarly, it is best to treat residual or recurrent tumours after chemo-radiation with total laryngectomy although select early stage of such cases may be still considered for partial laryngectomy.

6.12 Near Total Laryngectomy (NTL)

Near total laryngectomy was initially described from Mayo Clinic. It preserves the speech, but the patient has to live with permanent tracheostome. The speech is preserved by creating a myomucosal shunt that diverts the pulmonary air from the lungs to the pharynx. The main indications for near total laryngectomy include select T_3 and T_4 lateralized glottic lesions that don't involve the interarytenoid region or the contralateral vocal cord. The resection on the involved side is similar to the total laryngectomy. However, the uninvolved side, the recurrent laryngeal nerve with the arytenoids, the cricoarytenoid joint along with the segment of the cricoid and a strip of posterior tracheal wall, is preserved to create a dynamic myomucosal shunt bridging the tracheostome and pharynx. The shunt diverts the pulmonary air from the trachea to the pharynx. However, it acts like a sphincter and prevents aspiration because it preserves the nerve and mobile cricoarytenoid joint.

The chief advantage of the procedure is its simplicity and avoidance of tracheo-oesophageal prosthesis with its recurring costs and maintenance. However, patient has to occlude the tracheostoma.

6.13 Total Laryngectomy

Total laryngectomy is still the gold standard of treatment for most T_4 cancers, select T_3 transglottic lesions and majority of the residual or recurrent carcinoma after failed chemo-radiation.

6.14 Surgical Principle

Patient is operated under general anaesthesia via oro- or nasotracheal intubation. However, if airway obstruction is present, a prior tracheostomy is performed under local anaesthesia. A modified Sorenson ('U'-shaped) incision is made in the neck including the tracheostome, or the latter may be fashioned separately in the inferior flap. The skin flaps are elevated. If the patient has N+ disease, concurrent comprehensive neck dissection is performed. However, if patient has clinically negative neck (No), bilateral internal jugular clearance (or selective neck dissection) with clearance of levels II, III and IV is performed. The strap muscles are divided low down in the neck.

Both the superior and inferior thyroid vessels are ligated and divided, and the ipsilateral thyroid gland on the affected side is included in the specimen. Usually the contralateral (normal) side thyroid gland is preserved along with the para-thyroids and its blood supply from the inferior thyroid vessels.

The inferior constrictor muscle is divided on both sides along with the posterior surface of the thyroid lamina. The mucosa of the pyriform fossa is separated from the thyroid lamina. It is useful to remember the location of the tumour and whether there is any extra-laryngeal spread of disease. The resection can be tailored accordingly. The suprahyoid muscles are divided close to the hyoid bone avoiding injury to the lingual vessels. The larynx is skeletonized on both sides. The tracheostoma is created by dividing the trachea in the third or fourth ring, maintaining a close coordination with the anaesthetist, and ventilation is resumed via the tracheostome. The pharynx is entered through the vallecula, and the epiglottis is held with the Babcock's forceps. The mucosal cuts are carried along the aryepiglottic and then through the superior part of the post-cricoid mucosa. The separation of the larynx from the hypopharynx and cervical oesophagus is continued inferiorly until the tracheostome is reached and the larynx is delivered.

A cricopharyngeal myotomy may be carried out along with primary tracheo-oesophageal puncture. The wound is irrigated, and the pharynx is closed with 2-0 or 3-0 Vicryl suture in two layers. The wound is closed in two layers after taking care of the tracheostoma. The suction drains are applied on either side, and feeding tube (nasogastric tube) is usually kept for 10–14 days.

It is useful to raise pectoralis major myofascial flap to augment the pharyngeal closure, in case laryngectomy is being carried out in salvage setting in radiation failed cases. It is preferable to plan secondary voice restoration later (Figs. 6.7 and 6.8).

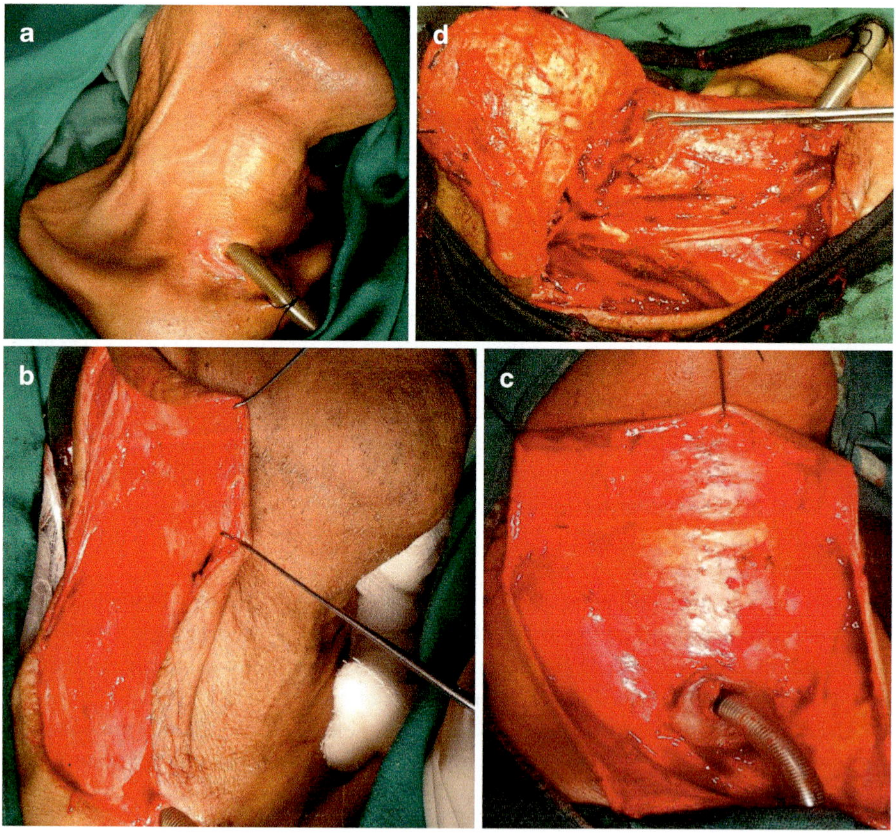

Fig. 6.7 (**a**) Patient preparation. Preoperative tracheostomy. (**b, c**) Raising of the skin flap in sub-platysmal plane up to the level of the hyoid bone. (**d**) Completion of neck dissection with the carotid artery being exposed. The hyoid bone has been grasped with Ellis forceps after the division of strap muscles and suprahyoid muscles. (**e**) Inferior constructor muscle has been divided. Sup. thyroid vessels ligated and divided, with the thyroid gland being preserved on the healthy side. (**f, g**) The larynx has been opened from above and from the contralateral side. Tumour is visible in the pyriform fossa. (**h**) Surgical specimen has been removed after transecting trachea mucosa of the hypopharynx is ready for repair. Ryle's tube is in situ

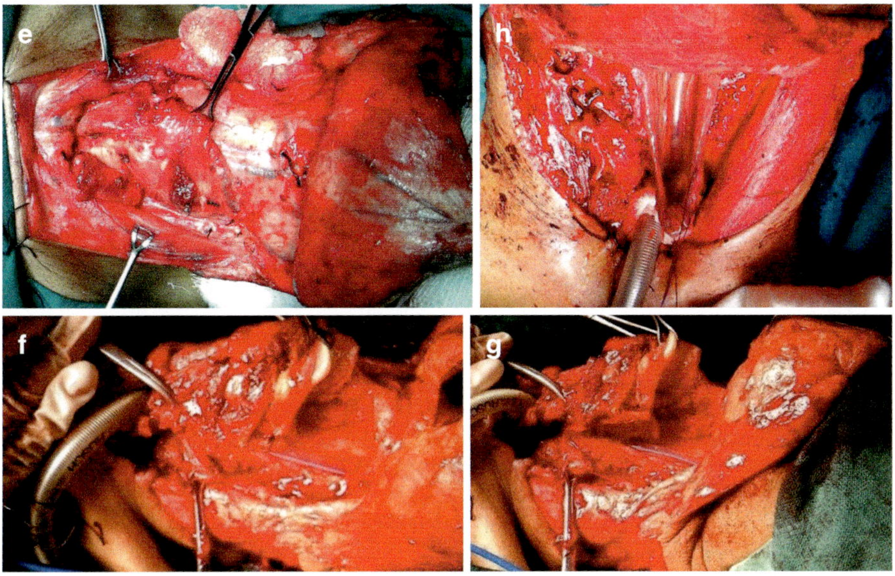

Fig. 6.7 (continued)

Fig. 6.8 Laryngectomy patient at follow-up. Narrow tracheostoma would require revision

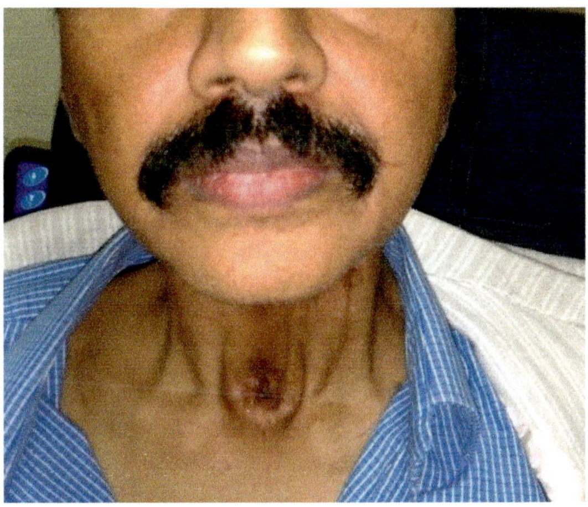

References

1. Dinshaw KA, Sharma V. Radiation therapy in early glottic carcinoma. Significance of prognostic factors and dose fractionation. Indian J Cancer. 1990;27:143–53.
2. Bahadur S, Iyer S. The results of surgery in advanced carcinoma of the larynx. Indian J Otolaryngol Head Neck Surg. 1985;37:131–4.
3. Bahadur S, Amatya RC, Kacker SK. Primary surgery versus radiation failed salvage surgery in advanced carcinoma of the larynx and hypopharynx. Indian J Cancer. 1986;23:89–93.

4. Chen AY, Sehrag H, Hao Y, et al. Changes in treatment of advanced laryngeal cancer 1985–2003. Otolaryngeal Head Neck Surg. 2006;35:831–7.
5. Bahadur S, Amatya RC, Iyer S, et al. Study of distribution of lymph node metastasis from squamous cell carcinoma of head and neck. Indian J Cancer. 1983;20:143–6.
6. Myers EN, Swen JY, Myers JN. Cancer of the head and neck. 4th ed. Philadelphia: Saounders; 2003.
7. Piccinilo JF. Importance of co-morbidity in head and neck cancer. Laryngoscope. 2000;110:593–602.
8. Hong WK, Lippman SM, Itri LM, et al. Prevention of second primary tumors isotretinoin in squamous cell carcinoma of the head and neck. N Engl J Med. 1990;323:795–801.
9. Breithart W, Holland J. Psychosocial aspects of head and neck cancers. Semin Oncol. 1988;15:61–9.
10. Dropkin MJ. Body image and quality of life after head and neck surgery. Cancer Pract. 1999;7:309–13.
11. Steiner W. Results of curative laser micro surgery of laryngeal carcinoma. Am J Otolaryngology. 1993;14:116–21.
12. The Department of Veterans Affairs Laryngeal Cancer Study Group. Induction chemotherapy plus radiation compared with surgery plus radiation in patients with advanced laryngeal cancer. N Engl J Med. 1991;324:1685–90.
13. Forastiere AA, Geopfert H, Maor M, et al. Concurrent chemotherapy and radiotherapy for organ preservation in advanced laryngeal cancer. N Engl J Med. 2003;349:2091–8.
14. Ferlito A, Rianaldo A, Silver CF, et al. Neck dissection for laryngeal cancer. J AM Coll Surg. 2008;207:587–97.
15. Leyland MK, Sessions DG, Lenox J. The influence of lymph node metastasis in treatment of squamous cell carcinoma of oral cavity, oropharynx, larynx and hypopharynx. Larynscope. 2005;115:629–39.
16. Weber PC, Johnson JT, Myers E. The impact of bilateral neck dissection on pattern of recurrence and survival in supraglottic carcinoma. Arch Otolaryngol Head Neck Surg. 1994;120:703–6.
17. Brazilian Head and Neck Cancer study group. End results of a prospective trial on elective lateral neck dissection vs type III modified radical neck dissection in management of supraglottic and transglottic carcinomas. Head Neck. 1999;21:694–702.
18. Lefebvre JL. What is the role of primary surgery in the treatment of laryngeal and hypopharyngeal cancer – Hays-Martin lecture. Arch Otolaryngol Head Neck Surg. 2000;126:285–8.
19. Zhang SY, Lu ZM, Luo XN. Retrospective analysis of prognostic factors in 205 patients with laryngeal carcinoma who underwent surgical treatment. PLoS One. 2013;4:e60157. www.plos.org
20. Bahadur S, Kumar S, Tandon DA, et al. Combined therapy in advanced head and neck cancer. J Laryngol Otol. 1992;106:243–9.
21. Berniere J, Domenge C, Ozsahin M, et al. Post operative irradiation with or without concurrent chemotherapy for locally advanced head and neck cancer. N Engl J Med. 2004;350:1945–52.
22. Tupchang L, Phil D, Scott CB, et al. Randomized study of pre-operative versus post – operative radiation therapy in advanced head and neck carcinoma long term follow up of RTOG study 73-03. Int J Radiat Oncol Biol Phy. 1991;20:21–8.
23. Krstevska V, Stojkovski J, Lazarevska E, Crrenkova S. Radical surgery and post operative radiotherapy in patients with advanced squamous cell carcinoma of the larynx. Arch Otolaryngol. 2011;19:1–2.
24. Spector GJ. Distant metastasis from laryngeal and hypopharyngeal cancer. ORL. 2001;63:224–8.
25. Yimaz T, Hosal S, Ozyar E, Akyol F, Gursal B. Post operative radiotherapy in advanced laryngeal cancer: effect on local regional recurrence, distant metastasis and second primaries J. Laryngol Otol. 2005;119:784–90.
26. Nguyen Tan PF, Le QT, Quivery M, et al. Treatment results and prognostic factors of advanced T3-T4 laryngeal carcinoma: the University of California San Francisco (UCSF) and Stanford university hospital (SUH) experience. Int J Radiat Oncol Bio Phys. 2001;50:1172–80.

27. Gounn CG, Conger BT, Shails WC, et al. The effect of treatment on survival in patients with advanced laryngeal carcinoma. Laryngoscope. 2009;119:1312–7.
28. Karatzanis AD, Psychogios G, Waldfaher F, et al. Management of locally advanced laryngeal cancer. J Otolaryngol Head Neck Surg. 2014;43:4–7.
29. Megwaln UC, Sikora AW. Survival outcomes in advanced laryngeal cancer. JAMA Otolaryngeal Head Neck Surg. 2014;140:855–60.
30. Cooper IS, Pajak TE, Forastiere A, et al. Precisely defining high risk operable head and neck tumors based on RTOG 85-03 and 88-24: targets for post operative radiotherapy. Head Neck. 1998;20:588–94.
31. Pearson BW, Salassa JR. Transoral laser microresection for cancer of the larynx involving the anterior commissure. Laryngoscope. 2003;113:1104–12.
32. Hinni ML, Salassa JR, Grant DG, et al. Transoral laser microsurgery for advanced laryngeal cancer. Arch Otolaryngeal Head Neck Surg. 2007;133:1198–204.
33. Strong MS, Jako GJ. Laser surgery in the larynx early: clinical experience with continuous CO_2 laser. Ann Otol Rhinol Laryngol. 1972;81:791–8.
34. Rudert HH, Warner JA, Hoft S. Transoral carbon dioxide laser resection of supraglottic carcinoma. Ann Otol Rhinol Laryngol. 1999;108:819–27.
35. Steiner W, Ambrosh P. Endoscopic laser surgery of the upper aerodigestive tract with special emphasis on cancer surgery. Stuttgart: Thieme; 2000.
36. Canis M, Martin A, et al. Organ preservation in T4 a laryngeal cancer: is transoral laser microsurgery an option? Eur Arch Otolaryngol. 2013;270:2719–27.
37. Pignon JP, Le Maltre E, Bourhis J, Match NC. Collaborative group. An update on 93 randomized trials and 17346 patients. Radiother Oncol. 2009;92:4–14.
38. Richard JM, Sancho Garniere H, Passey JJ, et al. Randomized trial of induction chemotherapy in larynx carcinoma. Oral Oncol. 1998;34:224–32.
39. Forastiere AA, Zhang Q, Weber RS, et al. Long term results of RTOG 91-11, a comparison of three non surgical treatment strategies to preserve the larynx in patients with advanced larynx cancer. J Clin Oncol. 2013;31:845–52.
40. Machtay M, Monghan J, Trotti A, et al. Factors associated with severe late toxicity after concurrent chemo-radiotherapy for locally advanced head and neck cancer: an RTOG analysis. J Clin Oncol. 2008;26:3582–9.
41. Wang JJ, Goldsmith TA, Holman AS, et al. Pharyngo-oesophageal stricture after treatment of head and neck cancer. Head Neck. 2012;34:967–73.
42. Pfister DG, Ridge JA. Induction chemotherapy for larynx preservation: patient selection or therapeutic effect? J Clin Oncol. 2006;26:540–2.
43. Vokes E. Competing roads to larynx preservation. J Clin Oncol. 2013;31:833–5.
44. Lefebvre JL, Pointreau V, Rolland F, et al. Induction chemotherapy followed by either chemoradiotherapy or bio radiotherapy for larynx preservation: the tremplin randomized phase II study. J Clin Oncol. 2013;31:853–9.
45. Posner MR, Norris CM, Wirth LJ, et al. Sequential therapy for locally advanced larynx and hypopharynx cancer sub group in Tax 324; survival surgery and organ preservation. Ann Oncol. 2009;20:921–7.
46. Brochstein B, Haraf DJ, Rademaket AV, et al. Patterns of failure prognostic factors and survival in loco-regionally advanced head and neck cancer treated with concurrent chemo radiotherapy a 9 year 337 patients multi institution of experience. Ann Oncol. 2004;15:1179–86.
47. Silver CE, Beither JJ, Shaha AR, et al. Current trends in initial management of laryngeal cancer; the declining use of open surgery. Eur Arch Otolaryngol. 2009;266:1332–52.
48. Cmelak AJ, Li S, Meredith SL, et al. Phase III trial of chemo-radiation for organ preservation in resectable stage III or IV squamous cell carcinoma of the larynx or oropharynx. Results of Eastern Co-operative Oncology Group study E2399. J Clin Oncol. 2007;25:3971–7.
49. Chen AV, Halpern M. Factors predictive of survivals in advanced laryngeal cancer. Arch Otolaryngol Head Neck. 2009;31:429–41.
50. Hoffman HT, Porter K, Karnell LH, et al. Laryngeal cancer in United States: changes in demographics patterns of care and survival. Larynscope. 2006;116:1–13.

51. Thakar A, Bahadur S, Mohanti BK, Nivsarkar S. Clinically staged T3NoMo laryngeal cancer: how is it best treated? Definitive radiotherapy with salvage surgery versus combined surgery and radiotherapy. J Laryngol Otol. 2000;114:108–12.
52. Thakar A, Bahadur S, Tandon DA, Ranganathan A, Rath GK. Laryngeal preservation by treatment with induction chemotherapy and radiotherapy protocol for stage III and IV carcinoma of larynx. J Laryngol Otol. 1999;113:433–8.
53. Mohanti BK, Umapathy U, Thakar A, Pathy S. Short course palliative radiotherapy of 20 Gyin 5 factions for advanced and incurable head and neck cancer. Radiother Oncol. 2004;71:275–80.

Trans-oral Laser Microsurgery

7

Alok Thakar and Kapil Sikka

7.1 Introduction

The CO_2 laser is a tool to enable endoscopic surgical treatment of laryngeal cancers. Minimally invasive trans-oral endoscopic treatment is obviously attractive to both patients and physicians and has been attempted for over a century. It was however the development of surgical innovations such as suspension laryngoscopy, microlaryngeal surgery, and the use of operating microscope for laryngeal surgery supplemented with their coupling with the CO_2 laser which has enabled a new paradigm in laryngeal surgical oncology wherein surgery can be simultaneously minimally invasive and also oncologically appropriate [1–3].

Though such surgical treatments are loosely termed as "laser resections", it is important to remember that the technique derives its advantages not only from the use of the laser but also by the nature of the resections being entirely endoscopic and the resections being undertaken under magnification with a microscope. The appropriate term for such resections therefore remains "trans-oral laser microsurgery (TLM)" [4].

The major advantage of trans-oral laser microsurgery stems from the procedure being undertaken endoscopically and so causing no disruptions to the pharyngeal muscles, motor and sensory innervation, and the laryngopharyngeal architecture. This preservation of the laryngopharyngeal architecture in relation to the hypopharynx and oropharynx, the preservation of laryngopharyngeal mucosal sensations, and the preservation of the coordinated motor movements of the pharynx ensure that the reflex and automatic pharyngeal phase of swallowing is minimally disrupted. Aspiration is thus significantly reduced, especially so in comparison to the open partial laryngectomy [4]. The preservation of swallowing and minimizing of aspiration enables the safe use of such endoscopic resections in the specific

A. Thakar (✉) · K. Sikka
Department of Otolaryngology and Head-Neck Surgery, All India Institute of Medical Sciences, New Delhi, India
e-mail: drathakar.orlhns@aiims.edu

S. Bahadur et al. (eds.), *Carcinoma of the Larynx and Hypopharynx*,
https://doi.org/10.1007/978-981-13-3110-7_7

Table 7.1 Technical advantages offered by each of the three components of trans-oral laser microsurgery which additively contribute to the improvement in functional outcomes with the technique

TLM—***T****rans-oral* ***L****aser* ***M****icrosurgery*
T*rans-oral* • Avoidance of disruption of laryngeal and pharyngeal muscles and cartilage • Less physiological disruption • Better functional outcomes
L*aser* (CO_2) • Surgical haemostasis • Improved margin assessment • Improved postoperative healing
M*icrosurgery* • Magnification • Better tumour delineation/improved margin assessment

population of laryngeal cancer patients who have generally been chronic smokers and so have compromised lung function. Physiological organ preservation can thus be achieved for these physiologically compromised patients.

Trans-oral robotic surgery (TORS) is an extension of the same concept with functional advantages being derived again from the trans-oral nature of the operation. It is important to emphasize that in both situations the functional and physiological advantages are derived primarily from the trans-oral nature of the procedure, and the laser and robot are but tools to achieve this objective.

Advantages are also gained from the use of the laser and the microscope. Both enable better appreciation of surgical margins and so enable close margin excisions. The advantages offered by each component of TLM are summarized in Table 7.1. It is however imperative to iterate that the advantages of the laser are specific to the CO_2 laser and may not be seen with other lasers which have differing wavelengths and so differing laser-tissue interactions.

The indications and enthusiasm for TLM have fluctuated over time. It was introduced in the early 1980s by Jako and Strong for early laryngeal lesions [2–3]. It was applied for tumour debulking in an effort to avoid tracheotomy in situations of tumours causing airway obstruction [5]. Great enthusiasm and interest were generated in the late 1990s, fuelled mainly by Steiner and other colleagues in Germany, for its application in advanced T_3/T_4 tumours wherein it offered the possibility of cure with laryngeal preservation [6–8]. Recent years have thrown up other non-surgical options for organ preservation by concurrent chemo-radiation, and in current times the technique is mainly applied to early and intermediate laryngeal cancers (T_1, T_2, selected T_3) [8, 9].

7.2 Lasers: Applied Physics

Laser is an acronym for "*L*ight *A*mplification by the *S*timulated *E*mission of *R*adiation". Albert Einstein postulated the theoretical foundation of laser action, stimulated emission of radiation, in 1917. A laser is an electro-optical device that emits organized light (rather than the random pattern light emitted from a light bulb) in a very narrow, intense beam by a process of optical feedback and amplification. The most versatile laser used in ENT and head and neck surgery is the carbon dioxide laser although ND Yag, Argon, and KTP lasers have also found the place. CO_2 lasers produce light with a wavelength of 10.6 μ in the infrared (invisible) range of the electromagnetic spectrum.

The CO_2 laser beam being an invisible laser, a second, built-in, coaxial helium-neon visible laser is necessary to indicate with its red colour the site where the invisible CO_2 laser beam will impact the target tissue. This laser, then, acts as an aiming beam for the invisible CO_2 laser beam.

The radiant energy produced by the CO_2 laser wavelength is strongly absorbed by pure, homogeneous water and by all biological tissues high in water content. The extinction length of this wavelength is about 0.03 mm in water and in soft tissue; reflection and scattering are negligible. It is these properties of minimal depth penetration and minimal scatter which give the CO_2 laser its unique property of precise surgical incisions on water-rich tissues with minimal damage to the deeper or lateral surrounding tissues.

7.3 Case Selection

Our current indications for TLM in the larynx are chiefly restricted to glottic or supraglottic tumours which are endolaryngeal and not associated with arytenoid fixation (T_1, T_2, selected T_3). Tumours classified as T_3 because of radiological evidence of paraglottic space involvement or pre-epiglottic space involvement are considered suitable for laser resections/partial laryngectomy, but cases classified as T_3 consequent to vocal cord fixation are generally not considered appropriate for partial resections. Superficial T_1 lesions of the subglottis and hypopharynx may sometimes be amenable to TLM if they are endoscopically accessible, but such lesions are rare.

A distinction has to be made between vocal cord fixation which may be secondary to tumour bulk and is amenable to TLM and partial laryngectomy resections and arytenoid fixation which is often consequent to cricoarytenoid joint or muscle involvement and may not be amenable to such resection. Pre-epiglottic and paraglottic extensions can be adequately excised with TLM. Subglottic mucosal involvement can be excised. The principles of partial laryngeal surgery indicate that the arytenoid is the main structure preventing aspiration and care has therefore to be exercised in its excision. The confidence of improved functional and swallowing results with TLM has however allowed a pushing of limits in this area, and arytenoid excision can be safely undertaken with far less concern than in an open partial laryngectomy.

The literature reports of experience with selected lesions with fixed vocal folds and cartilage involvement [9–11], but this is not universally accepted as suitable for TLM [11]. Situations wherein endoscopic exposure is poor (the "5 Ts"—*t*rismus, large *t*eeth, bulky *t*ongue, limited neck extension-*t*ilt, and very proliferative *t*umours) are also a relative contraindication and may be treated by open surgical approaches or non-surgical means. In salvage situations following failed radiation for early laryngeal cancer, there is a suggestion that open partial laryngectomy may offer better local control rates than TLM [12].

A pragmatic approach to patient workup keeping in mind the patient factors, surgeon's skill and experience, and assessment of disease is essential for deciding the candidacy for TLM. Candidacy is assessed in two broad categories—oncologic and functional.

It is imperative that practitioners of conservation laryngeal onco-surgery—whether undertaken by TLM or by one of the open partial laryngectomies—are very well versed with the anatomical barriers to cancer spread and also the preformed pathways to cancer spread. Laryngeal cancer has well defined and predictable patterns of spread and lends itself well to partial resections with minimal margins. In current times oncologic assessment is greatly supplemented by sectional imaging (thin section, contiguous, contrast enhanced CT or MR) and by high-resolution endoscopy, and these are essential aids to contemporary practice.

While consideration of the proposed resection's adequacy for oncologic clearance is paramount, consideration also has to be given to its impact on functional aspects of voice and swallowing. Though not as much as open partial laryngectomy, the concerns with postoperative aspiration, risk of haemorrhage, and other airway issues mandate thorough evaluation of preoperative pulmonary and cardiac status of patients.

Currently, TLM has largely usurped the surgical space that was initially held by open partial laryngectomy. Open partial laryngectomy today is mainly reserved for situations wherein TLM may be considered less appropriate because of either limitations of endoscopic access (trismus, cervical extension limitations, etc.), thyroid cartilage involvement (T_4), or salvage situations.

A separate chapter in this text on early laryngeal cancers lists in detail the considerations for case selection between radiation therapy and TLM. Some of the chief merits and demerits of both modalities are reproduced in Table 7.2. TLM is compared and contrasted to open partial resections in Table 7.3.

Table 7.2 Trans-oral laser microsurgery compared and contrasted to radiation therapy

Radiation treatment	Trans-oral laser surgery
7-week treatment duration	Single surgical treatment—often day care
Better preservation of anatomy	Avoids overtreatment (tailored Rx as per disease extent)
Functional voice results better initially	Functional voice results equivalent after healing
	Avoids long-term radiation morbidity
Option of radiation Rx limited for subsequent recurrence/second primary (10%)	All treatment options including radiation Rx/laser surgery/conventional surgery preserved for subsequent recurrence/second primary (10%)
Recurrence may need total laryngectomy	Overall laryngeal preservation rates possibly better [13]

Table 7.3 Trans-oral laser microsurgery compared and contrasted to open partial laryngectomy

Trans-oral laser surgery	Open partial laryngectomy
En bloc excision and sectioned excisions	En bloc excision
Surgical access limitations	No such limitation
Technology and cost	No such limitation
Improved intra-op margin assessment	Inclusion of thyroid cartilage—added dimension of oncologic clearance
Superior functional results Minimal physiologic disruption Preservation of sensation	Swallow outcome erratic

7.3.1 Surgical Technique

TLM is an overall scheme or philosophy that encompasses variedly different excisions "tailored" to the extent of the lesion. The European Laryngological Society classification for glottic and supraglottic resections is commonly used for categorization of the extent of resection (Table 7.4, Figs. 7.1, 7.2, and 7.3). The improved margin assessment with the technique as alluded to previously enables margins of excision to be restricted to 2–3 mm in the glottis and 5–7 mm in the supraglottis. Alternatively, "compartmental excisions" may also be undertaken—e.g. type IV cordectomy/total cordectomy which includes the entire vocal fold and paraglottic space compartment inclusive of the inner perichondrium of the thyroid cartilage (Fig. 7.2a) wherein this inner perichondrium is a natural barrier to lateral spread and supraglottic laser laryngectomy (Fig. 7.3a) wherein the quadrangular membrane in the ventricular fold separates the supraglottic compartment from the glottis and offers an additional barrier to inferior tumour spread.

While early lesions may be excised by a traditional en bloc excision, larger tumours need to be removed after sectioning of the tumour so as to allow for adequate surgical manipulation and specimen delivery when working trans-orally through a laryngoscope. This deviation from the Halstedian concept of en bloc excision led to some justified apprehensions among workers with regard to the oncologic appropriateness of such "piecemeal" excision. A distinction however needs to be drawn between a piecemeal excision which is typically taken to mean random surgical bites and avulsions of a tumour and the situation with TLM wherein a planned sectioned excision is undertaken. Sectioned surgical excision involves an assessment with regard to tumour margins prior to excision. The pre-planned extent of excision is then "breadloaved" by one or two horizontal sections along the tumour so as to penetrate through its deepest extension and beyond and then removed in two or three separate slices. It has been conversely argued that sectioning of a tumour may lead to better appreciation of its depth and so improve margin assessment. The oncologic results published from Germany wherein this technique was initiated, and subsequently by other workers [7–11, 14], have demonstrated oncologic equivalence with the partial laryngectomy alternatives, and this has led to greater acceptance of sectioned excisions.

Table 7.4 European Laryngological Society (ELS) classifications for glottic and supraglottic resections

Cancer glottis (cordectomy)	
Type I	Subepithelial cordectomy
Type II	Subligamental cordectomy
Type III	Transmuscular cordectomy
Type IV	Total or complete cordectomy
Type V	Extended cordectomy encompassing
Type Va	Contralateral fold/anterior commissure
Type Vb	Arytenoids
Type Vc	Ventricular fold
Type Vd	Subglottis
Cancer supraglottis (Supraglottic resections)	
Type I	Limited excision of small superficial lesions of the free edge of the epiglottis, AE fold, ventricular fold, arytenoids, etc.
Type II—medial supraglottic laryngectomy without pre-epiglottic space	T_1 lesions of suprahyoid or infrahyoid laryngeal surface of the epiglottis)
IIa—superior hemi-epiglottectomy	
IIb—total epiglottectomy	
Type III—medial supraglottic laryngectomy with pre-epiglottic space	T_1–T_2 tumours of the infrahyoid endolaryngeal epiglottis
IIIa—without extension to ventricular fold	
IIIb—with extension to the ventricular fold	
Type IV—lateral supraglottic laryngectomy	Tumours of the threefolds' region (AE fold, PE fold, ventricular fold)
IVa—including the ventricular fold	
IVb—including arytenoid	

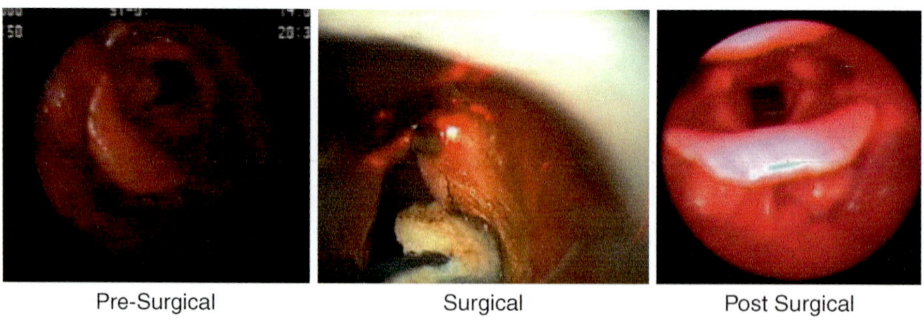

Fig. 7.1 Type I glottic resection—typical case with a mid-cordal superficial lesion being excised with resection through Reinke's space. Typical postsurgical healing with excellent anatomical and functional results

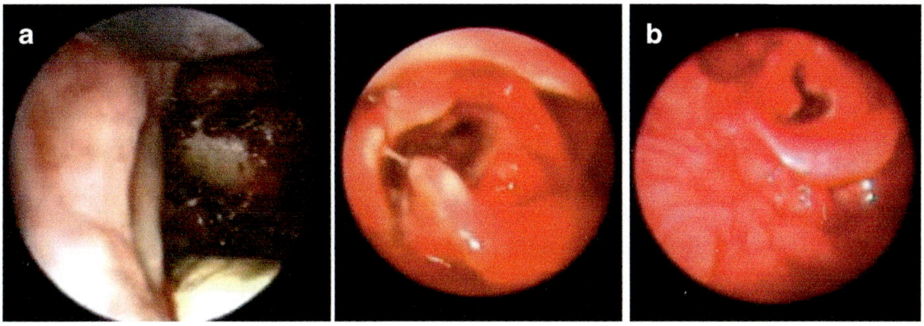

Fig. 7.2 (**a**) Type IV glottic resection (total cordectomy)—right. Intra-op and postop pictures demonstrating intact left vocal fold and ventricular fold. Complete absence of the right vocal and ventricular fold from arytenoid to anterior commissure and lateral extension till the thyroid cartilage. (**b**) Type Va glottic resection (anterior commissure resection)

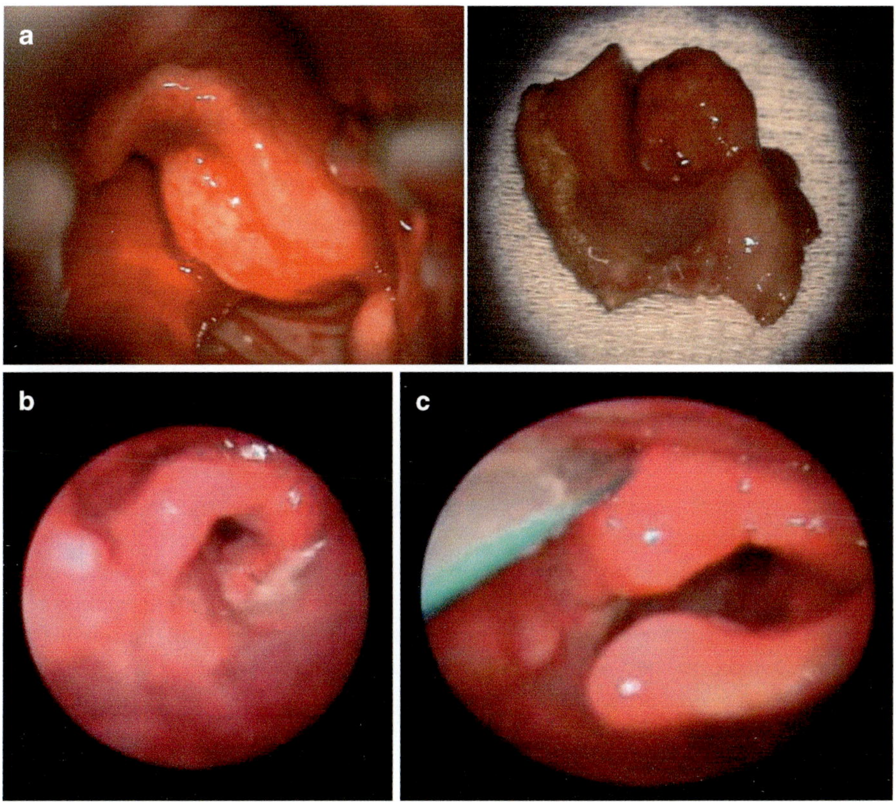

Fig. 7.3 (**a**) Type I supraglottic resection; (**b**) typical laser supraglottic laryngectomy with inclusion of pre-epiglottic space and ventricular folds (type IIIb); (**c**) lateral supraglottic laryngectomy of the "threefolds'" region (type IVa)

A corollary of the close excision margins is that histological assessment for margin positivity has to be meticulous. Positive margins are subjected to re-excision. Since the margin bed after initial surgery has not been closed but left open and undistorted, identification of the appropriate margin to be revised is straightforward. The literature typically indicates to excision margins being reported as involved or uncertain in 25–30% of cases. Re-excision is recommended but may not necessarily yield tumour, and this is to be expected as many re-excisions are undertaken for margins classified as uncertain rather than involved. The literature suggests that survival of patients is similar irrespective of whether a margin-free excision has been reached at the first or the second surgery [15].

The complication profile with TLM is quite different from open surgery, and surgical units undertaking major TLM resections have to be accordingly prepared. The most frequent complication following TLM is reactionary or secondary haemorrhage with its potential for aspiration and pulmonary complications [16]. Such complications are more common for supraglottic and hypopharyngeal resections. Such lesions also require a selective neck dissection for oncological sampling of lymph node regions at risk, and it has been the authors' practice to undertake this neck dissection concurrent to the TLM resection as it also allows the opportunity to ligate the ipsilateral superior thyroid artery supplying the tumour. Ligation of the superior thyroid artery minimizes surgical bleeding and also greatly reduces the risks of postsurgical secondary haemorrhage. Additionally, facilities have to be created for postsurgical care with personnel competent at airway management, as most such patients do not have a tracheotomy. Close co-operation with the anaesthesiology team is mandatory.

7.3.2 Precautions and Complications

Laser surgery is dangerous as the "invisible" beam misfiring can damage the vital organs and pose a serious health risk to patient, surgeon, and the OR staff. Precautions are necessary to prevent accidents, and it is the responsibility of the surgeon to exercise them.

All theatre staff must wear specialized eye protection, and the operator is only exempt if he/she is using the microscope as this confers eye protection to them. Warning signs must be visible inside and outside the theatre where a laser is being used. All metal equipment used throughout the operation must be minimal or non-reflective (Matt surface finish). All exposed patient surfaces in the surgical field (facial skin and especially eyes) should be covered with wet gauze.

Major airway fires are rare but have been reported. Surgeons and anaesthesiologists have to be obsessive about complications to prevent such a disaster [16, 17]. Endotracheal tubes used should be non-flammable, and the use of laser compatible endotracheal tubes is recommended. The surgical field should not have any gases that support combustion. Standard precautions to be taken by anaesthetic colleagues include the use of appropriate anaesthetic gases which do not support combustion (most currently used gases are appropriate), avoiding use of nitrous oxide which supports combustion (thus necessitating the use of an air-oxygen machine), avoiding high inspired oxygen concentrations (restrict to <30%), and avoiding the use of oil-based jelly or ointment in the surgical field [17].

As previously indicated wounds after TLM are left open for secondary intention healing. Since CO_2 laser inflicted incisions have little lateral thermal damage, wound healing is rapid with early epithelialization and a sensate and functional larynx. Tracheotomy is rarely required, and the lack of tracheotomy with the resultant maintenance of subglottic pressure and an effective cough further contribute to the little swallowing dysfunction seen in these patients. Unlike the situation with the partial supraglottic and supracricoid laryngectomies, equivalent resections can be undertaken by TLM with little risk for aspiration (Figs. 7.2 and 7.3). This is a significant advantage in patient populations which are often elderly and who have often been heavy smokers over several years.

Laryngeal oedema requiring tracheostomy, surgical emphysema, pharyngeal bruising, endotracheal tube cuff damage, glottis web, vocal cord granuloma, and laryngocele are other complications described though occur in less than 1% cases [16].

7.4 Special Situations

7.4.1 Anterior Commissure

The involvement of anterior commissure has been widely studied as a "danger zone" in otherwise indolent early-stage glottic cancers. The trepidation of rapid progression of early T_1 and T_2 cancers to stage 4 leaking through the weak point of attachment of vocal cords need not be overemphasized. It is well established that anterior commissure involvement is a poor prognostic indicator in such tumours. Whether or not trans-oral surgery should be offered to patients has been debated. A review put forward by Hoffmann [18] summarizes the literature as stating the anterior commissure as a poor prognostic site irrespective of modality used. Good oncologic outcomes, high laryngeal preservation rates, and availability of all salvage options make trans-oral surgery an attractive option for AC involved cases.

Voice results can be very disappointing in the immediate postoperative period as both vocal folds lose their anterior attachment and therefore lose tension leading to near total aphonia (Fig. 7.2b). It has however been the authors' experience that with subsequent healing and scar formation, vocal fold tension is restored and satisfactory voicing returns.

7.4.2 Salvage Settings

The most common treatment advocated throughout the world for radio-recurrent laryngeal cancer is total laryngectomy, which has been associated with good control rates. Many considerations indicate towards caution in undertaking conservation surgery. Radio-recurrent cancers can naturally be assumed to be more aggressive than similar tumours that have been cured by radiation. Radiation residual disease may also be multicentric and tumour margins less distinct. Further, post-radiation mucosal oedema and scarring and restrictions of laryngeal mobility may predispose to aspiration. A higher rate of surgical complications can be anticipated.

The above considerations notwithstanding some patients may be considered appropriate for conservation resections. The essential oncologic prerequisite in case selection is for the tumour extent to be amenable to a conservation resection both in its recurrent post-radiation extent and also in its previous pre-radiation initial assessment. Functional assessment of pulmonary and laryngeal function is also essential in case selection. As a general rule, previous treatment with chemo-radiation is often associated with significant oedema and laryngeal dysfunction, and such cases are almost never considered suitable for conservation resections. Radiation alone is however usually not so disabling to laryngeal function, and such patients may be amenable to conservation resections.

Salvage resections may be undertaken by TLM or by open partial laryngectomy. The authors' experience has been that in salvage situations, local control is better with open partial laryngectomy than with TLM. A recent meta-analysis has indicated similarly [12]. It is therefore recommended that extreme care be exercised in choosing TLM for salvage situations and a wider margin be undertaken than is usual for TLM.

7.5 Comparison with Other Modalities

7.5.1 Oncologic Outcomes

Though there are limited randomized controlled trials, there is abundant literature on prospective and retrospective studies comparing TLM with radiotherapy for early glottic cancer. The oncologic outcomes do not seem to be different considering the available literature. There is no evidence in favour of one treatment modality when considering the likelihood of local control or overall survival. The likelihood of laryngeal preservation may be higher when surgery can be offered as initial treatment [13, 12].

7.5.2 Voice and Quality of Life

The postsurgical voice following TLM is largely dependent on the extent of resection with type I and type II cordectomy being associated with excellent voices and type IV and Va cordectomy being associated with significant initial dysphonia. Postsurgical voice impact is worse in the immediate postsurgical period and tends to improve over time. Supraglottic resections naturally have minimal impact on phonation.

For cases with larger resections (cordectomy type III and IV), one of the key decisions in the postsurgical period is with regard to the choice of rehabilitating the voice by glottic phonation or supraglottic phonation. These decisions are taken jointly by the voice therapist and surgeon and based largely on the extent of resection, postsurgical laryngoscopy, and progress made with postsurgical speech therapy. Non-glottal voicing (supraglottic voicing) is gruff and low pitched in comparison to glottal voicing but nevertheless may need to be resorted to in situations with very poor glottic voice such as after some type IV cordectomies.

Although there are no direct comparisons by planned studies, the voice outcomes of TLM are believed better than open partial laryngectomy procedures.

It is generally stated that voice following radiation therapy may score over TLM in terms of objective assessment, but this is not so significant in terms of subjective patient perception. Recent systematic review on the subject has concluded that Voice Handicap indices are comparable following radical radiotherapy and TLM for T_1 glottic carcinoma [19]. A lack of randomized trials precludes any categorical conclusions.

References

1. Jako GJ, Kleinsasser O. Endolaryngeal micro-diagnosis and microsurgery. Reprint from the Annual Meeting of the American Medical Association. 1966.
2. Jako GJ. Laser surgery of the vocal cords. Laryngoscope. 1972;82:2204–15.
3. Strong MS, Jako GJ. Laser surgery of the larynx: early clinical experience with continuous CO_2 laser. Ann Otol Rhinol Laryngol. 1972;81:791–8.
4. Thakar A. Transoral laser microsurgery for moderately advanced cancers of the larynx. ENT NEWS. 2013;21(6):42–4.
5. Laccourreye H, Lacau Saint-Guily J, Brasnu D, et al. Use of the CO_2 laser in the emergency treatment of dyspnea in laryngeal cancer. Ann Otolaryngol Chir Cervicofac. 1984;101:39–42.
6. Canis M, Ihler F, Martin A, Wolff HA, Matthias C, Steiner W. Organ preservation in T4a laryngeal cancer: is transoral laser microsurgery an option? Eur Arch Otorhinolaryngol. 2013;270:2719–27. Full Text.
7. Steiner W, Vogt P, Ambrosch P, Kron M. Transoral carbon dioxide laser microsurgery for recurrent glottic carcinoma after radiotherapy. Head Neck. 2004;26:477–84.
8. Ambrosch P. The role of laser microsurgery in the treatment of laryngeal cancer. Curr Opin Otolaryngol Head Neck Surg. 2007;15:82–8.
9. Blanch JL, Vilaseca I, Caballero M, Moragas M, Berenguer J, Bernal-Sprekelsen M. Outcome of Transoral Laser Microsurgery for T2-T3 tumors growing in the laryngeal anterior commissure. Head Neck. 2011;33:2052–9.
10. Hinni ML, Salassa JR, Grant DG, Pearson BW, Hayden RE, Martin A, Christiansen H, Haughey BH, Nussenbaum B, Steiner W. Transoral laser microsurgery for advanced laryngeal cancer. Arch Otolaryngol Head Neck Surg. 2007;133:1198–204.
11. Suárez C, Rodrigo JP, Silver CE, Hartl DM, Takes RP, Rinaldo A, Strojan P, Ferlito A. Laser surgery for early to moderately advanced glottic, supraglottic, and hypopharyngeal cancers. Head Neck. 2012;34:1028–35.
12. Ramakrishnan Y, Drinnan M, Kwong FN, Grant DG, Mehanna H, Jones T, Paleri V. Oncologic outcomes of transoral laser microsurgery for radiorecurrent laryngeal carcinoma: a systematic review and meta-analysis of English-language literature. Head Neck. 2014;36:280–5.

13. Bron LP, Soldati D, Zouhair A, Ozsahin M, Brossard E, Monnier P, Pasche P. Treatment of early stage squamous-cell carcinoma of the glottic larynx: endoscopic surgery or cricohyoido-epiglottopexy versus radiotherapy. Head Neck. 2001;23:823–9.
14. Karatzanis AD, Psychogios G, Zenk J, Waldfahrer F, Hornung J, Velegrakis GA, Iro H. Comparison among different available surgical approaches in T1 glottic cancer. Laryngoscope. 2009;119(9):1704–8.
15. Jäckel MC, Ambrosch P, Martin A, Steiner W. Impact of re-resection for inadequate margins on the prognosis of upper aerodigestive tract cancer treated by laser microsurgery. Laryngoscope. 2007;117:350–6.
16. Lee M, Buchanan MA, Riffat F, Palme CE. Complications after CO_2 laser surgery for early glottic cancer: an institutional experience. Head Neck. 2016;38(Suppl 1):E987–90.
17. Ahmed F, Kinshuck AJ, Harrison M, O'Brien D, Lancaster J, Roland NJ, Jackson SR, Jones TM. Laser safety in head and neck cancer surgery. Eur Arch Otorhinolaryngol. 2010;267:1779–84.
18. Hoffmann C, Cornu N, Hans S, Sadoughi B, Badoual C, Brasnu D. Early glottic cancer involving the anterior commissure treated by transoral laser cordectomy. Laryngoscope. 2016;126:1817–22.
19. Greulich MT, Parker NP, Lee P, Merati AL, Misono S. Voice outcomes following radiation versus laser microsurgery for T1 glottic carcinoma: systematic review and meta-analysis. Otolaryngol Head Neck Surg. 2015;152:811–9.

Radiation/Chemoradiation in Treatment of Carcinoma of the Larynx

8

Bidhu K. Mohanti

8.1 Introduction

The larynx is, both anatomically and physiologically, an exquisite human organ. It performs the unique function of phonation and speech. Our deglutition is also intimately synchronized with the laryngeal mobility.

The anatomic parts of the larynx (Fig. 8.1) and its endoscopic picture as a correlate of the physiological function (Fig. 8.2) demand an intimate knowledge for the practice of radiation oncology. The endoscopic view is illustrative of the physiological functions of the larynx and its interrelationship to the hypopharyngeal (pyriform sinuses) swallowing activity.

The larynx is divided for clinical and treatment approaches into three subsites, supraglottis, glottis and subglottis, partially based on embryologic development. The supraglottis extends from the tip of the epiglottis to an artificial horizontal plane extending bilaterally across the apex of the laryngeal vestibule. The glottis extends from this plane to approximately 1 cm below the true vocal folds. The subglottis extends from this horizontal plane to the end of the cricoid cartilage.

The epithelium of the vocal folds consists of the stratified squamous epithelium which lies over the lamina propria. The lamina propria, a kind of layered gel-filled space, combined with the fat-filled pre-epiglottic and paraglottic spaces (on both sides) together allows for the free vibrations and phonation of the vocal folds. The mutual relationship between the speech function and the swallowing process is coordinated for a safe passage of the food bolus. This is almost like a musical

B. K. Mohanti (✉)
Department of Radiation Oncology, Manipal Hospital, New Delhi, India

S. Bahadur et al. (eds.), *Carcinoma of the Larynx and Hypopharynx*,
https://doi.org/10.1007/978-981-13-3110-7_8

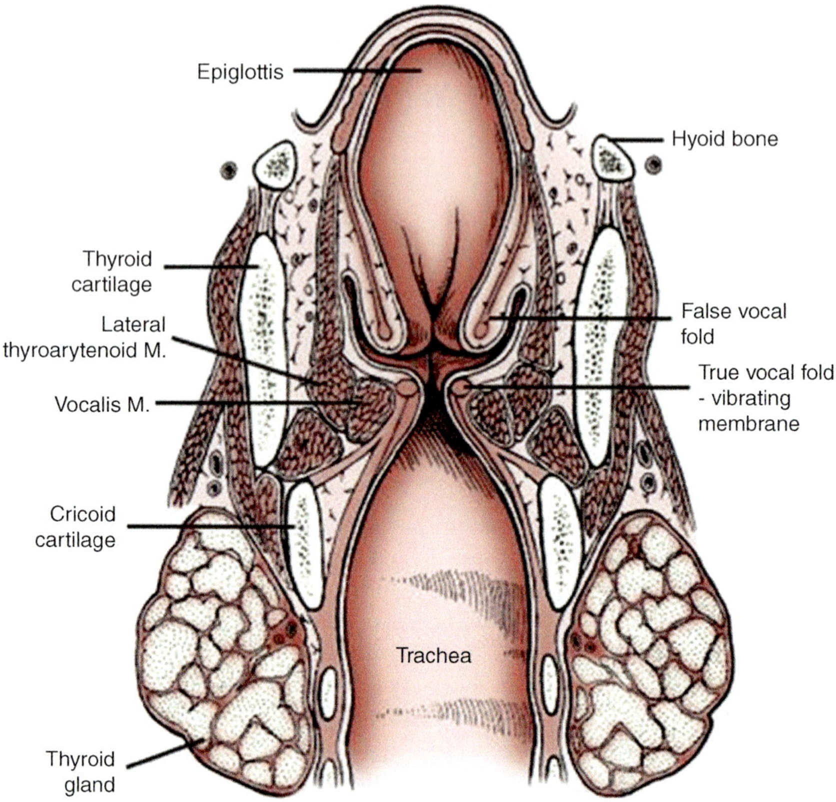

Fig. 8.1 The larynx with its surrounding structures in coronal plane (Ref. Med Clin N Am 1999; 83:115. Copyright 1999 W.B. Saunders Company)

concert. To create an adequate swallow, a concerted movement involving laryngeal elevation, tongue base protrusion of the epiglottis and closure of the rima glottis is critical. Inadequate function in any of these areas can result in persistent swallowing dysfunction after therapy. Moreover, inability to restore or preserve function during treatment in any of these areas can lead to persistent swallowing dysfunction after treatment. Tumours that invade either the glottis or the subglottis can severely affect a patient's swallow related to inability to close the glottis at the level of the epiglottis or the vocal cords [1]. These anatomic and physiologic correlations are relevant for the effects of radiation therapy (RT) or chemoradiotherapy (CRT) [2].

8.2 Evolution of Treatment Modalities for Laryngeal Cancer

Laryngeal cancer represents a model of multidisciplinary treatment approaches in HNC. Significant advances have contributed to the management.

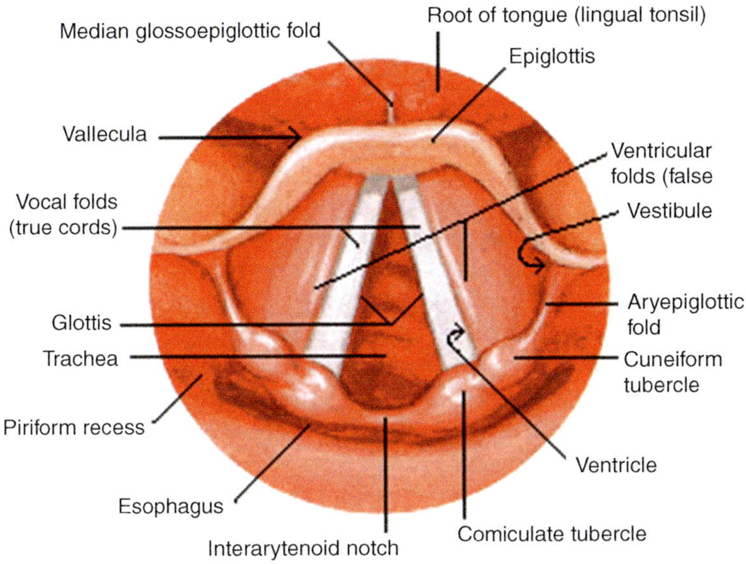

Fig. 8.2 Endoscopic view of the larynx (Courtesy: Department of Otolaryngology and Head-Neck Surgery, AIIMS, New Delhi)

In the progress made in cancer therapy over the centuries, the milestone description about the treatment for cancer of the larynx was recorded as the failure of Sir Morell Mackenzie, a British surgeon of high repute, to diagnose the throat cancer which had affected the crown prince of Germany (afterwards the Emperor Frederick III) in 1887. Within a year, the malignant growth progressed, leading to an acrimony between the German doctors and Sir Mackenzie, and the Emperor Frederick III died. The cellular pathology and tumour description were compiled by Rudolf Virchow at Berlin in 1858. The direct visualization of the voice box, precursor to the modern laryngoscopic examination, was made by Alfred Kirsten in 1895. The foundation for a curative approach was attempted by Theodor Billroth, the well-revered Viennese surgeon, when he completely removed the voice box and left a pharyngocutaneous fistula (the first total laryngectomy in medical history) on 31 December 1873. Neck dissection was later added to the primary surgery for laryngeal cancer. Considerable refinements in surgery for laryngeal tumours, both radical extirpative surgery and voice-preserving operations, have consistently improved the cure rates since the mid-twentieth century. In the last two decades, with the exciting strides through laser and robotic surgeries, the postoperative morbidities are declining in a sizeable manner [3].

Non-surgical methods to treat the cancer of the larynx were first tried with radiation therapy in the beginning of the twentieth century. In 1909, Finzi reported the first external beam radiotherapy delivery for laryngeal cancer [4]. From the encouraging results of the French group led by Coutard in the 1920s to the improvements conferred by megavoltage beams in the 1960s, radiation therapy alone as an alternative to surgery gained slow acceptance [5, 6]. In the 1980s, radiotherapy for laryngeal cancer became an established treatment modality, both for early and locally advanced tumours. Thus, radiotherapy has run parallel to surgery in its development and utilization during the last hundred years. As often happens in science, the early results were reported overenthusiastically. In one retrospective series of 67 patients, it was concluded that "Radical radiotherapy of laryngeal cancer produced results superior to those of radical surgery in patients seen and treated during the period under review in this hospital. The patients cured by radiotherapy have the advantage of salvage of voice and certain other functions" [7]. Towards the 1980s, surgeons came to appreciate the value and efficacy of modern radiotherapy techniques, more so, for the early stages I–II, where equivalent results could be obtained [8]. However, for the locally advanced stages III–IV, radiation therapy (RT) alone continued to show poorer overall survival (OS) and disease-free survival (DFS) compared to total laryngectomy (TL) or TL combined with postoperative radiotherapy (S+PORT). It became imperative that as a non-surgical approach and in order to avoid the long-term speech loss after laryngectomy, radiotherapy alone was not optimal to replace the standard practice of S+PORT.

In the post-World War II era, chemotherapeutic agents were developed for anticancer therapy for several solid and haematologic malignancies. Success rates with chemotherapy were published in the 1970s for breast cancer, lymphomas and leukaemia. Head and neck squamous cell carcinoma (HNSCC), in primary and recurrent status, were treated by single or multiple chemotherapy drug regimens. In the next decade, the chemotherapy showed partial and complete responses in a proportion of HNSCC patients [9]; adequate tumour downstaging was seen in preoperative schedule [10] and as induction therapy before definitive RT [11].

8.3 Radiation Sensitivity of Laryngeal Carcinoma

The cellular sensitivity of various epithelial carcinomas remains the basis of radiotherapy for clinical practice. Squamous cell carcinoma of the larynx is a relatively homogenous tumour which allows to study the dose-fraction parameters for local control. The earlier literature, with favourable result, used to deliver dose in range of 4500–6000 rads, which by modern SI unit of Gray (Gy) in clinical radiotherapy was considerably lower [7].

1. *Tumour and node*: According to clinical radiobiology, the early T1–T2 require a dose in range of 62–66 Gy. In our practice a moderate hypofractionation dose schedule of 60 Gy in 25 fractions, delivered as 5 fractions per week, is the most optimal for >80% local tumour control in the early stages. For the late stages, T3–T4 size tumours, conventional course of 70 Gy in 35 fractions over 7 weeks is recommended [12]. For negative and positive neck nodes, the dose prescriptions are in range of 50–54 Gy and 60–64 Gy, respectively.
2. *Dose fractionation*: The effect of fraction size is equally important in conventional RT course of five fractions per week. Ideally this should be 1.8–2.5 Gy [13].

Whereas hypofractionation is practised for early-stage laryngeal cancer, the late stages are usually delivered the conventional schedule concurrent with systemic chemotherapy. Accelerated and hyperfractionated RT regimens are recommended when CRT is not feasible due to any medical contraindication [14]. Postoperative radiotherapy in the S+PORT setting for advanced laryngeal stages is prescribed as 60–66 Gy to the loco-regional tumour bed, where the dose to negative lymph nodal region can be restricted to 54 Gy. Conventional schedule of 1.8–2.0 Gy per fraction in five fractions per week over a period of 6.5–7 weeks, to deliver the total postoperative dose, is preferred to minimize the tissue morbidities.

8.4 Radiotherapy Delivery

The equipment and techniques for delivery of RT have progressed with time, since the initial treatments with orthovoltage and cobalt between the 1920s and 1960s. In the present era, megavoltage linear accelerators with high-energy photons are the standard of external beam RT for laryngeal cancer, although in some low-resource countries cobalt therapy continues to be utilized. Since the 1990s, the modern linear accelerators are equipped with multileaf collimators, high-dose rate, precision techniques and on-board two-dimensional (2-D) and three-dimensional (3-D) imaging for a range of high-quality options in RT practices.

The techniques in RT delivery started with en face field marking and 2-D prescription of dose plan to the laryngopharyngeal (tumour) and neck (lymph nodes) regions during the first half of the nineteenth century. The dose delivery for laryngeal cancer was often imprecise in the 2-D era of radiotherapy practice, when substantial amount of normal tissues and vital organs surrounding the tumour region received the radiation dose, such as the parotid glands, oral cavity, oropharynx, spinal cord, etc.

The volumetric imaging (CT scan, MRI, PET-CT) ushered in the improvement, which is now broadly called the 3-D practice. This has laid the foundation for modern RT techniques, with accurate description of volumes for the RT dose prescriptions. The tumour region to which the radiation dose is aimed is called the *target volume* (GTV, CTV and PTV), and normal tissues and organs are called *organs at risk* (OARs). This concept was evolved in respect to the volumetric imaging, making it possible to an efficacious RT practice since the 1990s (Fig. 8.3).

The OAR is important in modern 3-D radiotherapy, in order to delineate those organs surrounding the PTV, which should ideally receive the least possible dose to minimize the radiation morbidities. These volume delineations are now mandatory.

In order to treat the laryngeal cancer, several techniques are well established, namely, intensity 3-D conformal radiotherapy (3-D CRT), intensity-modulated radiotherapy (IMRT), image-guided radiotherapy (IGRT), volumetric modulated arc therapy (VMAT) and stereotactic body radiotherapy (SBRT). Depending upon the facilities of imaging and the linear accelerator available in a particular centre, and the stage of disease, a particular technique is chosen. At our institute, we prefer VMAT technique, with adaptive imaging during the course of radiotherapy.

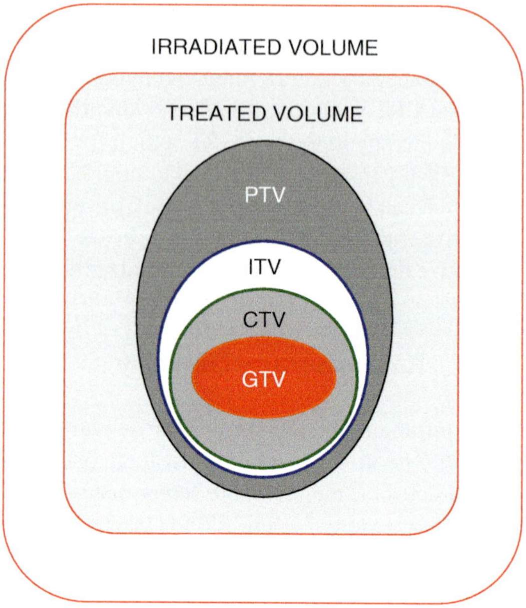

Fig. 8.3 Modern radiotherapy dose prescription volumes. *GTV* gross target volume, *CTV* clinical target volume, *ITV* internal target volume (CTV and ITV margins are given to include the subclinical disease and physiologic motion), *PTV* planning target volume (defined as the volume to which RT dose is prescribed for the optimal tumour coverage). From ICRU 50, 1993

The preparation for radiotherapy planning includes a proper thermoplastic immobilization, 3-D CT simulator image acquisition and contouring of the volumes as per the above-mentioned concepts. The dose planning is carried out on computerized radiotherapy planning system (RT-TPS) by the medical physicists, and then the dose prescription volumes are carefully evaluated by the radiation oncologists. In modern practice, these data are transferred from RT-TPS to the linear accelerator for daily treatments over the prescribed radiotherapy course of several weeks. Quality assurance at all steps of radiotherapy planning and delivery is essential.

8.5 Radiotherapy for Early Laryngeal Cancer

With satisfactory disease control and survival conferred by curative radiation therapy, the surgeons developed confidence to refer suitable patients [7]. In our experience, the multidisciplinary head and neck clinic helped our team to identify the patients and explain the options of surgery versus RT to the patient and accrued the study group who received curative RT. The initial results of definitive radiotherapy for T1-T2 glottic carcinoma gave our institutional practice the credence [15]. It is now established that 70–90% of early-stage laryngeal cancer show long-term disease control and the 5-year cancer-specific survival in 70–80% of radiotherapy-treated patients.

Usually the radiation therapy volume includes the primary disease with a margin to cover the nodal basin in immediate vicinity, such as level II–III and inter-jugular chain. In 2-D era of direct lateral portals to the neck, the field sizes used to be 5 × 5 cm to 8 × 8 cm. The 3-D image-based treatment requires immobilization for RT planning and a satisfactory scan sections for contouring the target volume and OARs. When the anterior commissure is involved, we place a wax bolus upon the

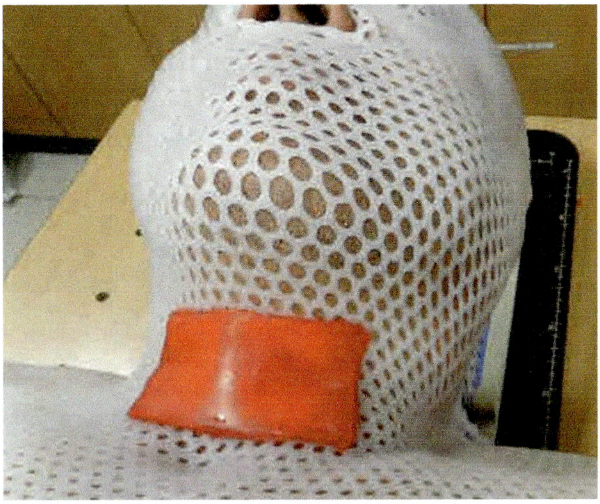

Fig. 8.4 Patient fitted with immobilization cast (with wax bolus anteriorly to increase dose to the anterior commissure)

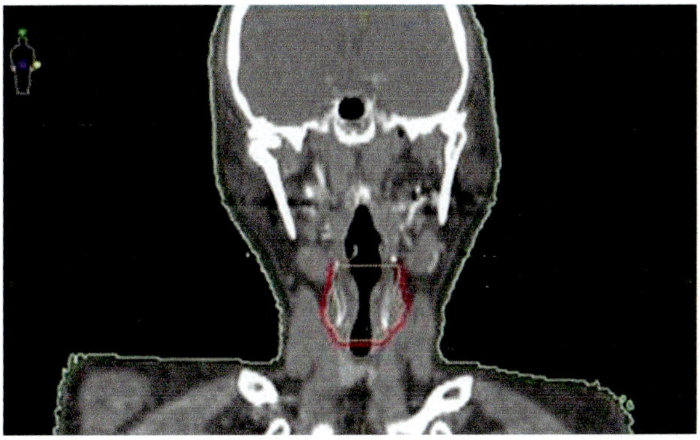

Fig. 8.5 Tumour volume contouring (red line) for glottic larynx

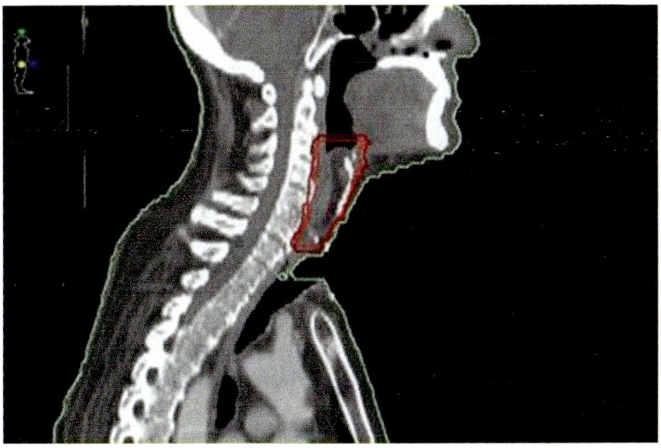

Fig. 8.6 Tumour volume contouring (red line) for supraglottic larynx

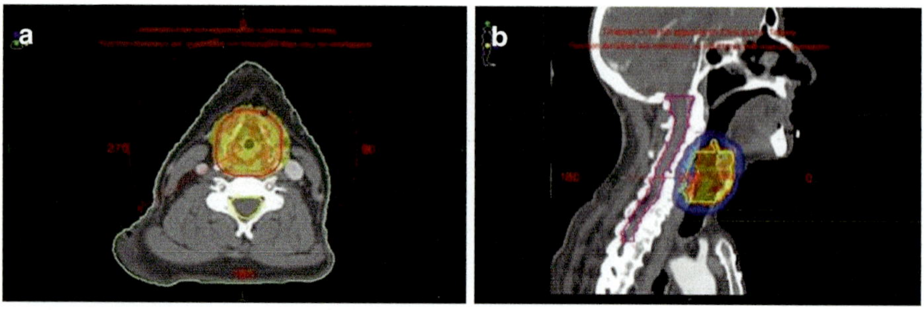

Fig. 8.7 Radiation therapy dose plan for early laryngeal cancer, (**a**) axial and (**b**) sagittal views (Author's note: Figures 8.4 to 8.7 were obtained from the Radiation Oncology, Fortis Memorial Research Institute, Gurgaon, India; the patient's identity is anonymized)

immobilization cast anteriorly to build up the dose (Fig. 8.4). The contouring will differ for glottic and supraglottic tumours (Figs. 8.5 and 8.6) [2].

The current techniques, such as IMRT, IGRT and VMAT, deliver the prescribe radiation dose to a much tighter volume and reduce the morbidities. In our practice, we utilize the VMAT for a more precise and faster delivery (Fig. 8.7).

As described in earlier section, conventional and hypofractionated radiotherapy at five fractions per week are routinely advised. A recent National Cancer Database analysis from the USA has shown that hypofractionation schedule is increasingly favoured in early stages. The data showed a comparison; the median conventional RT course was 66 Gy, at 2 Gy per fraction, over a period of 49 days, while the median hypofractionation patient received 63 Gy, at 2.25 Gy/fraction over a period of 41 days [16].

The voice and speech quality after treatment in early laryngeal cancer is another matter of concern for the patients and continues to remain an area of research. Curative radiotherapy, compared to open surgery, had shown better reported outcomes. A randomized study reported that the overall voice quality achieved was roughly similar after the treatments, but patients treated with radiation therapy had less breathy voice and experienced less inconvenience in their daily lives [17].

In summary, radiotherapy, open surgery and endolaryngeal excision (laser or robotic surgery) are all accepted modalities of treatment for early-stage cancer (T1–T2, N0). Over the years, results have shown equal results in terms of disease control, recurrence and overall survival. In choosing the treatment option, the patient should be adequately explained the options. Radiotherapy offers laryngeal preservation; however it is a prolonged treatment course and may be associated with unpleasant morbidities including oral mucositis, dysphagia, radiation dermatitis and xerostomia, more so when the irradiated volume includes oral cavity and oropharynx [18].

8.6 Advanced Laryngeal Cancer

Up until the early 1990s, total laryngectomy had historically been the mainstay of advanced-stage laryngeal cancer. The T3–T4 tumours, with extrinsic spread and nodal involvement, showed high failure rates and limited survival after radiotherapy alone [1, 6].

1. *Stage III laryngeal cancer*: The choice of definitive radiotherapy to a dose of 70 Gy in conventional schedule over 7 weeks or its equivalent in hyperfractionated regimen of 1.2 Gy per fraction delivered as two daily fractions for 5 days in a week up to 72–76.8 Gy over 6–6½ weeks can be decided for T3N0 or T3N1 disease status. Salvage surgery is reserved for loco-regional failure cases, because the organ preservation after radiotherapy alone for stage III is approximately 30% or less. However the cure rates are inferior to surgery with or without postoperative radiotherapy [19]. Actuarial 4-year disease-free survival rates were significantly better with combined treatment (79%) than with radical radiotherapy and surgical salvage (65%; $p = 0.024$). In the radical radiotherapy group, failure was almost always at the primary site, and the probability of surviving with an intact larynx was approximately half of the total survival. As per this study, a policy of radical radiotherapy (with salvage surgery for failure) for unselected clinically staged T3N0 cancer larynx does not provide for comparable cure rates or for satisfactory laryngeal preservation. Accordingly, our approach to select radiotherapy alone in stage III laryngeal cancer is limited to those patients who have medical contraindications, are elderly with poor performance status and decline the combined therapy [19]. The development of combined therapy in advanced cancer has gone through various stages. The gold standard is the TL or its modification in the form of partial/subtotal laryngectomy, combined with adjuvant radiotherapy for adverse histopathological features. Postoperative radiotherapy after the extirpative surgery is recommended for close or positive margins, node positive and extra-capsular spread and soft tissue or cartilage infiltration. The VA study from the USA in 1991 paved the way for the alternate combined therapy approach with CRT, in order to obviate the consequence of speech loss after S+PORT [20]. In the last 25 years, confirmation of the VA study results has come from European (EORTC) and American (RTOG) cooperative groups, where the trial designs of the CRT used different drug regimens in advanced laryngeal cancer. A recent paper excellently reviews the CRT data of larynx preservation [1].
2. *Stage IV laryngeal cancer*: The gold standard of S+PORT has been slowly replaced by CRT in the T4 and N+ stages. The two drug regimens of cisplatin plus 5-FU or cisplatin as single agent are combined with radical dose of radiotherapy. Some studies as well have used taxane with cisplatin and 5-FU (TPF), claiming the superiority over single or two drugs [1, 21, 22]. Further attempts to avoid the toxicities of systemic chemotherapy used the trial design of bio-radiotherapy, when targeted drugs are combined with radiotherapy [21]. Cetuximab is the favoured targeted drug. The major randomized studies CRT for larynx preservation are shown in Table 8.1.

According to our current knowledge, in the stage III–IV laryngeal cancer, the overall 5-year survival rates range from 35% to 65%, with the laryngeal preservation maintained in approximately 40% of the CRT-treated patients. Controversy still persists regarding the best practice for operable T4a laryngeal tumour. Studies of (non-T4a) locally advanced larynx cancer showing no difference in survival between larynx preservation CRT and TL plus postoperative radiotherapy (S+PORT) may not apply to T4a disease. Using the National Cancer Database of the USA [23], the

Table 8.1 Larynx preservation studies, randomized controlled trials

Study/author year [Reference]	Number of patients	Study arms	DFS	OS	Larynx preservation
VA study, 1991 [20]	332	1. PF × 3 then RT (66–70 Gy) 2. S+PORT (50.4–60.4 Gy)	– –	68% (2-year) 68% (2-year) ($p = 0.98$)	66% (2-year) –
Lefebvre, 2013 GORTEC [21]	116	1. ICT(TPF) × 3 then CRT(P) 2. ICT × 3 then RT+Cet	– –	75% (3-year) 73% (3-year)	95% (3 months) 93% (3 months)
Forastiere, 2013 RTOG [22]	547	1. PF × 3 then RT (70 Gy) 2. CRT(P) 3. RT alone (70 Gy)		39% (10-year) 28% (10-year) 32% (10-year) (p = NS)	67% (10-year) 81% (10-year) 63% (10-year)

Note: PF, cisplatin plus 5-FU (3 weekly); ICT, TPF, docetaxel (T) + platinum (P) + 5-FU(F) as induction; CRT(P), concurrent RT 70 Gy plus platinum; RT+Cet, concurrent RT 70 Gy plus cetuximab

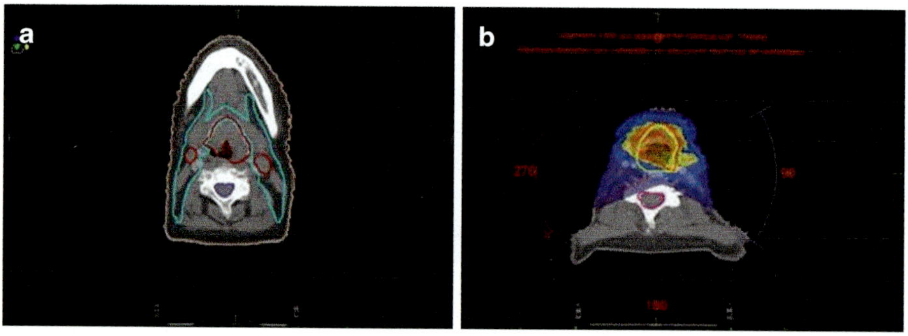

Fig. 8.8 (**a**) Stage III–IV laryngeal cancer, contouring of primary and nodal region; (**b**) dose plan showing dose prescriptions for primary (yellow) and nodes (blue)

T4a patients showed lower median overall survival in the larynx preservation CRT protocol compared to the gold standard S+PORT (39 months versus 61 months). Accordingly, the operable stage IV laryngeal cancer patients should be adequately counselled.

3. *Radiotherapy policy in advanced laryngeal cancer*: In the present 3-D era, accurate delineation of target volume and OAR needs to be emphasized both in the gold standard postoperative (S+PORT) setting and for the CRT practice of organ preservation [2]. The primary plus nodal region contouring for stages III–IV and the dose plan to the two different volumes by VMAT technique (our practice) are shown in Fig. 8.8a, b.

Radiotherapy treatment planning system (RT-TPS) is capable of demonstrating the dose-volume histogram (DVH), where the radiation oncologist, physicist and technologist can analyse the dose to primary tumour, nodes and OARs. This is very helpful to

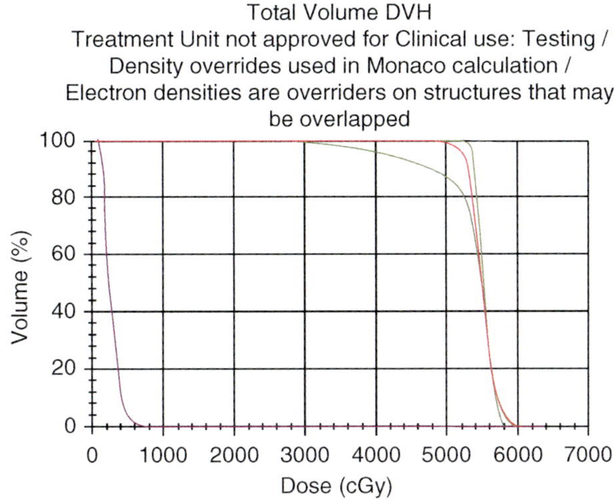

Fig. 8.9 The dose-volume histogram (DVH) for postoperative radiotherapy dose of 60 Gy

optimize the treatment delivery and limit the doses to OARs within the tolerance limits. The DVH for postoperative case to deliver 60 Gy is shown in Fig. 8.9. After the dose prescription and DVH are approved, the treatment parameters are placed for computerized delivery of the RT course daily to the patient on linear accelerator. RT delivery for the patient's set-up on a linear accelerator couch with immobilization cast, on-board cone beam CT imaging apparatus, etc. shown in Fig. 8.10.

8.7 Summary

The advancements in radiotherapy equipment and delivery techniques have significantly improved the role of radiotherapy since the 1990s.The volumetric imaging with CT, MRI and PET-CT, immobilization with CT simulation, contouring and 3-D dose-volume estimates and on-board imaging and morbidity assessments are some of the key developments in radiotherapy practice. The modern linear accelerator is the backbone in treatment delivery.

The early stages I–II can be treated by the modern 3-D planning to a limited volume. High long-term cure rates in range of 70–90% with larynx preservation in more than two-thirds of the patients make the choice of curative radiotherapy a suitable option for these patients. The morbidities related to speech and swallowing can be easily managed and recover in more than 80% of the treated patients. Definitive radiotherapy is shown to give rise to better quality of voice compared to open voice-preserving laryngeal surgery. In recent years, the voice-preserving laser or robotic surgery show the promise that the speech quality can be better by these tools of surgical excision, compared to the RT.

In stage III–IV laryngeal cancer patients, total laryngectomy or its modification of partial laryngectomy remains the standard of anticancer therapy for disease control. Often, the surgery for primary tumour is combined with neck dissection. Postoperative radiotherapy (S+PORT) improves the loco-regional control and disease-free survival.

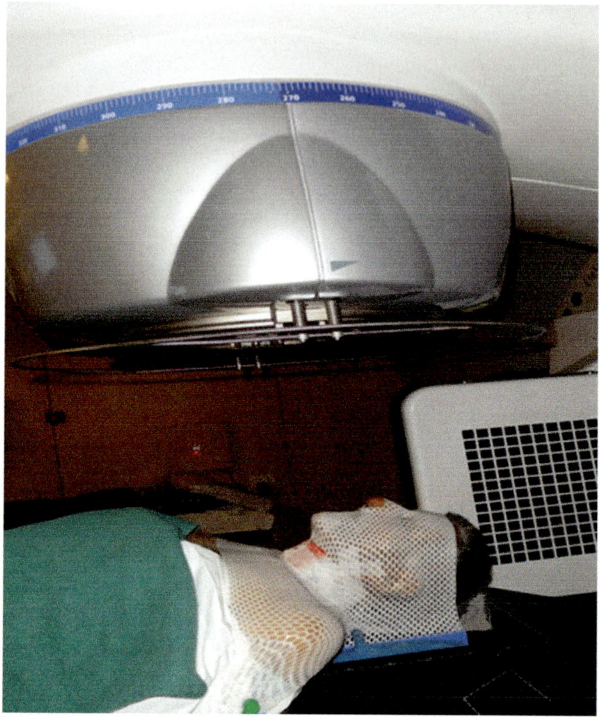

Fig. 8.10 Patient set-up on linear accelerator couch for treatment delivery and on-board cone beam CT imaging (Author's note: Figures 8.8 to 8.10 were obtained from the Radiation Oncology, Fortis Memorial Research Institute, Gurgaon, India; the patient's identity is anonymized)

Chemoradiotherapy, as induction or concurrent schedule, has become the alternative approach in the last 25 years. The CRT option has emerged mainly with the objective to avoid the permanent speech loss after laryngectomy. On the long term, the morbidities after CRT are substantial. Nearly 15–20% patients who may have disease control can continue to have poor speaking and swallowing abilities. The improvements in radiotherapy practice and chemotherapy drug regimen have resulted in incremental benefits. Nearly 50% of the locally advanced patients live beyond 5 years with well-maintained speech and swallowing. In recent years, the emphasis is on the rehabilitation and long-term quality of life of these patients.

References

1. Steuer CE, El-Deiry M, Parks JR, Higgins KA, Saba NF. An update on larynx cancer. CA Cancer J Clin. 2017;67:31–50.
2. D'Souza L, Jaswal J, Chan F, Johnson M, Tay KY, Fung K, Palma D. Evaluating the impact of an integrated multidisciplinary head & neck competency-based anatomy & radiology teaching approach in radiation oncology: a prospective cohort study. BMC Med Educ. 2014;14:124.
3. Cocek A. The history and current status of surgery in the treatment of laryngeal cancer. Acta Med (Hradec Kralove). 2008;51:157–63.
4. Finzi N. Untitled letter to Lancet. Lancet. 1909;1:868.
5. Lederman M. History of radiotherapy in the treatment of cancer of the larynx, 1896–1939. Laryngoscope. 1975;85:333–53.

6. Fletcher GH. History of irradiation in squamous cell carcinomas of the larynx and hypopharynx. Int J Radiat Oncol Biol Phys. 1986;12:2019–24.
7. Garland LH. Cancer of the larynx; results of surgical and radiological treatment in one institution. Calif Med. 1966;105:8–10.
8. Genden EM, Ferlito A, Silver CE, Jacobson AS, Werner JA, Suárez C, Leemans CR, Bradley PJ, Rinaldo A. Evolution of the management of laryngeal cancer. Oral Oncol. 2007;43:431–9.
9. Glick JH, Zehngebot LM, Taylor SG 4th. Chemotherapy for squamous cell carcinoma of the head and neck: a progress report. Am J Otolaryngol. 1980;1:306–23.
10. Norris CM Jr, Clark JR, Frei E, Ervin TJ, Fallon B, Tuttle SA, Fabian RL, Miller D. Pathology of surgery after induction chemotherapy: an analysis of resectability and locoregional control. Laryngoscope. 1986;96:292–302.
11. Demard F, Chauvel P, Santini J, Vallicioni J, Thyss A, Schneider M. Response to chemotherapy as justification for modification of the therapeutic strategy for pharyngolaryngeal carcinomas. Head Neck. 1990;12:225–31.
12. Robertson AG, Robertson C, Boyle P, Symonds RP, Wheldon TE. The effect of differing radiotherapeutic schedules on the response of glottic carcinoma of the larynx. Eur J Cancer. 1993;29A(4):501–10.
13. Le QT, Fu KK, Kroll S, Ryu JK, Quivey JM, Meyler TS, Krieg RM, Phillips TL. Influence of fraction size, total dose, and overall time on local control of T1-T2 glottic carcinoma. Int J Radiat Oncol Biol Phys. 1997;39:115–26.
14. Overgaard J, Mohanti BK, Begum N, Ali R, Agarwal JP, Kuddu M, Bhasker S, Tatsuzaki H, Grau C. Five versus six fractions of radiotherapy per week for squamous-cell carcinoma of the head and neck (IAEA-ACC study): a randomised, multicentre trial. Lancet Oncol. 2010;11:553–60.
15. Mohanti BK, Tandon DA, Bahadur S, Rath GK, Tanwar RK, Lal P, Biswal BM. Results of definitive radiotherapy in T1 and T2 glottic carcinoma: Institute of Rotary Cancer Hospital experience. Australas Radiol. 1996;40:287–90.
16. Stokes WA, Abbott D, Phan A, Raben D, Lanning RM, Karam SD. Patterns of care for patients with early-stage glottic cancer undergoing definitive radiation therapy: a national cancer database analysis. Int J Radiat Oncol Biol Phys. 2017;98:1014–21.
17. Aaltonen LM, Rautiainen N, Sellman J, Saarilahti K, Mäkitie A, Rihkanen H, Laranne J, Kleemola L, Wigren T, Sala E, Lindholm P, Grenman R, Joensuu H. Voice quality after treatment of early vocal cord cancer: a randomized trial comparing laser surgery with radiation therapy. Int J Radiat Oncol Biol Phys. 2014;90:255–60.
18. Warner L, Chudasama J, Kelly CG, Loughran S, McKenzie K, Wight R, Dey P. Radiotherapy versus open surgery versus endolaryngeal surgery (with or without laser) for early laryngeal squamous cell cancer. Cochrane Database Syst Rev. 2014;12:CD002027. https://doi.org/10.1002/14651858.CD002027.
19. Thakar A, Bahadur S, Mohanti BK, Nivsarkar S. Clinically staged T3N0M0 laryngeal cancer: how is it best treated? Definitive radiotherapy with salvage surgery v/s combined surgery and radiotherapy. J Laryngol Otol. 2000;114:108–12.
20. The Department of Veterans Affairs Laryngeal Cancer Study Group. Induction chemotherapy plus radiation compared with surgery plus radiation in patients with advanced laryngeal cancer. N Engl J Med. 1991;324:1685–90.
21. Lefebvre JL, Pointreau Y, Rolland F, et al. Induction chemotherapy followed by either chemoradiotherapy or bioradiotherapy for larynx preservation: the TREMPLIN randomized phase II study. J Clin Oncol. 2013;31:853–9.
22. Forastiere AA, Zhang Q, Weber RS, Maor MH, Goepfert H, Pajak TF, Morrison W, Glisson B, Trotti A, Ridge JA, Thorstad W, Wagner H, Ensley JF, Cooper JS. Long-term results of RTOG 91-11: a comparison of three nonsurgical treatment strategies to preserve the larynx in patients with locally advanced larynx cancer. J Clin Oncol. 2013;31:845–52.
23. Grover S, Swisher-McClure S, Mitra N, Li J, Cohen RB, Ahn PH, Lukens JN, Chalian AA, Weinstein GS, O'Malley BW Jr, Lin A. Total laryngectomy versus larynx preservation for T4a larynx cancer: patterns of care and survival outcomes. Int J Radiat Oncol Biol Phys. 2015;92:594–601.

9 Tumours of the Hypopharynx: Diagnosis, Assessment and Staging

Sudhir Bahadur and Arun Sharma

9.1 Introduction

The hypopharynx extends from the level of the hyoid bone to inferiorly the cervical oesophagus at lower border of cricoid cartilage. Tumours arising from the hypopharynx are generally aggressive and present late partly because of few symptoms. Most patients have lymph node metastasis at presentation and generally have worse prognosis as compared with 'intrinsic' laryngeal tumours. Smoking and alcohol consumption are important factors in aetiology [1].

The pyriform fossa is the commonest of the three sites in the hypopharynx accounting for 65–70% cases of malignant neoplasms, followed by post-cricoid region, comprising of 20% lesions. The posterior pharyngeal wall and cervical oesophagus account for 5% cases each. Post-cricoid cancers are more commonly seen in women and are linked to Patterson-Brown-Kelly syndrome.

The diagnosis and management of hypopharyngeal cancer are complex and difficult because of the surgical anatomy, its proximity to the larynx and tumour behaviour. Newer imaging techniques, however, have improved the case selection for treatment.

Lesions when diagnosed early respond well to radiation. However, most patients with advanced disease probably would require surgery and postoperative radiotherapy. Role of chemo-radiation primarily for organ preservation has not been clearly defined as in laryngeal lesions.

S. Bahadur (✉)
Department of Otolaryngology and Head-Neck Surgery, Formerly at All India Institute of Medical Sciences, New Delhi, India

A. Sharma
Department of Otolaryngology and Head-Neck Surgery, Hamdard Institute of Medical Sciences and Research, Jamia Hamdard, New Delhi, India

S. Bahadur et al. (eds.), *Carcinoma of the Larynx and Hypopharynx*,
https://doi.org/10.1007/978-981-13-3110-7_9

9.2 Surgical Anatomy

The hypopharynx is part of the pharynx which extends superiorly from the oropharynx to inferiorly the cervical oesophagus that reaches to the thoracic inlet. The superior extent roughly begins at level of hyoid bone or at level of pharyngo-epiglottic fold. The larynx is located anterior to the hypopharynx, and retropharyngeal space is behind it. The hypopharynx is subdivided into three: the pyriform fossa on either side, the post-cricoid region and the posterior pharyngeal wall.

The pyriform fossa is composed of anterior, medial and lateral walls that form inverted pyramid with its base at the level of pharyngo-epiglottic fold and the apex reaching to just below the cricoid cartilage. This region is lateral to the aryepiglottic folds and medial to the thyroid lamina. The medial pyriform fossa mucosa forms the posterior wall of the paraglottic space, and thus because of close anatomic relationship, tumours can invade the larynx, the arytenoid cartilages and the cricoarytenoid joint [1]. The apex of the pyriform fossa extends to the level of the cricoid cartilage and corresponds to the level of the vocal cord.

The post-cricoid region is located in the anterior wall of the hypopharynx, extending from just below the arytenoid cartilages to the oesophageal introitus. The posterior pharyngeal wall is separated from the vertebral and prevertebral structures by potential retropharyngeal space. Posterior pharyngeal wall extends from level of the hyoid bone to superior aspect of cricopharyngeus muscle.

The aryepiglottic folds separate the endolarynx from medial wall of the pyriform fossa bilaterally and from the marginal zone (part of the supraglottic region). However, tumours arising from this site behave more aggressively like the hypopharyngeal cancers [2]. There are four layers in the hypopharynx.

(a) The inner mucosal lining composed of stratified squamous epithelium
(b) The fibrous layer of pharyngeal aponeurosis
(c) The muscular layer formed by the inferior and middle constrictors
(d) An outer layer of fascia derived from buccopharyngeal fascia

The muscular layer is composed of the posterior cricoarytenoid muscles anteriorly and middle-inferior constrictor muscles posteriorly. The constrictor muscles are thin, especially the superior constrictor, and they offer little resistance to spread of the tumour. At the junction of the inferior constrictor and the cricopharyngeus is an area of relative weakness known as Killian's triangle, through which posterior pharyngeal wall tumours can extend outside the hypopharynx. Just inferior to the hyoid bone, at the thyrohyoid membrane, is another potential area of weakness through which tumours can extend along the vascular pedicle and superior laryngeal nerve.

Posteriorly, the hypopharynx is separated from the prevertebral fascia which covers the longitudinal spine muscles (longus colli and longus capitis) by thin layer of the fascia and the retropharyngeal space.

The blood supply to the hypopharynx is from the branches of the superior thyroid and lingual and ascending pharyngeal arteries. The sensory nerve supply to the hypopharynx is primarily from the internal branch of the superior laryngeal nerve which runs along the anterior wall of the pyriform fossa.

The lymphatics that drain the pyriform fossa traverse the thyrohyoid membrane by following the superior laryngeal nerve and vessels and drain primarily into jugulo-digastric lymph nodes and the middle deep cervical nodes. The drainage from posterior wall of the hypopharynx occurs to the midjugular chain and retropharyngeal lymph nodes. Lower portion of the hypopharynx and post-cricoid region drain to nodes along the recurrent laryngeal nerve, paratracheal nodes, paraoesophageal nodes and supraclavicular nodes [2].

Locoregional spread of hypopharyngeal cancer within the hypopharynx is less well defined than the neoplasm within the larynx mainly because the latter has well-defined structures and potential spaces that dictate the spread of tumour. The pattern of tumour spread is more difficult to determine. Several authors have described spread of the tumour based upon serial section studies [3, 4].

The pyriform fossa is the most frequently involved site in the hypopharynx accounting for approximately 65% or more of hypopharyngeal tumours. These tumours are known for aggressive behaviour with early metastasis. These lesions may also show extensive submucosal spread with an average of 10 mm of submucosal extent [5]. Tumours that involve the medial wall may spread to involve the aryepiglottic fold, or the tumour may spread medially to invade the paraglottic space. The lesion then behaves as a transglottic carcinoma and extends inferiorly along medial surface of the thyroid cartilage [5, 6]. The vocal cord may become fixed because of invasion of cricoarytenoid muscles or because of tumour invasion of the cricoarytenoid joint, the vocalis muscle or the recurrent laryngeal nerve. Tumours of the lateral wall of the pyriform fossa may spread over the mucosal surface and extend superiorly along the lateral pharyngeal wall. They may grow posteriorly to involve the posterior wall of the hypopharynx and may reach the opposite pyriform fossa.

Tumour extension to the apex of the pyriform fossa is also associated with thyroid cartilage invasion [6–8]. Thyroid gland may also become involved either as a result of direct extension through the thyroid cartilage or tumour extension through cricothyroid membrane.

Tumours arising from lateral pharyngeal may spread laterally through the weakness in area of thyrohyoid membrane to metastasize early into deep cervical lymph nodes and into other soft tissues of the neck.

9.3 Regional Metastases

The hypopharyngeal cancers are associated with regional lymph node involvement in approximately 60–80% of patients which can be detected on physical examination or by imaging at first presentation [9, 10]. Drainage to involve level II, III and

IV lymph nodes may occur frequently. The lymphatic drainage of the posterior pharyngeal wall occurs mainly into the retropharyngeal lymph nodes and accounts for nearly 40% of cases [11].

The risk of contralateral metastasis is high in hypopharyngeal cancer because of the risk of lesion crossing the midline and accounts for nearly 20% [11, 12]. It is, therefore, suggested to treat both sides of the neck, either by surgery or by radiotherapy.

9.3.1 Distant Metastasis

The incidence of distant metastasis on presentation was reviewed by Merino et al. [12] and found to be 11% of all head and neck squamous cancers. In hypopharyngeal cancers, however, the figure is 24% distant metastasis seen generally to the lungs, liver and bone, though other sites such as the adrenals, kidney, brain and bowel have also been described. The majority of patients at presentation have advanced disease when diagnosed.

9.3.2 Second Primary Cancer

Patients of hypopharyngeal cancer have the potential to develop a synchronous or metachronous cancer [13–15]. Several studies have pointed to the fact that there is high risk for hypopharyngeal cancers to develop multiple primary cancers. The prevalence rate of 15.9% of metachronous oesophageal carcinoma has been reported in hypopharyngeal cancer [16]. Nearly half of all patients will develop a second primary cancer within 2 years of the initial index primary lesion. There is also suggestion that there is increased risk of second primary cancer in the upper aerodigestive tract and lungs following initial hypopharyngeal cancer.

9.4 Diagnosis

9.4.1 Clinical Assessment

Most patients of carcinoma of the hypopharynx are diagnosed when the disease is far advanced. This may be because there are a few symptoms at the early stage of disease and even these generally receive little attention. Therefore, index of suspicion should be high while examining these patients who are in the middle or elderly age group and give history of consumption of tobacco and/or alcohol. Their level of nutrition is adversely affected because of the progressive difficulty in swallowing.

The cardinal clinical features of hypopharyngeal carcinoma include slowly increasing dysphagia, hoarseness, sore throat and weight loss with or without a lump in the neck. Similarly pain during swallowing tends to occur early in the disease. Altered sensation during swallowing such as gastro-oesophageal reflex is a common non-specific symptom [17, 18].

Otalgia has been described both in early disease in 25% cases and in advanced disease (in 75% cases) and is due to referred pain. This pain is referred via a small branch of vagus nerve and Arnold nerve which supplies sensation to external ear. The glossopharyngeal nerve supplies the base of tongue mucosa, which may be involved in high pyriform fossa cancer. Pain may again be referred to the ear, in this case by Jacobson's nerve supplying sensation to the middle ear mucosa.

Dysphagia occurs early in post-cricoid carcinoma but is a late symptom in pyriform fossa lesions. Hoarseness is due to various mechanisms involving the laryngeal fixation either due to tumour invasion of cricoarytenoid muscle, cricoarytenoid joint or the recurrent laryngeal nerve or even spread to the paraglottic space.

The nodal metastasis in the neck usually at level 2 is noted in nearly 75% of pyriform fossa cancers when first seen [19]; however, only 20–40% patients of post-cricoid carcinoma present with nodal mass in the neck at presentation, but mediastinal nodes and retropharyngeal nodes may be involved [20] and can be seen on MRI. However, it should be remembered that a significant number of patients of hypopharyngeal carcinoma with clinically negative neck (No) contain occult metastatic disease.

9.4.2 Physical Examination

Complete head and neck examination should be carried out including the indirect laryngoscopy and the use of fibre-optic endoscope. Once the tumour is seen, it should be photographed and recorded with the case file (Fig. 9.1). Most post-cricoid and posterior pharyngeal wall lesions may not be visualized unless these extend superiorly. Fixation of ipsilateral hemilarynx may be seen in nearly half of the

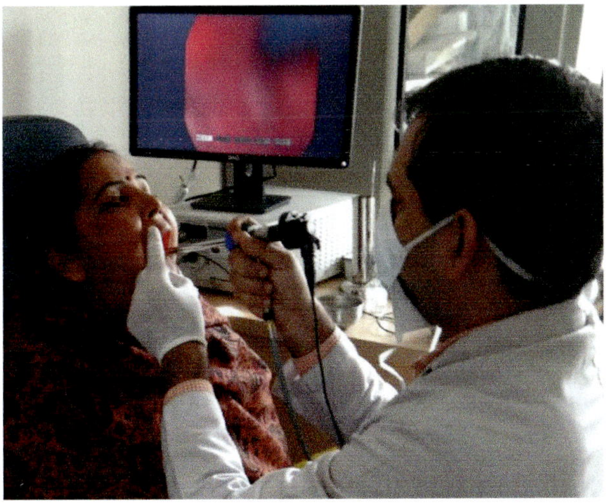

Fig. 9.1 Examination of the larynx and hypopharynx with rigid 90° telescope

patients. However, occasionally only pooling of saliva may be noted. There may be loss of laryngeal crepitus in large post-cricoid tumours. Detailed examination of the neck should be done for assessment of cervical lymphadenopathy in terms of size, number and level of lymph nodes involved, whether on ipsilateral side or both sides.

Stridor is uncommon in early stage of disease but, when present, suggests extensive involvement of the larynx, or it may be due to bilateral recurrent nerve involvement resulting in vocal cord fixity.

9.4.3 Imaging Studies

Diagnostic imaging is extremely important for assessment of extent and staging of disease. The aim of imaging is to determine the three-dimensional extent of the tumour [21, 22]. The imaging studies also help in detecting the neck metastasis, chest metastasis or synchronous second primary. Besides, the imaging is important for the surgeon to decide about the extent of resection and/or radiotherapy planning (Fig. 9.2a–c).

The X-rays of the lateral soft tissue of the neck may be a good screening image to begin with and rule out any increase in the prevertebral shadow, indicating a post-cricoid neoplasm. Similarly, a barium study may have limited role because of

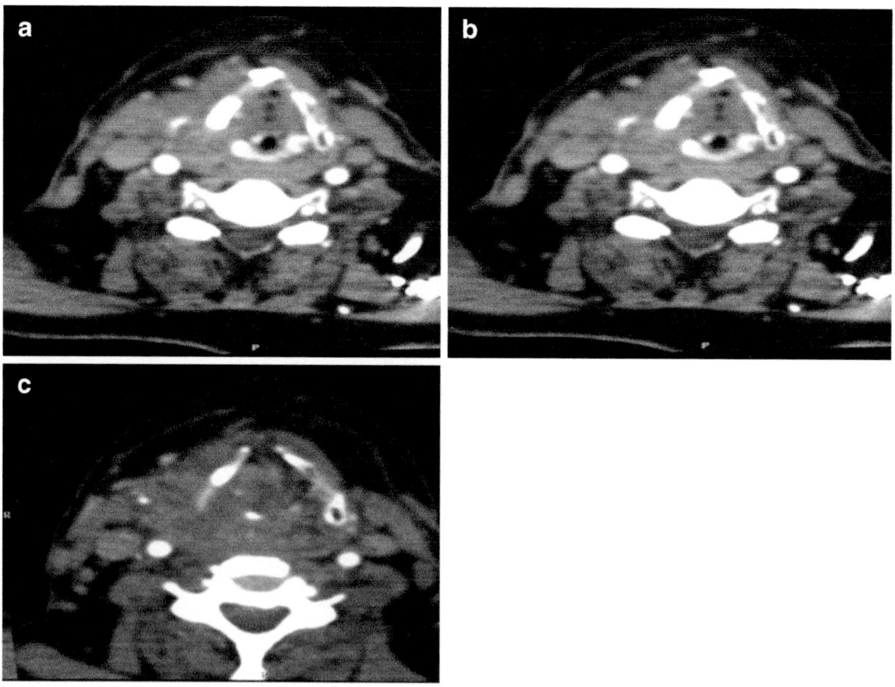

Fig. 9.2 (**a–c**) CT scans of a patient with extensive pyriform fossa (right) cancer T_4N_1

potential risk of aspiration and that it may not accurately identify the mucosal irregularities.

However, both the computed tomography (CT) and magnetic resonance imaging (MRI) are adequate imaging and serve different purposes. There is debate whether CT or the MRI is superior for assessment of primary neoplasm; the computed tomography visualizes and assesses the bone better. However, the MRI is more sensitive and produces magnetically image protons that largely reflect the water content of tissues.

The MR images also show peritumoural oedema which tend to overestimate the size of the tumour. On the other hand, it is difficult to differentiate the tumour from the soft tissue oedema on the CT scan. Incidentally both imaging modalities are complimentary to each other in assessment of disease. However, it is sometimes because of cost factors in our country that the choice is made in favour of one over the other.

There is large amount of literature in recent years on positron emission tomography (PET) [23, 24]. The isotope usually used 18F-fluoro-2-deoxy-D-glucose (FDG), and technique is essentially a measure of tissue metabolic rate. It is a sensitive tool for detecting primary lesion and metastatic spread. It is well realized that possibility of distant metastasis should be excluded before contemplating doing major resection and reconstructive surgery. It is also known that patients with neck nodal metastasis are more likely to develop chest metastasis and second primary cancers than patients with clinically negative neck. CT scan of the chest is useful in these cases. Nevertheless, PET scan is not carried out routinely in the initial workup of the patient partly because of the cost involved. However, the combination of PET and CT scan increases the specificity and is being increasingly used to image the post-treatment cases.

9.4.4 Endoscopy

Application of transnasal flexible fibre-optic oesophagoscopy has been advised in diagnosis of hypopharyngeal cancer under local anaesthesia and also to rule out presence of multiple primary cancer [25]. Muto et al. [26] laid stress on the importance of endoscopic detection of superficial carcinoma at various mucosal subsites in the hypopharynx. These authors also suggested the use of a novel optical technique called narrow band imaging (NBI) that allows non-invasive visualization of microvascular structure using reflected light thus identifying disease of an early stage during routine endoscopic examination.

The direct laryngoscopy and hypopharyngoscopy are carried out under general anaesthesia to visualize the extent and stage of disease. Further, the tumour extension into the subsites of the hypopharynx is noted. It is also important to appreciate if the lesion is circumferential or confined to one to the half of the hypopharynx, as it will help in deciding the subsequent surgical technique. It is also useful to note the vertical extent of the tumour and assess the vocal cord mobility. Finally, biopsy is taken from the lesion. However if a punch biopsy is inconclusive, trucut biopsy is reported to yield promising results [27].

9.4.5 Diagnosis of Recurrent Lesion

The diagnosis of residual or recurrent disease following initial treatment with radiation or chemo-radiation is difficult because of anatomic changes, fibrosis and post-radiation oedema. Advocates of PET scanning suggest that two scans performed in sequence with a gap of minimum of 1 year have 97% sensitivity. It is suggested that if scans are negative, no biopsy is necessary [23]. Although the sensitivity of CT or MRI scans is considerably higher, their specificity is lower [24]. It is also suggested that panendoscopy should be carried out in all hypopharyngeal cancers not only to assess the primary tumour but also to exclude multiple primary cancers [28].

9.4.6 Classification

T_1	Tumour limited to one subsite of hypopharynx and 2 cm or less in greatest diameter
T_2	Tumour invades more than one subsite of hypopharynx or an adjacent site or measures more than 2 cm but not more than 4 cm in greatest diameter
T_3	Tumour more than 4 cm in greatest dimension or with fixation of the hemilarynx
T_{4a}	Tumour invades one of the following: thyroid/cricoid cartilage, hyoid bone, thyroid gland, oesophagus, central compartments of soft tissue (pre-laryngeal strap muscles and subcutaneous fat)
T_{4b}	Tumour invades prevertebral fascia, encases carotid artery or invades mediastinal structures

The nodal classification for the hypopharynx is the same as in other regions in the head and neck, resulting in similar stage groupings of disease into early and late stage.

9.5 Author's Comment

Most hypopharyngeal cancers are diagnosed at an advanced stage. Usually the symptoms include gradually progressive dysphagia, hoarseness and otalgia. Often the patients present with neck node metastasis, sometimes, bilaterally and thus usually have guarded prognosis. Initial examination with indirect laryngoscopy and flexible fibre-optic endoscopy with or without 90° Hopkin's telescopic examination will reveal the lesion and exclude multiple primary cancers. Subsequent imaging techniques and hypopharyngoscopy and biopsy will reinforce the clinical findings and confirm the diagnosis. It is important to assess the location, stage and extent of disease and to note if the lesion is confined to one side (pyriform fossa) or it is circumferential as it will have a bearing on subsequent surgical planning. However, the assessment based on factors concerning tumour, patient and physician should help the surgeon to first decide if the treatment offered is going to be curative or palliative.

References

1. Thawley SE, Sessions DC, Genden EM. Surgical therapy of hypopharyngeal tumour. In: Thawley SC, Panje WR, Batsakis JG, Lindberg RD, editors. Comprehensive management of head and neck tumours. Philadelphia: W.B. Saunders Company; 1999: p. 876–933.
2. Uppaluri R, Sunwoo JB. Neoplasms of the hypopharynx and cervical oesophagus. In: Cummings C, editor. Cummings otolaryngology head and neck surgery. Philadelphia: Elsevier Mosby; 2005: p. 1899–931.
3. Kirchner JA. Pyriform fossa cancer: a clinical and laboratory study. Ann Otol Rhinol Laryngol. 1975;84:793–803.
4. McDonald TJ, Desanto LW, Weiland LH. Supraglottic larynx and its pathology as studied by whole laryngeal sections. Laryngoscope. 1976;86:635.
5. Harrison DFN. Pathology of hypopharyngeal cancer in relation to surgical management. J Laryngol Otol. 1970;84:349.
6. Kirchner JA. One hundred laryngeal cancers studied by serial section. Ann Otol Laryngol Rhinol. 1969;78:689.
7. Harrison DFN. Significance and means by which laryngeal cancer invades thyroid cartilage. Ann Otol Rhinol Laryngol. 1984;93:293.
8. Som ML, Nusspaum M. Surgical therapy of carcinoma of the hypopharynx and cervical oesophagus. Otolaryngol Clin North Am. 1969;2:631.
9. Bahadur S, Thakar A, Mohanti BK, Lal P. Results of radiotherapy with or without salvage surgery versus combined treatment in carcinoma of the hypopharynx. J Laryngol Otol. 2002;116:29–32.
10. Bradley PJ, Beasly N. Hypopharyngeal cancer. In: Watkinson J, Gilbert RW, editors. Stell and Maran's test book of head and neck surgery and oncology. Boca Raton: Hodder Arnold; 1011: p. 629–44.
11. Buckley JG, Maclenan K. Cervical node metastasis in laryngeal and hypopharyngeal carcinoma. Clin Otolaryngol. 1991;22:380–5.
12. Merino OR, Lindberg RD, Fleteher GH. An analysis of distant metastasis from squamous cell carcinoma of upper respiratory and digestive tracts. Cancer. 1977;40:145–51.
13. Martins AS. Multicentricity in pharyngoesophageal tumours. Argument for total laryngopharyngo-oesophagectomy and gastric transposition. Head and Neck. 2000;22:156–63.
14. Raghvan U, Quanishi Q, Bradley PJ. Multiple primary tumours in patients diagnosed with hypopharyngeal cancer. Otolaryngol Head Neck Surg. 2003;128:419–25.
15. Dikshit RP, Boffeta P, Bouchardy C, et al. Risk factors for development of second primary tumours among men in laryngeal & hypopharyngeal carcinoma. Cancer. 2005;103:2326–33.
16. Wang CP, Lee C, Tang TL, et al. Application of unsedated transnasal oesophagus duodenoscopy in the diagnosis of hypo-pharyngeal cancer. Head Neck. 2009;31:153–7.
17. Hoffman HT, et al. The national cancer data base report on cancer of the head and neck. Arch Otolaryngol Head Neck Surg. 1988;124:951–62.
18. Hoffman HT, et al. Hypopharyngeal cancer patient care evaluation. Laryngoscope. 1997;107:1005–17.
19. Bahadur S Amalya RC, Iyer S, et al. Study of distribution of cervical lymph node metastasis in squamous cell carcinoma of the head and neck. Indian J Cancer. 1983;20:142–6.
20. Jones AD, Phillips DE, Helliwell TR Roland NJ. The level of cervical lymph node metastasis. Their prognostic relevance and relationship with head and neck carcinoma – primary sites. Clin Otolaryngol. 1994;19:63–9.
21. Curtin HD, Ishwaran H, Mancuso AA, et al. Comparison of CT and MRI imaging in staging of neck metastasis. Radiology. 1998;207:123–30.
22. Jones A. Tumours of the hypopharynx and cervical oesophagus. In: Gleeson M, editor. Scott-Browns otolaryngology, vol. 2. London: Hodder Arnold; 2008: p. 2633–61.

23. Terhaard CH, Benger V, Van-Rijk PP, et al. F-18 Fluoro-deoxy-glucose positron -emission-tomography scanning in detection of local recurrence after radiotherapy for laryngeal and pharyngeal cancer. Head Neck. 2001;23:993–41.
24. Voldes Olmos RA, Balm AJ, Hilgers FJ, et al. Thallium 201 SPECT in diagnosis of head and neck cancer. J Nucl Med. 1997;38:873–9.
25. Su YY, Fang FM, Chuang HC, Luo SD, Chien CY. Detection of metachronous esophageal squamous carcinoma in patients with head and neck cancer with use of transnasal esophagoscopy. Head Neck. 2010;32:780–5.
26. Muto M, Nakane M, Katada C, et al. Squamous cell carcinoma in situ at oropharyngeal and hypopharyngeal mucosal sites. Cancer. 2004;101:1375–80.
27. Gandhi S, Bhowmick NP, Kelkar DS, Chandorker A. Trucut biopsy – an effective diagnostic tool in laryngeal and hypopharyngeal cancer. J Laryngol Voice. 2012;2:85.
28. Haughey BH, Gates GA, Arfken CL. Meta-analysis of second malignant tumours in head and neck cancer: the cases for endoscopic screening protocol. Ann Otol Rhinol Laryngol. 1992;101:105–12.

10 Guidelines in Management of Carcinoma of the Hypopharynx

Sudhir Bahadur

10.1 Introduction

Carcinoma of the hypopharynx is a difficult disease to treat. Most patients on presentation have a few symptoms but have advanced stage of disease, often with cervical lymphadenopathy resulting in poor prognosis. Besides, airway and nutritional status are other important issues. Nearly 60–80% of patients are diagnosed to have stage III or IV disease at presentation [1–3]. Besides the high incidence of lymph node metastasis, another factor which contributes to poor prognosis is the significant rates of distant metastasis [4]. Nearly 60–80% patients of hypopharyngeal cancer present with clinically palpable nodal metastasis and often in contralateral neck. The distant metastasis may be seen in up to 40% and 60% cases [5]. Predominant sites for distant metastasis are the lung, mediastinal lymph nodes, liver and bone.

It has been observed that almost 50% patients develop recurrences within a year of completing treatment and nearly half of these are in the form of distant metastasis. Besides, other adverse characteristics of hypopharyngeal cancer are multicentricity and submucosal spread of disease with soft tissue extension to involve the constrictor muscle and parapharyngeal space [6].

10.2 Treatment Options

Over the past few decades, there has been significant improvement in the management of hypopharyngeal cancer. The imaging has improved a great deal resulting in better delineation of tumour extent and staging. This also helps in better case

S. Bahadur (✉)
Department of Otolaryngology and Head-Neck Surgery, Formerly at All India Institute of Medical Sciences, New Delhi, India

S. Bahadur et al. (eds.), *Carcinoma of the Larynx and Hypopharynx*,
https://doi.org/10.1007/978-981-13-3110-7_10

selection for specific treatment. It is known that radiation techniques have also improved significantly leading to better disease control and less damage to vital surroundings.

The aim of treatment is to control disease at locoregional level while attempting to improve disease-free survival. Besides, it is important to maintain good quality of life with minimum of morbidity and treatment duration.

Often the choice of treatment depends upon the stage and extent of disease (tumour factors), patients' age and Karnofsky's scale and their preference for treatment (patient factors) and facilities available in the treating centre (physician factors). In general, stages I and II (with negative neck), regarded as early disease, are treated by external radiotherapy. Early lesions may also be treated by surgical resection with adequate margin while preserving the larynx. Transoral resection with a carbon dioxide laser has been equally found to be effective in early and select exophytic lesions not invading the cartridge [7]. Both modalities of treatment usually produce satisfactory results. However, the precise choice of treatment depends on the experience of physician.

However, for advanced lesions of the hypopharynx (T_3 and resectable T_4 No/N_+), the debate is between performing radical surgery including laryngopharyngectomy with or without the neck dissection (and postoperative radiotherapy) and organ preservation using chemoradiotherapy. Traditionally, surgery is the preferred option for advanced lesions but is at the expense of sacrificing the larynx and permanent stoma (Fig. 10.1a, b). However even chemoradiation may have severe toxic effects, and even though larynx may be preserved, it may not always be functional. Careful case selection is necessary, and follow-up compliance is almost mandatory.

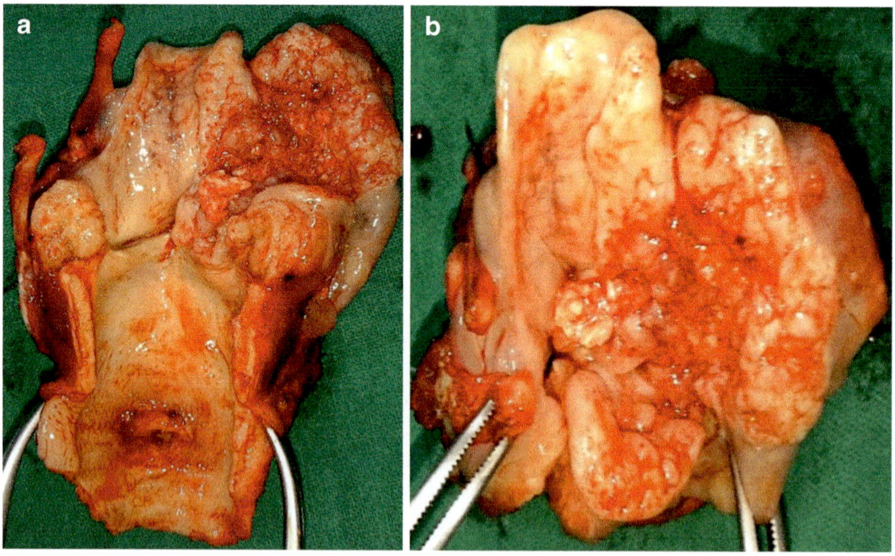

Fig. 10.1 (**a**, **b**) Advanced pyriform fossa cancer, involving the aryepiglottic fold

10.3 Surgical Treatment

10.3.1 Management of Neck Metastasis

Buckley and MacLennan noted in patients with clinically negative necks that 36% of neck nodes on the side of primary tumour and 27% of contralateral nodes contained metastatic disease [9]. Most of the positive nodes were located in levels II, III and IV.

The neck, therefore, requires some form of treatment electively in clinically negative situations (No). If surgery is used in the treatment of primary tumour, selective neck dissection for levels II, III and IV should be performed. However, for clinically positive neck nodes, radical neck dissection or modified neck dissection on side of the lesion is performed with resection of primary neoplasm. On the other hand, if radiotherapy is employed, radiation field should cover the neck.

When a small hypopharyngeal cancer is present and suitable for radiotherapy, the neck may be treated in two ways: if node is less than 2 cm, radiotherapy may be given and the likelihood is that it will be sterilized, but in case the node persists for 2 months after radiation, the neck dissection should be performed. On the other hand, if the node is larger than 2 cm, a neck dissection may be required first and subsequent radiation to primary site [6].

10.3.2 Surgical Management of Primary Neoplasm

10.3.2.1 Advanced Resectable Disease (T_3/T_4 No/N+)

Total Laryngectomy and Partial Pharyngectomy

The ultimate goal of surgery is to carry out adequate curative resection while preserving as much of the normal tissue as possible to minimize morbidity and mortality [10]. It is important to understand the tumour behaviour in terms of high incidence of nodal metastasis and extensive submucosal spread. The latter should be taken into account when resection of primary tumour is planned (Figs. 10.2a–b). It has been suggested that resection margin in patients without prior radiation should be 15 mm superiorly, 30 mm inferiorly and 20 mm laterally [10]. However, for patients with previous radiation, it should be 20 mm, 40 mm and 30 mm, respectively. The deep margin should be greater than 1 mm (Figs. 10.3a–d).

Tumour-free margins are further confirmed by frozen section during surgery, and appropriate reconstruction is carried out. When a partial pharyngectomy is carried out for tumour excision (for pyriform fossa cancer), pharyngeal defect may be closed primarily (if enough contralateral mucosa is available—more than 2 cm to cover around size 18 feeding tube) or by 'patched' pectoralis major myocutaneous flap. The latter flap is extremely useful particularly if the surgery is carried out in radiation-failed case (Figs. 10.4a–d).

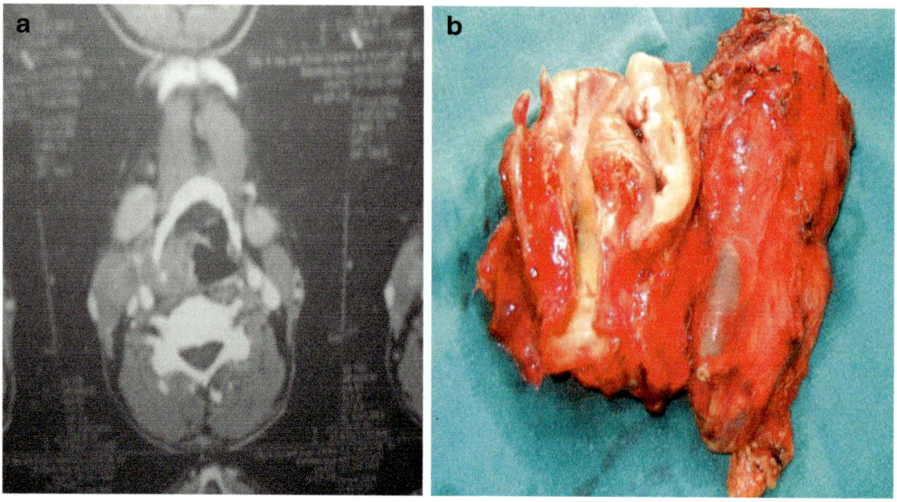

Fig. 10.2 (**a**, **b**) CT scan and surgical specimen of carcinoma pyriform fossa (T_4N_1). CT scan is almost mirror image of the specimen

In suitable cases of T3 or select T4 pyriform fossa cancer, near-total laryngectomy may be considered. Although the patient is left with a permanent stoma, he retains the voice because of the creation of myomucosal shunt between the trachea and pharynx.

10.3.2.2 Circumferential Lesions

Total Laryngopharyngectomy

However, when adequate tumour resection results in circumferential pharyngeal defects that require reconstruction, institutional preferences usually depend upon the training and expertise of the surgical team [11]. There has been a major debate on methodology of reconstruction of the hypopharynx. The use of deltopectoral flap enjoyed limited success before the myocutaneous flaps became the workhorse in reconstruction of defects created by tumour excision of lesions slightly extending into the cervical oesophagus. This flap has been useful even today in elderly patients or with poor nutrition [12, 13].

Recently, for both patch and circumferential defects, pharyngeal repair is carried out by using microvascular free flap using either jejunum [14] or radial forearm flap or anterolateral thigh flap. Still fasciocutaneous free flap, radial forearm flap and anterolateral thigh are being increasingly preferred over jejunal flap because of reliability, technical accessibility and popularity with surgeons [6, 15]. Also the functional outcomes have been better with the former flaps than with jejunal flaps [15]. However, the morbidity after flap reconstruction is considerable. According to one series, fistulas and wound complications were seen in 33% and 25% cases, respectively. The late complication and stricture rates were 26% and 15%, respectively, and 16% of patients required permanent feeding through a gastrostomy tube [16].

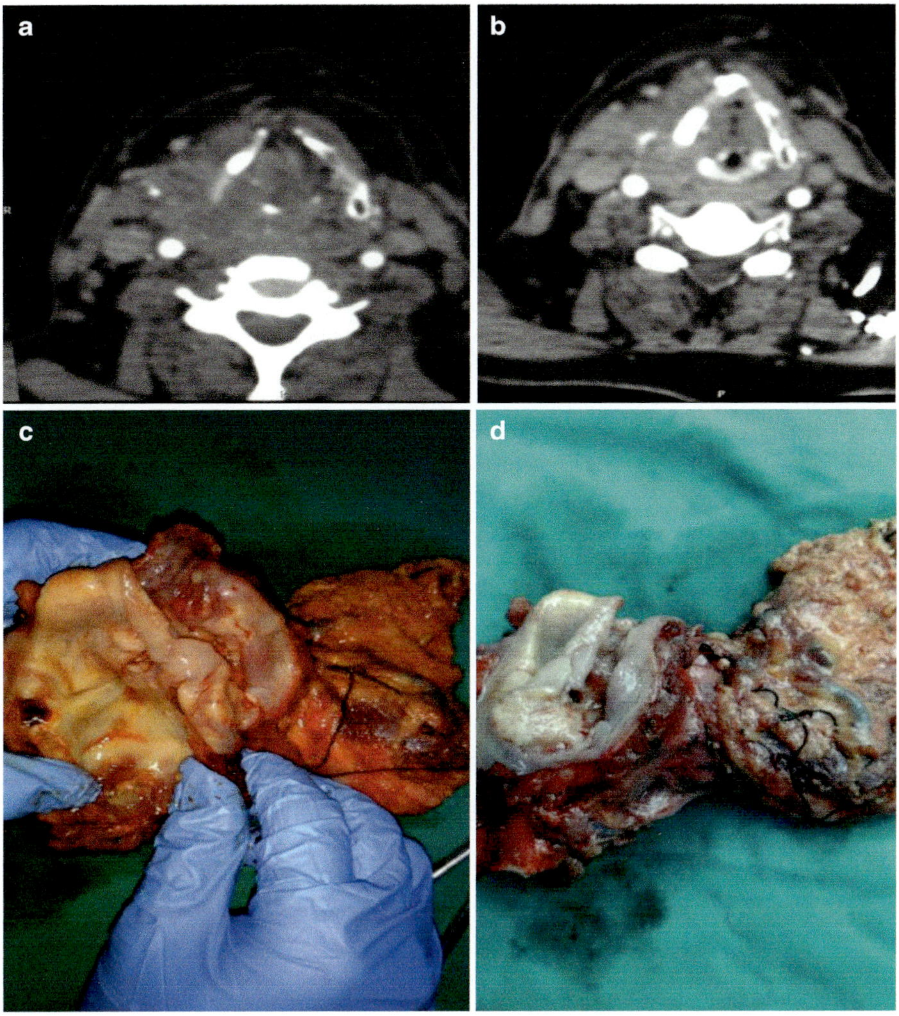

Fig. 10.3 (**a–d**) CT scans and surgical specimen of extensive pyriform fossa cancer (T_4N_1) with adjacent base of tongue involvement

When the hypopharyngeal cancer extends inferiorly to involve the cervical oesophagus, it may be important to do tumour excision with the removal of the oesophagus to achieve adequate resection margins (Fig. 10.5). The resultant defect following total laryngopharyngo-oesophagectomy, thus, created may be reconstructed by mobilizing the stomach for a single pharyngo-gastric anastomosis [10–17]. The single-stage procedure, however, produces significant trauma to patients who may be otherwise elderly and nutritionally deficient with poor chest condition. The resultant morbidity may be severe enough to produce mortality [6, 10, 17]. Nevertheless, when surgical procedure is successful and the patient tolerates it well,

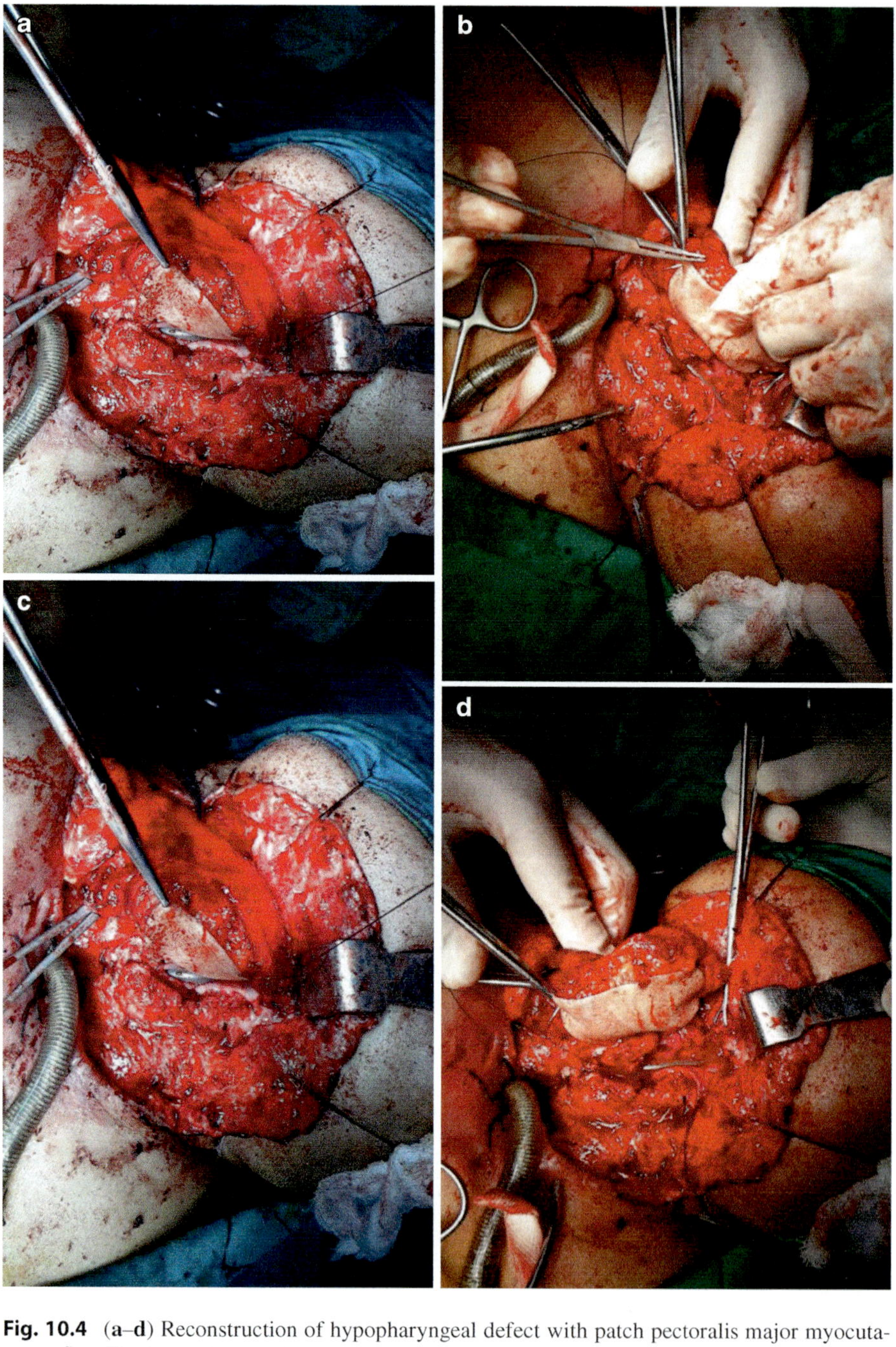

Fig. 10.4 (**a**–**d**) Reconstruction of hypopharyngeal defect with patch pectoralis major myocutaneous flap. The latter also provides cover for the exposed carotid artery

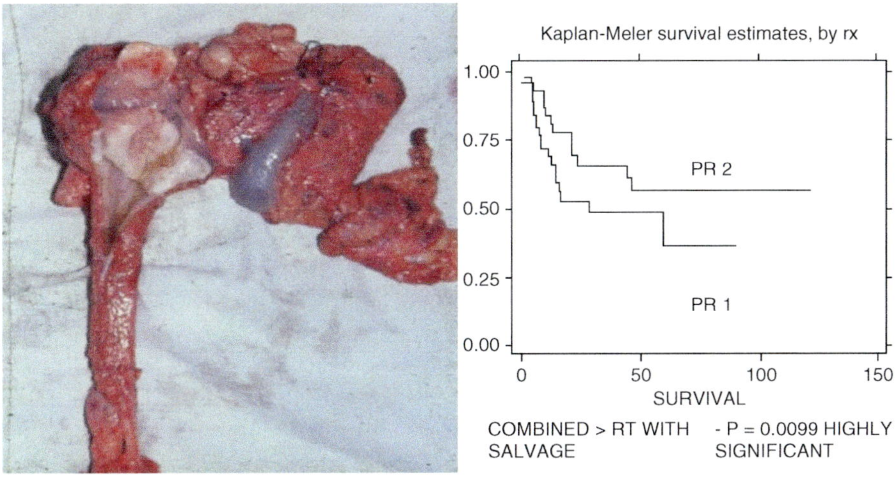

Fig. 10.5 Surgical specimen of total laryngopharyngo-oesophagectomy and radical neck dissection for a patient of circumferential lesion of the hypopharynx. Graph shows survival estimates in post-cricoid cancer [33]

he shall benefit with excellent palliation in terms of easy swallowing and long-term good functional results [10, 16, 17].

The gastric 'pull-up' surgery is performed by two surgical teams. The head and neck team completes the resection of primary neoplasm with or without a radical neck dissection, whereas the second surgical team prepares the stomach in the abdomen. The oesophagus is mobilized transhiatally by blunt dissection and removed along with primary tumour and neck dissection specimen. The stomach is subsequently 'pulled up' to the neck through the posterior mediastinum and anastomosed to the oropharynx *complications*: Major complications that are known to occur relate to vessels, posterior tracheal wall and pleura. The bleeding can be severe when azygos vein is damaged during blunt dissection and will require immediate thoracotomy to secure haemostasis. Similarly, injury to upper tracheal wall may be repaired through the neck, whereas a large tear involving the posterior tracheal wall in lower trachea may need thoracotomy for repair. Over the years, mortality rate after surgery has declined from nearly 30% to 8%, and anastomotic leaks have been reduced from 22% to 9% [10, 16]. The other complications include pneumonia, graft necrosis and occasionally cerebrovascular accidents.

10.3.3 Surgery for Early Disease (T_1/T_2 No)

Conservation surgery for early hypopharyngeal cancer is less well established as compared to similar procedures for carcinoma of the larynx. This organ (larynx)-preserving surgery may be carried out as either endoscopic (laser) microsurgery or endoscopic robotic surgery or as open hemilaryngopharyngectomy procedures.

However, these procedures are designed for usually select early T-stage hypopharyngeal cancer. It may be noted that disease at this site has a propensity for extensive submucosal spread.

10.3.3.1 Open Conservation Surgery

One of the large series published by Ogura et al. [18] included supraglottic laryngectomy and partial pharyngectomy in 175 cases treated for cancers of pyriform fossa. The actuarial 3-year survival rate was 59% for PLP group and 36% for TLP-treated group. The case selection was based on the tumour stage. Laccourreye et al. [19, 20, 21] reported results of supracricoid hemilaryngopharyngectomy (SCI+LP) in selected T_2 pyriform fossa cancer. This technique was found to be a safe method of voice preservation, respiration and swallowing while achieving a 5-year disease-specific survival rate of 56%. Another series involving 48 pyriform sinus cancers of select cases work treated with induction chemotherapy followed by surgery resulting in 5-year survival rate of 47% [22].

10.3.3.2 Transoral Laser Surgery (TOLS)

Transoral laser surgery was initially employed for carcinoma of the larynx. Its use was extended to tumours of the hypopharynx [23, 24]. Steiner et al. [24] reported on 129 cases of pyriform sinus cancer treated by TOLS. Sixty-eight percent had nodal metastasis. Overall, 24 tumours were T_1, 74 were PT_2, 17 were PT_3 and 14 were PT_4. Of these, treatment consisted of TOLS and neck dissection in 42%, and 58% also were treated with postoperative radiotherapy. The 5-year overall survival rate was 71% for stage I and II disease and 47% for stage III and stage IV disease. The reported 5-year recurrence-free survival rates for stage I/II and stage III/IV were 95% and 69%, respectively.

Martin et al. [25] reported 172 patients with hypopharyngeal cancer treated with TOLS and 91% underwent neck dissection. The 5-year overall survival rate was 68% for stages I and II, 64% for stage III and 41% for stage IV. Besides, 52% patients also received postoperative chemoradiation.

Overall, TOLS appear to give comparable results with open partial surgery with a 5-year overall survival rate of around 50–70% in stage I and II disease and 40–50% in stage III and IV disease. These are still select patients. However, early cancers that may be suitable for few such treatment may also respond to radiotherapy and chemoradiotherapy, and as such the place of transoral endoscopic laser surgery for treatment of hypopharyngeal cancer still remains to be established.

10.4 Patterns of Failures and Survival Outcome

Most authors have noted that hypopharyngeal cancer is an aggressive disease and a majority of patients present with advanced disease and have poor prognosis. The early lesions (T_1 and T_2) are usually treated by irradiation. Also the primary site recurrence rate is higher in radiotherapy-treated group than in similar surgical group. Most radiation failures (if proper follow-up is maintained) may be suitable for salvage surgery, and final survival rates are calculated on results of radiotherapy with or without salvage surgery.

Advanced lesions (T_3/T_4), however, tend to be treated with surgery and postoperative radiotherapy. The skip lesions in oesophagus are common in post-cricoid carcinoma. Higher rates of locoregional failures have been reported when advanced T_3 and T_4 lesions have been treated with radiotherapy and failure rates have varied from 34% to 85% [17, 26, 27, 28, 29]. Spector et al. [30] reviewed charts of 2500 patients of hypopharyngeal cancer and noted high incidence of delayed regional metastasis (2 years after treatment) and distant metastasis, and these parameters were found to be associated with advanced primary disease, positive neck node metastasis and locoregional recurrences.

In a large series, Hoffman et al. [31] compiled data from 769 hospitals, representing 2939 patients of carcinoma of the hypopharynx. These authors reported 5-year disease-specific survival of 33.4% which segregated to 83% for stage I, 57.8% for stage II, 41% for stage III and 22% for stage IV lesions.

Jones et al. [27] noted overall 27% of hypopharyngeal cancers were not suitable for curative treatment. Of 32% patients treated with curative radiotherapy and salvage surgery, 5-year survival was 46%. Of the remaining 41% patients treated with surgery and postoperative radiotherapy, 5-year survival was 42%. There was no significant difference in survival between two groups.

Many other authors have similarly noted 5-year disease-free survivals to be 20–47% following treatment [27, 29, 35–38]. The survival rates have been reported to be best when these cases have been treated with planned combined treatment of surgery and postoperative radiotherapy or with surgery alone [31–34, 39]. The results have been worse when patients with advanced disease have been treated with radiotherapy alone [28, 29, 33]. Bahadur et al. [33] compared the results of 195 cases of hypopharyngeal cancer treated with either curative radiotherapy and surgical salvage in reserve for radiation failures or combined treatment of surgery and postoperative radiotherapy. Actuarial 2-year disease-free survival rates were significantly better with combined treatment when stage III and IV lesions (164 patients) were compared to those treated with curative radiotherapy without salvage (p-0.000) or by radiotherapy with surgical salvage for residual and recurrent tumours ($p = 0.0021$).

10.5 Non-surgical Treatment Options for Hypopharyngeal Cancer

Radiotherapy is a good treatment option for early hypopharyngeal cancer to preserve the larynx. However, for advanced lesions, treatment with radiotherapy usually has poor outcome, and surgery is the preferred option, though it carries morbidity in terms of loss of the larynx. It has been suggested that the addition of chemotherapy to primary radiotherapy produces results that are comparable to surgery and postoperative radiotherapy, but with advantage of larynx preservation in a significant number of patients [38, 39]. However, unlike advanced laryngeal cancer, the question of organ preservation in hypopharyngeal cancer has not been adequately studied.

Besides, terms such as organ preservation and larynx preservation have not been always clearly defined, indicating the anatomic integrity, through remaining silent on functional aspects, which include both voice and swallowing. Therefore, so long as laryngeal functions are preserved and the survival of patient is not compromised, using chemoradiation is fine. However, in some cases, the functions are seriously compromised, or if the survival is inferior to surgery, then it may be argued that it is better to sacrifice the organ and allow the patient to live with aspiration-free deglutition and prosthetic rehabilitation, than by retaining intact but functionless larynx [40, 41].

Besides, treatment strategy of laryngeal preservation following chemoradiation includes the option of surgical salvage in cases of persistent or recurrent disease in order to optimize the survival rate and is thus nor entirely non-surgical. There have been a few randomized phase III trials in hypopharyngeal cancer [42, 43].

One study was carried out by the European Organisation for Research and Treatment of Cancer (EORTC) [8]. Patients were randomly assigned to one of two treatment arms: (1) immediate surgery with postoperative radiotherapy (50–70 Gy) or (2) induction chemotherapy (cisplatin, 100 mg/m^2) given as bolus intravenous injection, followed by infusion of fluorouracil (1000 mg/m^2/day on days 1–5).

The 3- and 5-year estimates of retaining a functional larynx in patients treated with induction chemotherapy arm were 42% and 35%, respectively. Lefebvre et al. [8] concluded that larynx preservation without jeopardizing survival appears feasible in patients with cancer of hypopharynx. These observations were similar to other studies [4]. The larynx preservation rate in hypopharyngeal cancer appears to be inferior to that obtained with concurrent chemoradiotherapy in laryngeal cancer. However, two points are worth mentioning: firstly in the Veterans Affairs Laryngeal Cancer Study Group trial [42, 43], the larynx preservation rate was reported at 2 years instead of 5 years as in EORTC study. Besides, in the latter study, the end point was noted as survival with a functional larynx (i.e. without local disease, tracheostomy and gastrostomy).

However, in India the follow-up is often poor, and the lesion may continue to grow and become unresectable. As such even the results of residual resectable lesions of hypopharynx are poor following salvage surgery.

Pignon et al. [44] conducted the meta-analysis of chemotherapy with 87 trials between 1965 and 2000 with a total of 16,486 patients. An absolute survival benefit of 4.5% at 5 years was confirmed, as did pronounced benefit in concomitant trials (6.5 at 5 years). No survival advantage was shown for induction chemotherapy. The beneficial effect of the addition of concomitant chemoradiotherapy versus radiotherapy above was similar in patients with hypopharyngeal cancer.

Posner et al. [45] reported a similar phase III trial of sequential therapy comparing docetaxel, cisplatin and fluorouracil against cisplatin and fluorouracil, followed by chemoradiotherapy with weekly carboplatin. Surgery-free survival was significantly greater with docetaxel, cisplatin and fluorouracil at 5 years, 52% vs 32% with cisplatin and fluorouracil. Another important aspect of non-surgical approaches is their potential ability to decrease the development of distant metastasis [42–44]. However, patients with M1 disease have a very poor prognosis.

10.6 Toxicity of Chemoradiation, Prognosis and Quality of Life

Important morbidity following chemoradiation includes both acute and late toxicity such as xerostomia, skin reaction, cervical fibrosis, lymphoedema and ototoxicity [46–48]. However, significant swallowing dysfunction is a common finding after intensive chemoradiotherapy. The rate of symptomatic strictures is nearly 20% [49].

Probably, the most important factors resulting in morbidity in these patients are dysphagia and aspiration because of chemoradiotherapy. There is a suggestion in literature that patients treated with intensity-modulated radiotherapy (IMRT) had fewer swallowing problems after completion of radiotherapy or chemoradiotherapy than patients treated with conventional three-dimensional radiotherapy [50]. There is some promise in the role of targeted systemic therapies in combination with chemoradiotherapy, but it remains to be established in treatment of hypopharyngeal cancer.

10.7 Salvage Surgery

The importance of salvage surgery in cases of persistent or recurrent disease cannot be minimized to improve the patient survival in larynx preservation protocol with chemoradiation/radiation alone. Adequate and timely salvage surgery (good follow-up is essential) is, therefore, important to achieve good locoregional control; 5-year control rates of nearly 70% have been reported following salvage surgery [51, 52]. However, other authors have not reported good results with such surgery in radiation-failed cases [28, 33, 53].

Besides, rates of complications have been shown to be high following salvage surgery with regard to wound breakdown and pharyngocutaneous fistula formation. Surgical complications occurred in 30–75% cases [32, 50–52] depending on the interval between completion of radiotherapy and subsequent surgery. Also, long-term stricture formation may occur following salvage surgery in approximately 15% cases [51, 52].

10.8 Conclusions

Most patients of hypopharyngeal cancer present when the disease is advanced when first seen. Radical surgery including a total laryngectomy with partial or total pharyngectomy ± oesophagectomy with postoperative radiation is the gold standard treatment.

In early cases partial laryngopharyngectomy as an open procedure or performed endoscopically with laser as minimal invasive procedure has offered the opportunity of preserving the larynx in select patients of hypopharyngeal cancer. The treatment may be equally effective with radiotherapy. However, the choice of treatment may depend on patient-related factors like age, co-morbidity, occupation and patient preferences and tumour-related factors such as size and location and also the facilities available. However in advanced disease (stage III and resectable IV), most patients will be treated with TLP followed by (chemo)radiotherapy or upfront chemoradiation. Facilities available in a given centre and quality to monitor and treat complications are extremely important aspects of treatment strategy. Besides, patient's preference and compliance for regular follow-up go a long way in influencing the choice of treatment.

When comparison between the two treatment modalities of surgery and non-surgical treatment options are done, survival outcomes are important, but functional results and quality of life are important as well. It is well realized that the role of radiotherapy alone in preserving the laryngeal functions in advanced lesions is poor, although chemoradiotherapy has gained acceptance and is an important treatment option in carcinoma of the larynx. However in hypopharyngeal cancer, the role of chemoradiation has been less clearly established in terms of oncologic cure and functional outcome.

The severe toxic reactions and morbidity resulting from chemoradiation is a serious consideration. Similarly, concern for regular follow-up and difficulty in diagnosis of residual and recurrent disease are important issues. Besides, morbidity and prognosis of possible salvage surgery have to be explained beforehand.

Thus, the role of the surgeon in the treatment and follow-up remains important [54]. Also despite the current declining use of open surgery, the role of primary surgery in advanced hypopharyngeal cancer is probably still relevant.

10.9 Surgical Techniques

10.9.1 Near-Total Laryngectomy

This procedure is advised for select T_3 and T_4 lateralized lesions of the pyriform fossa. It is part of conservation surgery which combines the virtues of total laryngectomy (along with stoma) but with preservation of voice by creation of myomucosal shunt between the trachea and pharynx [55–58].

However, case selection is extremely important based upon careful clinical and radiological workup and discussion with colleagues in the tumour clinic, and patient's concurrence for a particular treatment protocol is extremely important.

An extensive primary tumour with cartilage destruction or functional impartment of the larynx may be treated initially with surgery. On the other hand, large bulky tumour without obvious destruction and impaired laryngeal functions may be considered for chemoradiation. Tumour volume may be a better predictive factor [54]. Most trials consider overall staging for specific treatment protocol rather than primary tumour (T) and neck metastasis (N) separately. Also a small primary lesion such as T_1 and T_2 may be associated with large nodal metastasis (staged N) and may be considered differently than a large T_4 which is also a stage IV lesion [6].

10.9.2 Pharyngolaryngectomy With or Without Reconstruction with Pectoralis Myocutaneous Flap

Total laryngectomy with partial pharyngectomy usually with ipsilateral neck dissection is required for locally advanced carcinomas of the hypopharynx. Similar surgical procedure may be needed for primary disease in the larynx extending to involve the pyriform fossa, lateral pharyngeal wall and post-cricoid area with suitable reconstruction.

The general anaesthesia is administered by endotracheal intubation so long as the airway is adequate. However, if the airway is compromised, a preliminary tracheostomy should be performed first under local anaesthesia before general anaesthesia is induced. It is extremely important to check the disease status again before starting the major surgery by performing endoscopic evaluation of primary tumour and its extension. The areas of interest include the base of the tongue, apex of the pyriform fossa, lateral pharyngeal wall post-cricoid area, cervical oesophagus and interior of the larynx. It is useful to assess if the disease is circumferential or it is confined to one half the hypopharynx because this will help plan surgical resection and subsequent reconstruction.

The surgical procedure shall include either a radical or modified radical neck dissection (N+ disease) or selective neck dissection (clearance of levels II, III and IV for No disease). The technical details have been described elsewhere. The neck dissection specimen is left attached medially to the larynx and hypopharynx. The strap muscles are divided low in the neck exposing the thyroid gland. The isthmus of the latter is divided, and the contralateral (normal) lobe with its blood supply (inferior thyroid vessels) and intact parathyroids are separated from the trachea and retracted laterally. The thyroid lobe on the ipsilateral side is included in the surgical specimen after the superior and inferior thyroid vessels have been ligated and divided.

The trachea is divided at the appropriate level in a bevelled fashion, and tracheostome is sutured to the skin edges with interrupted nylon sutures. The suprahyoid muscles are divided from the superior surface of the hyoid bone with the help of an electrocautery. Similarly the inferior constrictor muscle on the healthy side is divided on the thyroid cartilage with the electrocautery. The mucosa is mobilized and incised and preserved. Subsequently, entry is made into the pharynx by incising the muscle of the vallecula. The epiglottis is grasped with Babcock's forceps, and by visualizing the tumour from above as well as from contralateral (healthy) pyriform fossa side, adequate margins that can be obtained around the tumour resection can be carried out under direct vision according to the tumour extent into the apex of the pyriform fossa or beyond and on the midline of posterior pharyngeal wall on ipsilateral side. Thus, full-thickness resection of the pharyngeal wall (lateral and middle half of affected post-pharyngeal) is carried out. The surgical specimen consisting of neck dissection, the larynx and adjacent pharynx are excised in a monobloc fashion. The specimen is then assessed for adequacy of margins. Haemostasis is secured and wound is irrigated with saline. Frozen sections are obtained from the peripheral margins of the surgical defect.

The assessment is made of the resultant defect, whether sufficient healthy mucosa is available for closure without tension around a 16 G feeding tube, connecting the oropharynx to the cervical oesophagus. However, if it is not the case, it is better to use the patch pectoralis myocutaneous flap.

10.9.3 Reconstruction with Pectoralis Myocutaneous Flap (PMMF)

The dimensions of pharyngeal defect are carefully measured and matched against the previously outlined markings of pectoralis major myocutaneous flap, and necessary corrections are carried out.

The PMMF is raised off the chest in the usual manner and its vascular pedicle isolated and the flap turned 180° so as to bring the skin side in. The vascular pedicle which is on deep surface of the muscle is now outside. The flap is elevated into the neck, and closure of the pharyngeal defect begins with approximation of lateral edge of the remaining pharyngeal mucosa, with the lateral edge of the myocutaneous flap using 2-0 Vicryl sutures. The closure begins at lower most part of defect near the cervical oesophagus in the form of a racquet. The apex of the myocutaneous flap is then inserted into the narrow angle of racquet-shaped pharyngeal defect to avoid concentric stricture formation; the lateral vertical suture line is continued until the upper end of flap reaches the upper and defect of posterior pharyngeal wall.

The flap is then turned over, and suture line continues between the mucosa of base of the tongue and the distal margin of the myocutaneous flap. The vertical suture line between the opposite edge of remaining pharynx and contralateral edge of the myocutaneous flap continues interiorly until the whole pharynx is fully reconstructed. A feeding tube is inserted and passed into distal oesophagus before complete closure of the pharyngeal defect. Tension on the vascular pedicle should be avoided by measuring the length of the flap and the pharyngeal defect to be covered prior to elevation and rotation. The vascular pedicle of the myocutaneous flap lies beneath the skin overlying the clavicle.

Suction drains are applied one in the neck and the other in the chest. The nasogastric feeding is started 24 h after surgery and continued for 7–14 days till the healing is complete, and no salivary leaks are detected. Suction drains are kept until they drain for 3–5 days. The PMMF is an excellent technique for repair of partial pharyngeal defects.

10.9.4 Total Laryngopharyngo-oesophagectomy and Reconstruction with Gastric Transposition

10.9.4.1 Indications

One of the important indications for carrying out total laryngopharyngectomy is for a circumferential lesion of the hypopharynx such as the post-cricoid carcinoma extending to the cervical oesophagus. Total oesophagectomy is suggested in these cases because of (a) multiple skip lesions in the submucosal plane, (b) multiple clinically apparent primary cancers in the oesophagus, and (c) extension of distal margin of the lesion behind the manubrium sterni (d) where facilities of microvascular techniques are not available to carry out free jejunal flaps for reconstruction and total oesophagectomy may be combined with gastric transposition. It is important that the entire oesophagus and stomach should be carefully studied radiologically to rule out the presence of any other lesion.

10.9.4.2 Surgical Technique

Ideally two surgical teams need to work simultaneously and thus require collaboration of a head and neck team and a thoracic surgical team to cut down on the operating time and expertise in their respective fields. Two separate sets of instruments and scrub nurses are required to help carry out surgical procedure simultaneously. However, the head and neck surgical team begins the procedure first to assess the resectability of the lesion before the abdominal team.

The patient is placed in a supine position with extension of the neck. Sorenson's u-shaped incision is marked overlying the anterior border of the sternomastoid muscle on both sides, and the permanent tracheostome is similarly marked in the suprasternal notch. The skin flap is raised in the subplatysmal plane superiorly until the hyoid bone is exposed. The fascia on the anterior border of sternomastoid muscle is divided to expose the strap muscles. The latter are divided low in the neck exposing the thyroid gland.

The middle thyroid vein on the left side is identified, ligated and divided. The exposure to the trachea-oesophageal groove and access to the prevertebral plane are thus obtained behind the cervical oesophagus to assess the resectability of the lesion. Once this has been established, the thoracic team is allowed to start the surgery in the abdomen. In the meantime, dissection is carried forwards in the exposed thyroid gland, preserving the thyroid gland on the normal side with parathyroids and its blood supply through the inferior thyroid vessels. The isthmus is divided in midline, and the normal thyroid gland is dissected from the trachea with the electrocautery into the lateral side, whereas the gland on the diseased side will be sacrificed with the specimen (after ligating the superior and inferior thyroid vessels). The stump of the isthmus is sutured with 3-0 Vicryl for haemostasis.

The trachea is divided in a bevel-shaped manner at the appropriate level, slightly lower to the palpable tumour (through the third ring or lower), and a permanent tracheostome is created. The orotracheal tube is now removed, and a fresh flexible endotracheal tube is inserted for direct tracheal intubation, and anaesthesia is thus transferred. Dissection is now continued in the trachea-oesophageal plane in the superior mediastinum, separating the posterior membranous trachea from the anterior upper thoracic oesophagus. This step should be done carefully so as to avoid injury to membranous trachea.

The suprahyoid muscles are divided from the hyoid bone with an electrocautery, and the pharynx is entered through the vallecula and glossoepiglottic fold. The remaining circumference of the pharynx is divided under direct vision remaining well above the tumour with a healthy margin; the pharynx is thus circumferentially transected while mobilizing the pharynx over prevertebral fascia with the finger dissection.

The superior laryngeal vessels and superior thyroid vessels are ligated and divided, if not already done so. The specimen mobilized now consists of the larynx, hypopharynx and cervical oesophagus. Further, the mobilization of upper thoracic oesophagus continues under direct vision with the help of digital dissection and long instruments (DeBakey forceps and Metzenbaum scissor) in a circumferential fashion all around the upper thoracic oesophagus. The upper thoracic oesophagus receives its segmental blood supply from the branches of intercostal vessels, and prevertebral vascular clips are useful, while mobilization proceeds inferiorly around the upper thoracic oesophagus reaching down to the level of the carina.

If the two surgical teams are working together, then mobilization of the upper and lower thoracic oesophagus is achieved almost at the same time. The abdomen is prepared in the usual fashion from the xiphisternum to the pubis. A midline skin incision is made in the upper abdomen exposing the rectus sheath. The abdomen is explored following the opening of the peritoneum, to exclude the presence of metastatic disease. The triangular ligament of the left lobe of the liver is divided, and the left lobe is retracted to the right-hand side, thus exposing the anterior aspect of the stomach.

The stomach is mobilized by dividing the gastrocolic and gastrosplenic ligaments by isolation and individual ligation of each of the branches of gastro-epiploic vessels. The left gastric vessels, the short gastric vessels and the left gastro-epiploic vessels are divided and ligated. The blood supply of the stomach comes from right gastric and right gastro-epiploic vessels which are preserved. Thus, the stomach is attached to the cardio-oesophageal junction at the diaphragmatic hiatus.

Since the patient needs to have a total oesophagectomy and bilateral vagectomy requiring a drainage procedure through the pylorus, a pyloroplasty, pyloromyotomy or pyloromyectomy is performed for adequate drainage of the stomach. The right crus of the diaphragm is divided, and the diaphragmatic hiatus is widened by digital dissection. Mobilization of the distal thoracic oesophagus is performed, under direct vision, with a long flexible light source and a single arm Hemoclip Applier. Digital mobilization of distal thoracic oesophagus is continued until the carina is reached in the posterior mediastinum. Once the oesophagus is completely mobilized with digital confirmation by two operating surgeons in the posterior mediastinum, one from above and the other from abdominal side, the stomach is ready for transfer into the neck.

The surgical specimen of the larynx, hypopharynx and upper thoracic oesophagus is pulled up with gentle pressure, while the lower oesophagus and stomach are slowly fed into the posterior mediastinum into the chest. The thoracic oesophagus and the stomach are gently delivered into the neck, as the pressure is slowly applied on the laryngectomy specimen from above. Fundus of the stomach is brought into the neck with the help of Babcock clamp, and adequate length should be available to allow a tension-free anastomosis between the upper border of fundus of the stomach and stump of the pharynx and base of the tongue.

The cardio-oesophageal junction is divided with a scalpel and the transected cardiac end of the stomach oversewn with interrupted inverting chromic catgut sutures and a second layer of interrupted serosal sutures with 3-0 silk. Once the cardiac end of the stomach is closed, a gastrostomy opening is created at the convex upper end of the stomach which should be wide enough to permit at least three fingers. The anastomosis is carried out between the stomach and the pharynx with a single layer of 2-0 chromium catgut or 2-0 silk interrupted sutures. The posterior lip of the opening in the stomach is sutured first with the posterior wall of the stump of the pharynx before closing the lateral and anterior walls. However, a nasogastric tube is inserted before closure, and neck wound is irrigated with saline. Two Hemovac drains are inserted and the incision is closed in two layers.

A large skin of 2 cm is excised to help in creating the permanent tracheostome by suturing the skin edges with the stump of the trachea. The abdominal wound is similarly closed after irrigation. Immediate postoperative X-rays are carried out to rule out pneumothorax. A chest tube is inserted with underwater seal drainage system if pneumothorax is detected on the X-ray. Both chest cavities may similarly be drained if pleural tear occurs on both sides. Periodic chest X-rays are performed to confirm expansion of the lungs. When this happens and drainage from pleural cavities becomes minimal, the chest tubes are removed.

In the postoperative period, the nasogastric tube is attached to suction drainage until peristalsis returns. Feeding is then started through the nasogastric tube. It is useful to keep the tracheostomy (laryngectomy) tube to maintain the patency of the airway in the immediate postoperative period.

Once the drainage from neck wound is minimal, the drains are removed. Similarly, the nasogastric tube can be removed after 10–15 days, and small but frequent meals may be permitted, if neck wound has healed and there is no fistula. However, in order to avoid regurgitation, patient is advised to remain in upright position. Some patients may have features of dumping syndrome, but these settle down spontaneously.

Total laryngopharyngo-oesophagectomy with gastric transposition is a safe oncologic procedure which helps in the resection of tumour of the hypopharynx and restores the continuity of alimentary canal in a single stage. It provides excellent palliation in terms of early swallowing and rehabilitation, though quality of gastric speech is usually poor and patient has to use artificial electronic larynx for communication. The operating time when two teams operate together is usually between 2.5 hours and 4 hours, and blood loss is minimal to moderate.

10.10 Authors' Comment

Management of carcinoma of the hypopharynx is a challenging issue. These are aggressive cancers and few cases are diagnosed at early stage. Most cases present with advanced disease often with metastatic neck disease and sometimes with evidence of distant metastasis. These cases need to be carefully worked up and staged.

Early lesions (T_1 and T_2) carry relatively better prognosis and should be treated with radiotherapy with preservation of the larynx. Alternatively, they may be treated with transoral endoscopic laser surgery with equal success provided facilities and expertise of laser are available.

However, most advanced lesions (T_3 and T_4 No/N+) do badly when treated with radiotherapy alone. Most cases should be treated with surgery followed by radiation/chemoradiation. The extent of surgery will depend upon whether the lesion is confined to one side (pyriform fossa) or it is circumferential pathology. In the former situation, total laryngectomy with partial pharyngectomy with concurrent neck dissection will suffice (use of PMMC flap may be necessary). However in the latter case, total laryngopharyngectomy is required. The reconstruction of the pharyngeal defect may be carried out either by (a) free jejunal or free radial or free anterolateral thigh flap or (b) gastric pull-up surgery if the lesion in the hypopharynx extends to involve cervical oesophagus. This surgical technique also takes care of multiple cancers (skip lesion in the oesophagus). The choice of technique depends on several factors including disease extent, institutional experience and expertise available. The gastric pull-up surgery, despite its morbidity, can provide excellent palliation.

Non-surgical treatment option of chemoradiation for organ preservation is less clearly established in hypopharyngeal cancer than in the larynx. The morbidity due to toxicity of concurrent chemoradiotherapy is a serious issue and requires careful institutional care and monitoring. Besides, regular follow-up to diagnose residual or recurrent disease is needed which is not always easy in Indian setting. The case selection is important, and this group should include young and otherwise fit patients (T_3 No/N+) who are willing to follow-up.

References

1. Hall SF, Groome PA, Irish J, O'Sullivan B. The natural history of patients with squamous cell carcinoma of hypopharynx. Larygngcope. 2008;118:1362–72.
2. Bahadur S, Amalya RC, Iyer S, et al. Study of distribution of cervical lymph node metastasis in squamous cell carcinoma of head and neck. Indian J Cancer. 1983;20:142–6.
3. Bahadur S, Kacker SK. Surgical treatment of pyriform fossa cancer. Indian J Otolaryngol. 1985;37:83–5.
4. Gourin CG, Terris DJ. Carcinoma of the hypopharynx. Surg Oncol Clin N Am. 2004;13:81–98.
5. Kotwalk C, Sako K, Razack MS, et al. Metastasis Patterns in squamous cell carcinoma of head and neck. Am J Surg. 1987;154:439–224.
6. Takas RP, Strigan P, Silver CE, Bradley PK, et al. Current trends in initial management of hypopharyngeal cancer: the declining use of open surgery. Head Neck. 2012;2:270–81.
7. Steiner W, Ambrosch P, Hess CF, Kron M. Organ preservation by trans oral laser microsurgery in pyriform sinus carcinoma. Otolaryngol Head Neck Surg. 2001;124:58–67.
8. Lefebvre IL, Chevtiar D, Luboinski B, et al. Larynx preservation in pyriform sinus cancer: preliminary results of a European organization for research and treatment of cancer phase III trial. J Natl Cancer Inst. 1996;88:890–8.
9. Buckley JG, MacLennan K. Cervical lymph node metastasis in laryngeal and hypopharyngeal cancer a prospective analysis of prevalence and distribution. Head Neck. 2000;22:380–5.
10. Wei WI. The dilemma of treating hypopharyngeal carcinoma: more or less. Arch Otolaryngeal Head Neck Surg. 2002;128:229–32.
11. Richman ID, Samji HA, Deschler DG. National laryngopharyngectomy and reconstructive surgery survival. Laryngoscope. 2009;119:1472–8.
12. Cusumano R, Silver C, Brauer R, Strauch B. Pectoralis myocutaneous flap for replacement of cervical oesophagus. Head Neck. 1989;11:450–6.
13. Lam K, Wei V, Lan V. Avoiding stenosis in tubed greater pectoral flap in pharyngeal repair. Arch Otolaryngol Head Neck Surg. 1996;83:1279–83.
14. Jones, AS, Roland NJ, Husband D, Hamilton JW, Gati I. Free revascularized jejunal loop repair following total pharyngolaryngectomy for carcinoma of the hypopharynx: Report of 90 patients. Br J Surg. 1996;83:1279–1283.

15. Rob GL, Larin J, Deschler DG, et al. Speech and swallowing outcomes in reconstruction of the pharynx and cervical esophagus. Head Neck. 2003;25:232–44.
16. Clark JR, Gilbert R, Irish J, et al. Morbidity after flap reconstruction of hypopharyngeal defects. Laryngoscope. 2006;116:173–81.
17. Bahadur S, Chatterjee TK. Repair of pharyngeal defect following pharyngolaryngectomy with special reference to gastric transposition. Indian J Otolaryngol. 1988;40:100–2.
18. Ogura JH, Marks JE, Freeman RB. Results of conservation surgery for supraglottic and pyriform sinus cancer. Laryngoscope. 1980;90:591–600.
19. Laccourreye O, Merite Drancy A, Brasnu D, et al. Supracricoid hemilaryngopharyngectomy in select pyriform sinus carcinoma staged T_2. Laryngoscope. 1993;103:1373–9.
20. Laccourreye O, Ishoo E, de Mones E, et al. Supracricoid hemilaryngectomy pharyngectomy in patients with squamous cell carcinoma of the pyriform sinus. Ann Otol Rhinol Laryngol. 2005;114:25–34.
21. Ferlito A, Silver CE, Doward DJ, et al. Role of partial laryngeal cancer. Acta Otolaryngol. 2000;120:456–65.
22. Chevalier D, Watelet JB, Darras JA, Piquet JJ. Supraglottic hemilaryngectomy plus radiation for treatment of early lateral margin and pyriform sinus carcinoma. Head Neck. 1997;19:1–5.
23. Zeital SM, Koufman JA, Davis RK, et al. Endoscopic treatment of supraglottic and hypopharynx cancer. Laryngoscope. 1994;104:71–8.
24. Steiner W, Ambrosch P, Hess CF, Kron M. Organ preservation by trans oral laser microsurgery in pyriform sinus cancer. Otolaryngol Head Neck Surgery. 2001;124:58–67.
25. Martin A, Jacket MC, Christiansen H, et al. Organ preservation with transoral laser microsurgery for cancer of hypopharynx. Laryngoscope. 2008;118:398–402.
26. Tandon DA, Bahadur S, Chatterjee TK, Rath GK. Carcinoma of the hypopharynx. Result of combined therapy. Indian J Cancer. 1991;28:131–8.
27. Jones AS. Surgery for hypopharyngeal cancer. In: Gleason M, editor. Scott-Brown otorhinolaryngology head and neck surgery, vol. 2. London: Hodder Arnold; 2008. p. 2633–62.
28. Vargees BT, Sebastian P, Mathew A. Treatment outcome in patients undergoing surgery for carcinoma of larynx and hypopharynx. Acta Otolaryngol. 2009;129:1480–5.
29. Johnson LV, Gran C, Overgeard J. Hypopharyngeal Squamous cell carcinoma treatment results in 138 consumptive advised patients. Acta Otolaryngol. 2000;39:529–36.
30. Spector JG, Sessions DG, Haughey BH, et al. Delayed regional metastasis distant metastasis and second primary malignancies in carcinoma of larynx and hypopharynx. Laryngoscope. 2001;111:1079–87.
31. Hoffman HT, Karnell LH, Shah JP, et al. Hypopharyngeal cancer. Patient care evaluation. Laryngoscope. 1997;107:1005–17.
32. Combe M, Jones AS. Radiotherapy complications following laryngectomy. J Laryngol Otol. 1993;107:130–2.
33. Bahadur S, Thakar A, Mohanti BK, Lal P. Results of radiotherapy with or without salvage surgery versus combined surgery and radiotherapy in advanced carcinoma of hypopharynx. J Laryngol Otol. 2002;116:29–32.
34. Kim S, Wu HG, Heo D, et al. Advanced hypopharynx carcinoma treatment results according to treatment modalities. Head Neck. 2001;23:713–7.
35. Pingree TF, Davis RK, Richman O, Derrick L. Treatment of hypopharyngeal carcinoma: a 10 year review of 1362 cases. Laryngoscope. 1987;97:901–4.
36. Kraus DH, Relefsky MJ, Brock HA, Huo J, Harrison LB, Shah JP. Combined surgery and radiotherapy for squamous carcinoma of the hypopharynx. Otolaryngol Head Neck Surg. 1997;116:637–41.
37. Wallberg PC, Anderson KE, Biorklund AT. Carcinoma of the hypopharynx: analysis of incidence and survival in Sweden over a 30 year period. Head Neck. 1998;20:714–9.
38. Forastiere AA, Geopfert H, Maor M, et al. Concurrent chemotherapy and radiotherapy for organ preservation in advanced laryngeal cancer. N Engl J Med. 2003;349:2091–8.
39. Gupta T, Chopra S, Agarwal JP, et al. Squamous cell carcinoma of the hypopharynx single institution outcome analysis of large cohort of patients treated with primary non-surgical approaches. Acta Oncol. 2009;48:541–8.

40. Eckel HE, Starr S, Volling P, Suttal C, et al. Surgical treatment for hypopharynx carcinoma: feasibility, mortality and results. Otolaryngol Head Neck Surg. 2001;124:561–9.
41. Lefebvre JL. What is the role of primary surgery in treatment of laryngeal and hypopharyngeal cancer- Harrys- Martin Lecture. Arch Otolaryngol Head Neck Surg. 2000;126:285–588.
42. The Department of veterans affairs Laryngeal cancer study group. Induction chemotherapy plus radiation compared with surgery plus radiation in patients with advanced laryngeal cancer. N Engl J Med. 1991;324:1685–90.
43. Lefebvre JL, Rolland F, Tessalar M, et al. Phase 3 randomized trial on larynx preservation comparing sequential vs alternating chemotherapy and radiotherapy. J Natl Cancer Inst. 2009;101:142–52.
44. Pignon JP, Le Maitre A, Maillard E, Bourhis J, MACH-NC collaborative Group. Meta-analysis of chemotherapy in head and neck cancer (MACH-NC): an update on 93 randomized trials and 17346 patients. Radiother Oncol. 2009;92:4–14.
45. Posner MR, Norris CM, Wirth LJ, et al. Sequential therapy for locally advanced larynx and hypopharynx cancer subgroup in Tax 324, survival, surgery and organ preservation. Ann Oncol. 2009;20:921–7.
46. Rades D, Fehlaur F, Sheikh Sharaf M, et al. Toxicity of two cisplatin-based radio-chemotherapy regimens for treatment of patients with stage III/IV head and neck cancer. Head Neck. 2008;30:235–41.
47. Zuur CL, Simmis YJ, Lahadaal PE, et al. Risk factors of ototoxicity after cisplatin based chemo-radiation in locally advanced head and neck cancer; a multivariate analysis. Int J Radiat Oncol Biol Phys. 2007;68:1320–5.
48. Sharma A, Mohanti BK, Thakar A, Bahadur S, Bhaskar S. Concomitant chemoradiation versus radical radiotherapy in advanced squamous cell carcinoma of oropharynx and nasopharynx using weekly cisplatin: a phase II randomized trial. Ann Oncol. 2010;21(11):2272–7.
49. Lee WT, Akst LM, Adelstein DJ, et al. Risk factors for hypopharyngeal/upper esophageal stricture formation after concurrent chemo-radiotherapy. Head Neck. 2006;28:808–12.
50. Vergeer MR, Doornaert PA, Reitveld DH, et al. Intensity induced morbidity and improves health related quality of life: results of a non-randomized prospective study. Int J Radiat Oncol Biol Phys. 2009;74:1–8.
51. Clark JR, de Almeida J, Gilbert R, et al. Primary and salvage hypopharyngectomy: analysis and outcome. Head Neck. 2006;28:671–7.
52. Relic A, Sleveict M, Stapf J, et al. Salvage surgery after induction chemotherapy with paclitaxel cisplatin and primary radiotherapy for advanced laryngeal and hypopharyngeal carcinoma. Ear Arch Otolaryngeal. 2009;206:1799–805.
53. Davidsom J, Briant D, Gullane P, et al. The role of surgery following radiotherapy failure for advanced laryngopharyngeal cancer. Arch Otolaryngol Head Neck Surg. 1994;120:269–76.
54. Wang RJ, Shah JP. The role of the head and neck surgeon in contemporary multidisciplinary treatment programme for advanced head and neck cancer. Curr Opin Otolaryngol Head Neck Surg. 2010;18:79–82.
55. Pradhan SA, D'Cruz AK, Pai PS, et al. Near total laryngectomy in advanced laryngeal and piriform cancers. Laryngoscope. 2002;112:375–80.
56. Shenoy AM, Pinkert PK, Nunjundappa N, et al. Functional utility and oncologic safety of near total laryngectomy with trachea-pharyngeal speech shunt in a Third World Oncologic Centre. Eur Arch Otolaryngol. 1997;254:128–32.
57. Thakar A, Bahadur S, Toran KC, et al. Oncologic and functional failures in near total laryngectomy. Otolaryngol Head Neck Surg. 2007;137:223.
58. Shah J. Hypopharynx and cervical oesophagus. In: Shah JP, Patel SG, editors. Head and neck surgery and oncology. 3rd ed. Philadelphia: Mosby; 2004. p. 235–66.

11 Treatment of Early-Stage Hypopharyngeal by Radiation Therapy

Shelley Hukku, Shikha Halder, and Bidhu K. Mohanti

Cancers arising from the hypopharynx are more commonly seen in developing countries including India, compared to the western countries. Out of all head and neck cancers (HNC), the reported incidence rates are 2–5% in the developed versus 15–30% in the developing countries [1]. In view of its anatomic location, the hypopharynx is a blind spot in the head and neck region of the human body. Unless the patient has serious compromise in the food swallowing activity, a gross change in voice or both, he/she does not report. Hence, more than 70% are diagnosed at an advanced stage, and the early stages I–II are reported in approximately 25% of all hypopharyngeal cancers [2]. Majority of these cancers arise from the pyriform sinus (PFS), whereas post-cricoid cancer is common in an anaemic female. Squamous cell carcinoma is the commonest histologic type. In India, hypopharyngeal cancers constitute more than 10% of all HNC [3].

The overall treatment results in hypopharyngeal carcinoma continue to remain lower than other subsites in the head and neck [1, 2]. Five-year survival is poor with overall survival at 30% for all stages together, although for T1 and T2 tumours, the survival is almost 60% [4]. In the early stages I–II, the treatment approaches can achieve good loco-regional control and long-term survival. In this context, the therapeutic goal is to maximize the preservation of deglutition, speech and breathing functions.

Since the 1990s, the treatment shift has occurred from a radical surgery towards preserving the physiologic functions [2].

S. Hukku · S. Halder
Department of Radiation Oncology, BLK Super Specialty Hospital, New Delhi, India

B. K. Mohanti (✉)
Department of Radiation Oncology, Manipal Hospital, New Delhi, India

S. Bahadur et al. (eds.), *Carcinoma of the Larynx and Hypopharynx*,
https://doi.org/10.1007/978-981-13-3110-7_11

11.1 Management of Early-Stage Hypopharyngeal Cancer

The clinical presentation includes dysphagia, hoarseness, neck mass and a referred pain in the ear while eating. Besides a thorough clinical examination of the head and neck region, the general physical assessment including performance and nutritional status should be documented. The diagnosis is directed by imaging, endoscopy and biopsy.

Currently the imaging should be good-quality three-dimensional CT or MRI; and in case of any suspicion, the 18F-FDG PET-CT scan can be helpful to detect the loco-regional and metastatic disease burden [4]. High-definition endoscopy and narrow-band imaging can be helpful to detect the early hypopharyngeal tumour, which may otherwise be missed by a routine rigid endoscopy [5]. It is recommended that endoscopic biopsy should be performed in the same sitting.

Early-stage cancers of hypopharynx constitute T1N0 and T2N0 tumours, without any evidence of systemic metastasis. In specialized cancer centres, the T3N0 tumour which has not grossly infiltrated into the larynx or oesophagus can be grouped in early stage for the similar treatment approaches. For patients presenting with early-stage resectable disease, voice-preserving surgery or definitive radiotherapy (RT) alone is a viable and acceptable treatment option [4]. In the early stages, the primary surgery is to be selected carefully so that the voice and swallowing functions are not grossly affected postoperatively. Tumours which grossly extend into the larynx and pharyngeal wall become unsuitable [6]. Published literature shows that there is no difference in survival for patients comparing primary surgery to primary radiotherapy [7].

The following description gives an overall picture about curative (definitive) radiotherapy for early-stage hypopharyngeal cancers.

11.2 Definitive Radiotherapy

The curative approach with radiotherapy for T1 and T2 lesions and in selected T3 tumours is a suitable alternative to primary surgery, where physiologic functions of speech and swallowing are likely to be well preserved in a patient who achieves the disease control.

11.2.1 Pre-RT Evaluation

Disease stage, comorbidities, oro-dental status and performance status should be carefully documented. The blood test parameters including complete blood counts and liver and renal function tests require to be checked before radiation therapy planning.

11.2.2 Dose and Fractionation

Published literature support the use of conventional radiotherapy fractionation schedule of 1.8–2.0 Gy per fraction, delivered as five fractions per week (from Monday to Friday) over a treatment course of 6.5–7.5 weeks. The total dose prescribed to the gross tumour volume ranges from 64 Gy to 72 Gy: lower dose of 64–66 Gy for T1 and 66–72 Gy for T2–T3 tumours [8]. Altered fractionation practices are utilized with an aim to improve the disease control and/or reduce the late morbidities. In early-stage hypopharyngeal carcinoma, hyperfractionation schedule of 1.2 Gy per fraction, delivered as 2 fractions per day, at interval of 6 h or more has been studied [9]. The hyperfractionated radiotherapy is prescribed to a dose range of (1) 72 Gy in 60 fractions over 6 weeks (2) up to 76.8 Gy in 64 fractions over 6.5 weeks.

11.2.3 Our Institutional Practice

In low-volume T1 and T2 tumours without neck nodes, our practice is to prescribe a moderate hypofractionated schedule of 45 Gy in 20 fractions over 4 weeks to the primary tumour plus nodal region II–IV levels as the PTV (planning target volume) followed by 22–24 Gy in 10–12 fractions over 2–2.5 weeks to the primary tumour with margin.

11.2.4 Neck Nodes

In clinically negative neck nodes, the bilateral neck levels II–IV including retropharyngeal nodes are prescribed the dose of 45–50 Gy. The N1–N2 nodal stages should be prescribed dose of 64–70 Gy [1, 8, 9]. Clinical decision to individualize the node prescription has become easier with 3-D image-based planning. For example, in a right-sided pyriform sinus cancer with T2N1 stage, the primary tumour and right neck will receive 66–70 Gy, whereas the left neck will be delivered 45–50 Gy. In this manner, the radiation morbidities to neck and lower pharynx-oesophagus can be minimized.

11.3 Radiation Therapy Technique

11.3.1 Conventional 2-D

Before the advent of 3-D imaging in radiotherapy, the 2-D planning with simulator was a standard practice. Radiation fields involve a shrinking field technique that initiates with two parallel opposing fields covering the primary and upper neck lymphatics (Fig. 11.1), and another single anterior field (Fig. 11.2) is used to cover lower neck lymphatics. The spinal cord is shielded at 45 Gy, final mucosal reduction is done at 54–60 Gy and the primary gross disease receives 70 Gy.

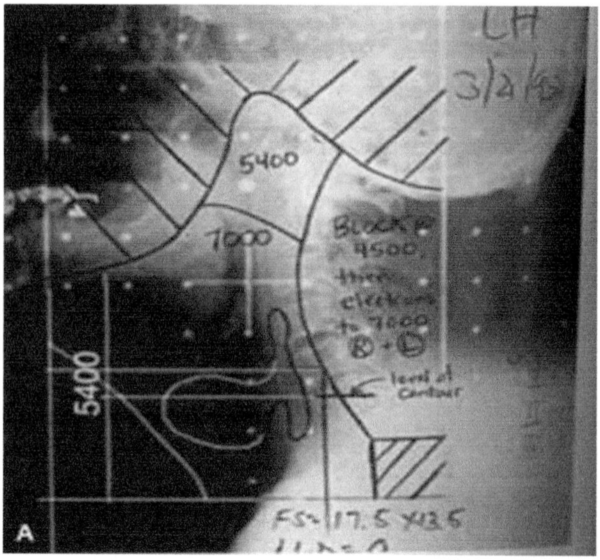

Fig. 11.1 The 2-D technique of parallel opposing lateral portals to cover the primary (hypopharynx) plus upper neck node levels

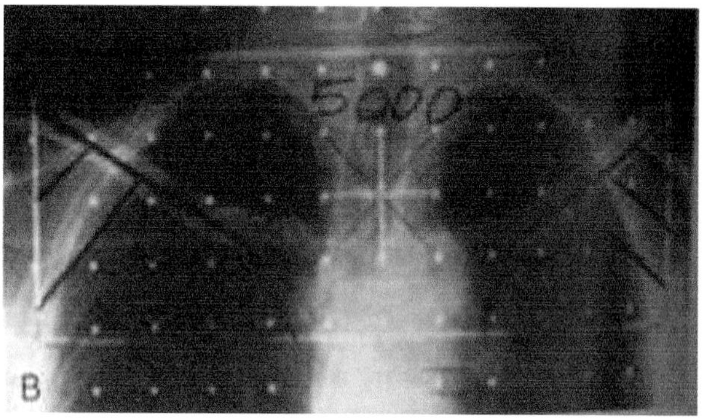

Fig. 11.2 The 2-D technique portal of single anterior field to cover lower neck nodes

For this 2-D setup, the treatment field margins or radiation portals are placed as below.

(a) Superior: mastoids and cranial base, including retropharyngeal lymph nodes
(b) Inferior: whole neck, by pulling shoulders down as much as possible (at least 1 cm below tumour)
(c) Posterior: spinous processes of vertebrae
(d) Anterior: 2–3 cm anterior to tumour (level IA and IB lymphatics are left outside if not involved).

11.3.2 Intensity-Modulated Radiation Therapy (IMRT)

During the last 10–15 years, IMRT is favoured to improve the dose distribution to the tumour and nodal region and to reduce the morbidities of the skin, mucosa and normal organ in the HN region. Towards the first decade of the twenty-first century,

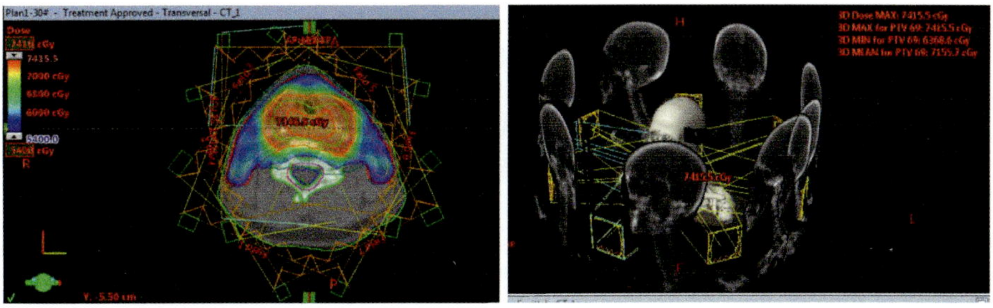

Fig. 11.3 Multiple noncoplanar beams using dynamic multi-leaf collimator in IMRT technique [Courtesy: BLK Hospital, Delhi, India]

the linear accelerator (Linac) incorporated the device called multi-leaf collimators (MLC), which made it feasible to shape the radiation fields and block unnecessary tissues into the clinical target volume (CTV) and PTV for primary and nodal areas. The MLC has moveable leaves of thin strips, which block/shape a fraction of radiation beam(s) through computerized control of the leaf movements [10]. This allows for better target/tumour region conformity, higher precision in dose delivery and lesser normal tissue morbidity. In recent years, IMRT is utilized to treat hypopharyngeal cancers [1, 11].

Each radiotherapy beam is divided into many small beamlets that can vary their intensity (Fig. 11.3). This allows different doses of radiation to be given across the tumour, node and normal tissue volumes. Accordingly, the dose prescription can be tailored to deliver 60–66 Gy in 30 fractions to the tumour volume (T1–T2) and 48–54 Gy to the neck node (N0) region for prophylactic irradiation. This type of dose delivery is called simultaneous integrated boost (SIB) technique.

11.3.3 Volumetric-Modulated Arc Therapy (VMAT)/RapidArc Radiotherapy

The VMAT technique is a novel improvement of the IMRT technique. It is realized that IMRT increases the treatment time on a Linac machine by requiring a larger number of beam directions, increased monitor units (MU) and, in the case of tomotherapy, a slice-by-slice delivery. The VMAT technique provides the solution to overcome the limitation of IMRT, by the process of a novel aperture-based algorithm for radiotherapy treatment plan optimization where dose is delivered during a single gantry arc of up to 360°. In VMAT (or RapidArc), multi-leaf collimator (MLC) leaf motion and number of monitor unit (MU) per degree of gantry rotation is restricted during the optimization so that gantry rotation speed, leaf translation speed and dose rate maxima do not excessively limit the radiation dose delivery efficiency [12]. During the last few years, IMRT is rapidly adopted into the treatment of head and neck cancers, because of the reduced treatment time and overall MU (which indirectly gives lower dose to surrounding normal structures) compared to IMRT [13]. It is observed that VMAT/RapidArc reduces the treatment delivery time by 50% in comparison with IMRT.

The radiotherapy for the hypopharyngeal cancer by VMAT/RapidArc technique, carried out by authors' institutions, is shown in Fig. 11.4. In the clinical practice, VMAT can be used to deliver a comprehensive radiotherapy course in SIB, similar to IMRT, to the different target regions of interest, as shown in Figs. 11.5 and 11.6. This has resulted in lower morbidities and better treatment tolerance.

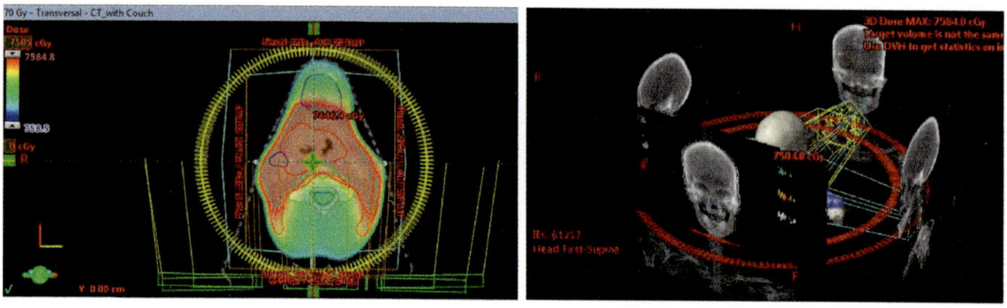

Fig. 11.4 IMRT using RapidArc [Courtesy: BLK Hospital, Delhi, India]

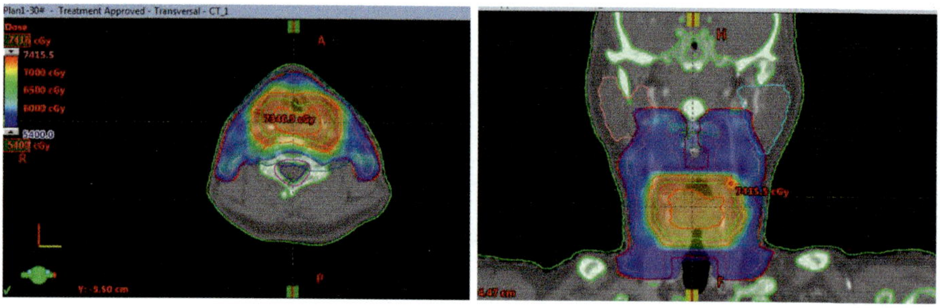

Fig. 11.5 Differential high doses to the target volume of N0 neck receiving 54 Gy and hypopharynx (gross disease) receiving 70 Gy by VMAT technique [Courtesy: BLK Hospital, Delhi, India]

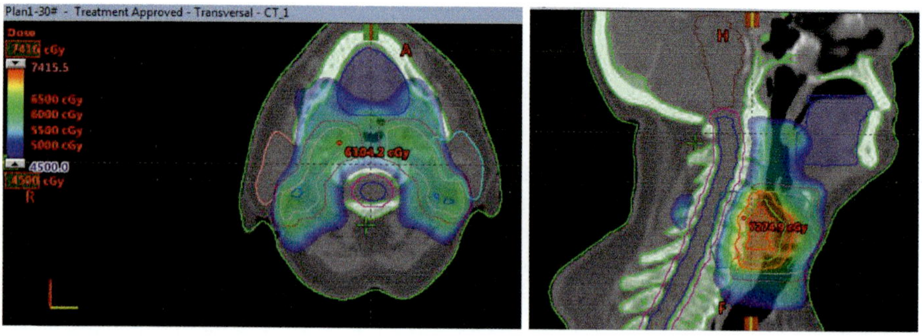

Fig. 11.6 Sparing of the parotid gland and spinal cord (VMAT technique) [Courtesy: BLK Hospital, Delhi, India]

11.4 Results and Salient Features of Early-Stage Hypopharyngeal Cancers

Author (Ref)	OS	DFS	LC	LP	Remark
Nishimura [8]	81% (5 year)	69% (5 year)	83% (5 year)	92% (5 year)	A proportion received chemotherapy
Amadur [14]	96% (5 year)	-	85% (5 year)	61% (5 year)	All PFS tumours
Nakajima [15]	70% (3 year)	-	85% (3 year)		PFS better control than PC
Gupta [1]	-	49.3% (3 year	49.7% (3 year)	-	

Note: *OS* Overall Survival, *DFS* Disease-Free Survival, *LC* Local Control, *LP* Laryngeal Preservation

- There is no difference between surgery and radiotherapy as regards treatment results; RT provides a better laryngeal preservation.
- Approximately 30–40% do harbour occult neck metastases.
- Infiltration into the apex and medial wall of pyriform fossa shows poorer disease control.
- Second cancers are higher in hypopharyngeal compared to laryngeal cancers.

References

1. Gupta T, Chopra S, Agarwal JP, Laskar SG, D'cruz AK, Shrivastava SK, Dinshaw KA. Squamous cell carcinoma of the hypopharynx: single-institution outcome analysis of a large cohort of patients treated with primary non-surgical approaches. Acta Oncol. 2009;48:541–8.
2. Petersen JF, Timmermans AJ, van Dijk BAC, et al. Trends in treatment, incidence and survival of hypopharynx cancer: a 20-year population-based study in the Netherlands. Eur Arch Otorhinolaryngol. 2018;275:181–9.
3. Mohanti BK, Nachiappan P, Pandey RM, Sharma A, Bahadur S, Thakar A. Analysis of 2167 head and neck cancer patients' management, treatment compliance and outcomes from a regional cancer centre, Delhi, India. J Laryngol Otol. 2007;121:49–56.
4. Pracy P, Loughran S, Good J, Parmar S, Goranova R. Hypopharyngeal cancer: United Kingdom national multidisciplinary guidelines. J Laryngol Otol. 2016;130(S2):S104–10.
5. Bok GH, Cho WY, Cho JY, Jin SY, Ahn JH, Chun CG, Lee TH, Kim HG. Endoscopic resection of hypopharyngeal squamous cell carcinoma. Clin Endosc. 2013;46:189–92.
6. Imanishi Y, Ozawa H, Sakamoto K, Fujii R, Shigetomi S, Habu N, Otsuka K, Sato Y, Watanabe Y, Sekimizu M, Ito F, Tomita T, Ogawa K. Clinical outcomes of transoral videolaryngoscopic surgery for hypopharyngeal and supraglottic cancer. BMC Cancer. 2017;17:445.
7. Hall SF, Groome PA, Irish J, O'Sullivan B. Radiotherapy or surgery for head and neck squamous cell cancer: establishing the baseline for hypopharyngeal carcinoma? Cancer. 2009;115:5711–22.
8. Nishimura H, Sasaki R, Yoshida K, Miyawaki D, Okamoto Y, Kiyota N, Saito M, Otsuki N, Nibu K. Radiotherapy for stage I or II hypopharyngeal carcinoma. J Radiat Res. 2012;53:892–9.

9. Kawashima M, Hayashi R, Tahara M, Yamazaki M, Miyazaki M, Arahira S, Ogino T. Accelerated radiotherapy and larynx preservation in favorable-risk patients with T2 or worse hypopharyngeal cancer. Jpn J Clin Oncol. 2007;37:345–52.
10. Boyer A, Biggs P, Galvin J, et al. Basic applications of multileaf collimators.AAPM Report No.72. Wisconsins: Medical Physics Publishing; 2001.
11. Studer G, Peponi E, Kloeck S, Dossenbach T, Huber G, Glanzmann C. Surviving hypopharynx-larynx carcinoma in the era of IMRT. Int J Radiat Oncol Biol Phys. 2010;77:1391–6.
12. Otto K. Volumetric modulated arc therapy: IMRT in a single gantry arc. Med Phys. 2008;35:310–7.
13. Holt A, Van Gestel D, Arends MP, et al. Multi-institutional comparison of volumetric modulated arc therapy vs. intensity-modulated radiation therapy for head-and-neck cancer: a planning study. Radiat Oncol. 2013;8:26. https://doi.org/10.1186/1748-717X-8-26.
14. Amdur RJ, Mendenhall WM, Stringer SP, Villaret DB, Cassisi NJ. Organ preservation with radiotherapy for T1-T2 carcinoma of the pyriform sinus. Head Neck. 2001;23:353–62.
15. Nakajima A, Nishiyama K, Morimoto M, Nakamura S, Suzuki O, Kawaguchi Y, Miyagi K, Fujii T, Yoshino K. Definitive radiotherapy for T1-2 hypopharyngeal cancer: a single-institution experience. Int J Radiat Oncol Biol Phys. 2012;82:e129–35.

Larynx Preservation in Hypopharyngeal Carcinomas

12

Shelley Hukku, Shikha Halder, and Bidhu K. Mohanti

12.1 Introduction

The larynx and hypopharynx are major crossroads for essential physiological functions such as swallowing, speech, and breathing. The hypopharynx is a rare cancer site for head and neck cancer (HNC) in the western countries, but hypopharyngeal cancers constitute a major disease burden in Asia, Africa, and South America [1, 2]. It is mostly associated with smoking and alcohol consumption. Hypopharyngeal cancers are characterized by aggressive disease biology and dismal treatment outcomes and are associated with one of the highest mortality rates in any HNC. The reasons for the poor prognosis are diverse. Hypopharynx is a silent site, patients usually present in advanced tumor stages, submucosal spread is a characteristic feature, and the tumors have a notorious propensity to metastasize to regional lymphatics and distant sites; and furthermore, hypopharyngeal cancers are associated with the highest incidence of second primary tumors which further reduces survival [3].

12.2 Management Principle for Advanced Stages of HPC

More than 80% of hypopharyngeal cancers present in locoregionally advanced stages of III and IV. For these patients, the treatment options have evolved over the years: (I) surgery alone, (II) combined modality surgery and postoperative radiotherapy (S-PORT), (III) radiotherapy alone, and (IV) combined chemoradiotherapy

S. Hukku · S. Halder
Department of Radiation Oncology, BLK Super Specialty Hospital, New Delhi, India

B. K. Mohanti (✉)
Department of Radiation Oncology, Manipal Hospital, New Delhi, India

S. Bahadur et al. (eds.), *Carcinoma of the Larynx and Hypopharynx*,
https://doi.org/10.1007/978-981-13-3110-7_12

(CRT). It has been realized from the long-term results that single modality of surgery or radiotherapy alone is inferior to combined modalities [4]. The present literature point to the fact that between S-PORT and CRT, it is difficult to identify the superiority of one arm of combined modalities over the other arm [5]. In view of this, the nonsurgical CRT practice has gained acceptance, and there is a decline in the use of surgery for stages III–IV HPC [6].

A multidisciplinary approach is crucial in the overall management of patients with advanced stage hypopharyngeal cancer in order to achieve the best results and maintain or improve functional results.

12.2.1 Larynx Preservation Strategies

Between the 1970s and 1980s, it was realized that surgery alone, even with extreme radical approach, was inadequate to control advanced stage HPC, and postoperative radiotherapy was added to improve the locoregional control and survival. Except for a small proportion of patients who present with T1–T2N1 disease where voice and swallowing preservation can be possible with surgery ± postoperative RT, the vast majority of HPC patients are diagnosed as T3–T4, N+ where the surgery will comprise of total laryngectomy, with partial/circumferential pharyngectomy and repair, with unilateral or bilateral neck dissection. Such extensive surgical procedure entails the loss of voice (with a permanent tracheostomy), compromise in swallowing capacity, and demands a long-term post-therapy rehabilitation, after the S-PORT treatment course [2, 4].

The shift from surgery as the upfront modality in the treatment of stage III–IV HPC to the nonsurgical modalities has taken place during the last 20 years, with the initial encouraging results coming from Europe and the USA [7, 8]. A few years earlier, the well-designed Veterans Affairs study on stage III–IV laryngeal cancer had established the new treatment strategy of induction chemotherapy and definitive radiotherapy as a suitable alternative to the surgery combined with radiotherapy [9]. These studies, published in the 1990s, have paved the way for "larynx preservation" in locoregionally advanced laryngeal and hypopharyngeal cancers.

In our current state of knowledge, the larynx preservation strategies for advanced HPC can be practiced with following options:

1. Induction chemotherapy followed by definitive radiotherapy (IC-RT)
2. Concurrent chemoradiotherapy (CCRT)
3. Induction chemotherapy followed by concurrent chemoroadiotherapy (IC-CCRT)
4. Induction chemotherapy followed by concurrent targeted drug bio-radiotherapy (IC-BRT)

However, for any of the above approaches, the provision of salvage surgery for the residual or recurrent primary and nodal disease should be in place.

12.2.2 Multidisciplinary Clinic or Team

The multidisciplinary head and neck clinic- and team-based comprehensive care for advanced stage HPC can show consistent good outcomes.

The complex management of these tumors creates an essential need for multidisciplinary team approach involving a head and neck surgeon, radiation oncologist, medical oncologist, radiologist, pathologist, nutritionist, dentist, speech and swallow therapist, and social worker [2, 3].

12.2.3 Nonsurgical Treatment Practices

12.2.3.1 Induction Therapy Followed by Radical Radiotherapy in Carcinoma of the Hypopharynx

One of the earliest studies on preservation of larynx in hypopharyngeal cancer was conducted by the European Organization for Research and Treatment of Cancer (EORTC) [7]. Patients were randomly assigned to one of the two treatment arms: (1) immediate surgery with postoperative radiotherapy (50–70 Gy) or (2) induction chemotherapy (cisplatin [100 mg/m^2] given as a bolus intravenous injection on day 1, followed by infusion of fluorouracil [1000 mg/m^2 per day] on days 1–5). An endoscopic evaluation was performed after each cycle of chemotherapy. After two cycles, only partial and complete responders received the third cycle. Patients with a complete response after two or three cycles of chemotherapy were treated thereafter by irradiation (70 Gy); nonresponding patients underwent conventional surgery with postoperative radiation (50–70 Gy). Salvage surgery was also performed when patients relapsed after chemotherapy and irradiation. The trial was designed to test the equivalence of the two treatment arms. The locoregional failure and survival rates were similar in the two arms, and the laryngeal function was preserved in one-third of the IC-RT-treated patients at 5 years. The study published in 1996, EORTC 24891, essentially concluded that LP was feasible in hypopharyngeal cancers with the use of induction chemotherapy and RT. Furthermore, the study established the chemosensitivity of hypopharyngeal squamous cell carcinoma (SCC), similar to the earlier reported benefit in laryngeal SCC [7, 9].

A recent update of the above EORTC 24891 trial showed that at longer follow-up of 10 years, the OS rate was 13.8% in the S-PORT arm and 13.1% in the IC-RT arm. The 10-year PFS rates were 8.5% and 10.8%, respectively. In the chemotherapy arm, functional LP was possible in 8.7% of cases [10].

The role of induction chemotherapy (IC-RT) for locally advanced laryngeal/hypopharyngeal cancers has been separately addressed within the meta-analysis of chemotherapy in head and neck cancer (MACH-NC) and has shown that the IC-RT practice has similar overall survival (39% vs. 45% in IC-RT vs. S-PORT) and event-free survival (34% vs. 40% in IC-RT vs. S-PORT) rates at 5 years when compared with combined S-PORT. The larynx preservation is seen in half of the patients [11].

12.2.3.2 Concurrent Chemoradiotherapy (CCRT)

Subsequent to the development of induction chemotherapy, aimed to avoid the need for surgery seen in the IC-RT trials, the use of chemotherapy concomitant with RT emerged. Since 2000, published single institution studies and meta-analyses have consistently shown the improved survival advantage of CCRT compared to IC-RT. The best superiority is seen when cisplatin as single agent or in combination regimen forms the treatment protocol of CCRT [11]. Most of the current studies have utilized (1) cisplatin (or carboplatin, in case of compromised renal function) as single agent weekly [1] or (2) cisplatin plus 5-FU (PF), as two-drug regimen every week [12], delivered concurrently during the 6–7 weeks of radiotherapy course.

The more intense drug regimen, TPF (docetaxel, cisplatin, and 5-FU), has been compared with PF, with higher response rates. However, the three-drug regimen is not routinely delivered due to higher toxicities. Secondly, the information has emerged that combined chemoradiotherapy has long-term harmful effects in older patients above the age of 70 years [13]. Thus, evidence-based medicine has shown that concurrent chemoradiotherapy without prolongation of overall treatment time and including cisplatin only or cisplatin-5-fluorouracil should be considered the treatment of choice for patients who are fit for chemotherapy (National Cancer Institute [NCI] Level 1 of evidence supporting recommendation) [14]. In most of the institutions in India, weekly cisplatin at 30–40 mg/m^2 is the current choice in comparison to three weekly practices favored in western world [1].

12.2.3.3 Induction Chemotherapy Followed by Concurrent Chemoradiotherapy (IC-CCRT)

During the last 15 years, improved drug delivery, refinement in radiotherapy techniques, and better understanding of morbidities related to chemotherapy and radiotherapy have come together in the nonsurgical modalities for head and neck SCC in general and in selected HPC. After the treatment approaches of IC-RT and CCRT, results have proven the efficacy of laryngeal preservation, and the newer trials have extended a more intense treatment approach. Can induction chemotherapy (IC) followed by CCRT (IC-CCRT) increase the outcomes?

A phase III randomized study utilized PF or TPF as IC for three cycles followed by three weekly cisplatins plus RT as CCRT [15]. In this study reported from Spain, patients received either CF (cisplatin 100 mg/m^2 on day 1 plus FU 1000 mg/m^2 continuous infusion on days 1 through 5) or PCF (paclitaxel 175 mg/m^2 on day 1, cisplatin 100 mg/m^2 on day 2, and FU 500 mg/m^2 continuous infusion on days 2 through 6); both regimens were administered for three cycles every 21 days. Patients with complete response (CR) or partial response of greater than 80% in primary tumor received additional CRT (cisplatin 100 mg/m^2 on days 1, 22, and 43 plus RT dose 70 Gy). This treatment approach had shown higher overall survival, more so with three-drug regimen in the unresectable patients [15].

Long-term results of IC-CCRT, from the French collaborative group, GORTEC (Groupe Oncologie Radiothérapie Tête et Cou), have recommended that TPF regimen as induction chemotherapy followed by RT or CCRT can show increased larynx preservation rate. At 5 years, two-thirds of the surviving patients maintained laryngeal dysfunction-free survival (LDFFS) [16]. The radiotherapy-related organ morbidities were lower in TPF compared to PF induction chemotherapy, but the grade 2–4 hematological toxicities were observed in more than 50% of the patients in TPF arm. The OS and DFS were not statistically different between the induction regimen of TPF vs. PF.

In a similar study from the USA, TAX 324, subgroup of laryngeal and hypopharyngeal cancers were treated by three cycles of IC (TPF vs. PF) at three weekly intervals, followed by carboplatin weekly concurrent with radiotherapy dose of 70–74 Gy (CCRT) or RT (70–74 Gy) over 7 weeks. The OS (52% vs. 42% at 5 years), DFS (45% vs. 34% at 5 years), and laryngeal preservation rate (52% vs. 32% at 3 years) showed superior results with TPF induction chemotherapy followed by CCRT [17].

Interest in neoadjuvant, or induction, chemotherapy has been renewed with the demonstrated efficacy of a three-drug regimen consisting of docetaxel, cisplatin, and fluorouracil (TPF) and a consistent reduction in distant failure. A study was conducted to evaluate the role of IC-CCRT in order to improve the disease control in N2 and N3 nodal status of HNSCC but failed to show any advantage of induction chemotherapy with three-drug regimen [18]. Addedly, toxicity, as measured by the adverse events, was higher in the IC arm. It is also observed that T4 hypopharyngeal cancer shows a poorer overall survival, functional, and oncologic outcomes after the IC-CCRT [19]. Hence, in view of the added toxicity of IC to CCRT, careful evaluation host and tumor factors will be required to utilize this treatment approach for larynx preservation in locoregionally advanced hypopharyngeal cancers.

12.2.3.4 Induction Chemotherapy Followed by Concurrent Targeted Drug Bio-radiotherapy (IC-BRT)

A newer treatment approach, called bio-radiotherapy (BRT), has emerged where biological modifier and targeted drugs are combined with radiation therapy in HNSCC. The BRT is aimed to be an alternative to CCRT, with a lower and lesser toxicity profile.

The cells of almost all epithelial neoplasms, including head and neck cancer, express high levels of epidermal growth factor receptor (EGFR), a member of the Erb B family of receptor tyrosine kinases. This EGFR expression in HNSCC is associated with a poor clinical outcome. Radiation increases the expression of EGFR in cancer cells, and blockade of EGFR signaling sensitizes cells to the effects of radiation. Cetuximab, an IgG1 monoclonal antibody against the ligand-binding domain of EGFR, is a tyrosine kinase inhibitor (TKI) drug which enhances the cytotoxic effects of radiation in squamous-cell carcinoma. The combined use of cetuximab and radiotherapy was studied in an international phase III trial. The results of this trial in stage III–IV HNSCC showed higher outcomes for cetuximab plus RT (BRT) versus RT alone at relevant end points of locoregional control (50% vs. 41% at 2 years), progression-free survival (46% vs. 37% at 2 years), and overall survival (55% vs. 45% at 3 years) [20].

The utilization of BRT for advanced laryngeal and hypopharyngeal cancers has the purpose of laryngeal preservation. Phase II and phase III clinical trials have been reported in the last 10 years. The most significant and cited study is the TREMPLIN trial from Europe [21]. In this study, previously untreated patients with stage III to IV larynx/hypopharynx squamous-cell carcinoma received three cycles of IC consisting of docetaxel and cisplatin 75 mg/m^2 each on day 1 and fluorouracil 750 mg/m^2 per day on days 1 through 5. Poor responders (<50% response) underwent salvage surgery. Responders (>50% response) were randomly assigned to conventional radiotherapy (RT; 70 Gy) with concurrent cisplatin 100 mg/m^2 per day on days 1, 22, and 43 of RT (arm A, CCRT) or concurrent cetuximab 400 mg/m^2 loading dose and 250 mg/m^2 per week during RT (arm B, BRT). The BRT showed results comparable with CCRT as regards laryngeal preservation (72% vs. 79% at 3 years). The grade 3–4 late toxicities were higher in the cisplatin (Arm A, CCRT) than cetuximab (Arm B, BRT), mucosal (3.5% vs. 1.8%), xerostomia (10.3% vs. 8.9%), and fibrosis (7% vs. 2%), whereas acute hematological toxicity was higher with cisplatin and the radiation-in-field morbidity was higher for cetuximab [21]. Thus, targeted drug therapy with radiotherapy (BRT) can be efficacious, in suitably chosen hypopharyngeal cancer, for larynx preservation.

The landmark studies involving above four treatment approaches are outlined in Table 12.1.

Table 12.1 Landmark studies in locally advanced hypopharyngeal cancers aimed at larynx preservation

Study	Treatment(s)	OS	DFS	LR failure	LP
EORTC 24891, 1996 [7]	Arm1 = Sx > PORT Arm2 = PF > RT	Arm1 = 32.6% Arm2 = 38% (5 years)	Arm1 = 26.4% Arm2 = 31.7% (5 years)	Arm1 = 31% Arm2 = 33% (5 years)	Arm2=35% (5 years)
GORTEC, 2016 [16]	Arm1 = TPF > CCRT/RT Arm2 = PF > CCRT/RT	Arm1 = 50.9% Arm2 = 41.9% (5 years)	Arm1 = 42.4% Arm2 = 31.4% (5 years)	Arm1 = 34% Arm2 = 45%	Arm1 = 67.2% Arm2 = 46.5% (5 years)
TAX 324 (subgroup) [17]	Arm1 = TPF > CCRT Arm2 = PF > CCRT	Arm1 = 52% Arm2 = 42% (5 years)	Arm1 = 45% Arm2 = 34% (5 years)	Arm1 = 32% Arm2 = 38%	Arm1 = 52% Arm2 = 32% (3 years)
TREMPLIN [21]	TPF > followed by Arm1 = CCRT (cisplatin) Arm2 = RT + cetuximab	Arm1 = 75% Arm2 = 73% (at 3 years)	-	Arm1 = 23% Arm2 = 30% (at 18 months)	Arm1 = 79% Arm2 = 72% (2 year)

Note (for Table 12.1): *Arm* denotes randomized group, *CCRT* concurrent chemoradiotherapy, *DFS* disease-free survival, *LP* larynx preservation, *LR* locoregional, overall survival, *PF* cisplatin+5-FU regimen, *PORT* postoperative radiotherapy, *RT* radiation therapy, *Sx* surgery, *TPF* docetaxel+cisplatin+5-FU

12.3 Radiation Therapy (RT)

Definitive primary radiotherapy for operable early and locally advanced stages of hypopharyngeal cancers has been in clinical practice since the 1950s [22]. As a treatment modality, RT alone was conceived to achieve disease control. Although the radiation response is consistent in HPC, the disease control reduces with higher tumor volume (T) and nodal burden (N). Whereas surgery or radical radiotherapy shows equal effectiveness for early-stage I-II HPC, RT alone gives a poorer outcome in terms of both OS and DFS for the higher stages III–IV [23].

Long-term results of radiotherapeutic practice were published in the 1970s and 1980s [24].

As an alternative to surgery, the locoregional radiotherapy received attention from head and neck surgeons, multidisciplinary tumor clinics, and patients. Whereas RT showed similar effectiveness to surgery in early-stage HPC, the outcomes with RT alone are inferior for stages III–IV. Since the 1990s, chemoradiotherapy has increasingly become an area of clinical research with an aim to (i) avoid surgery and (ii) achieve organ preservation. The chemoradiotherapy (CRT) and more recently bio-radiotherapy (BRT), as the nonsurgical approach described in the above four sections, have undergone considerable developments during the last two decades. The advancements of technique and technology in radiation therapy are becoming applicable in the management of HPC.

12.3.1 Techniques

In the initial period from the 1970s till the 1990s, the two-dimensional (2-D) technique was used in the reports and trials [1, 7–9, 24]. Three-dimensional conformal radiation therapy (3-DCRT) with computer-controlled radiation therapy planning system (TPS) was introduced into clinical radiotherapy after the advent of CT and MRI scan. The volumetric 3-D image data sets enable the delineation and contouring of the tumor, nodal regions, and surrounding organs (such as spine, orbit, parotid, etc.). Radiation therapy for head and neck cancer has benefited from the volumetric dose planning by TPS. With the 3-DCRT, it became possible to see and decide the amount of dose to be delivered to the locoregional tumor and to the surrounding normal tissues and organs. This has helped in minimizing the radiation morbidities. The treatment for HPC, by RT and CRT, has utilized volumetric image-based radiation therapy delivery in recent years [1, 3].

The linear accelerator machines with computer-controlled multi-leaf collimators (MLC) are now capable to deliver radiation beams shaped into a precise target volume. Since 2000, the MLC-based Linacs utilize the intensity-modulated radiation therapy (IMRT) and image-guided radiation therapy (IGRT) techniques. With these newer techniques, such as IMRT and IGRT which incorporate onboard imaging for target volume conformity, the organ sparing and morbidity control have improved considerably. It has been documented that IMRT carries the potential benefits to increase the tolerance to chemoradiotherapy and reduces the radiotherapy-/

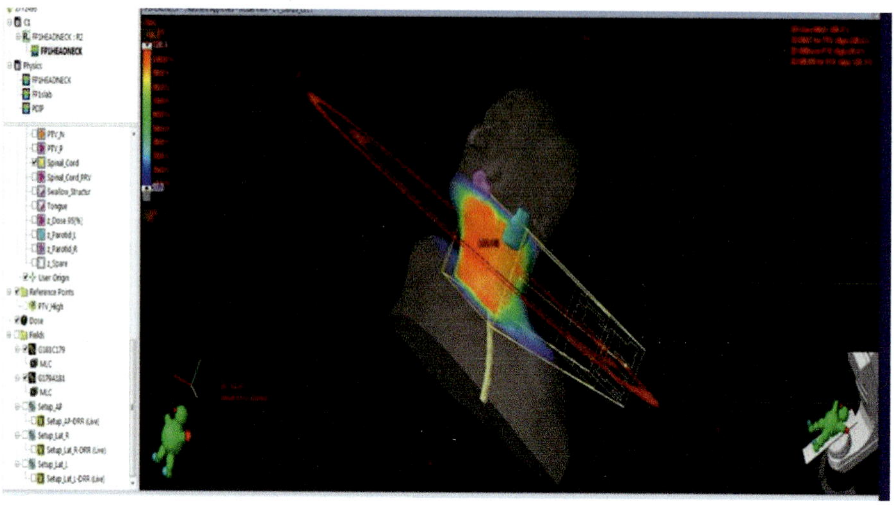

Fig. 12.1 Volumetric modulated arc therapy (VMAT) technique in hypopharyngeal cancer [Courtesy: Department of Radiation Oncology, Manipal Hospital, Delhi]

chemotherapy-related toxicities [3, 25]. With these newer techniques, simultaneous integrated boost (SIB) and adaptive radiotherapy can allow dose prescription in a deferential manner, such as primary tumor and palpable nodal area to receive 64–70 Gy, whereas prophylactic irradiation for microscopic node levels will receive 50–54 Gy.

From 2013 onwards, we have used the volumetric modulated arc therapy (VMAT) in the treatment of head and neck cancer patients. In comparison with multiple fixed fields of IMRT, the treatment delivery with arc technique of VMAT is relatively smooth and less time-consuming. The basic concept of arc therapy (VMAT), as shown in Fig. 12.1, is the delivery of radiation from a continuous rotation of the radiation source and allows the patient to be treated from a full 360° beam angle. Arc therapies have the ability to achieve highly conformal dose distributions and are essentially an alternative form of IMRT. The major advantages of VMAT, over fixed gantry IMRT, constitute (a) the improvement in treatment delivery efficiency, (b) reduction in treatment delivery time, and (c) the reduction in MU usage with subsequent reduction of integral radiation dose to the rest of the body [26]. Dose conformity for the tumor is similar or better to IMRT, and organ sparing shows a reduction in dose [27].

The treatment of one locoregionally advanced HPC, at our center, is shown in Fig. 12.2 for contouring and Fig. 12.3 for dose plan generated with VMAT technique.

12.3.2 Dose Prescription

The standard convention dose fraction of 5 fractions per week (Monday to Friday) is delivered, at a prescription dose of 66–70 Gy in 33–35 fractions to tumor (primary PTV) and to significant nodal burden (nodal PTV) and 50–54 Gy in 25–30 fraction to

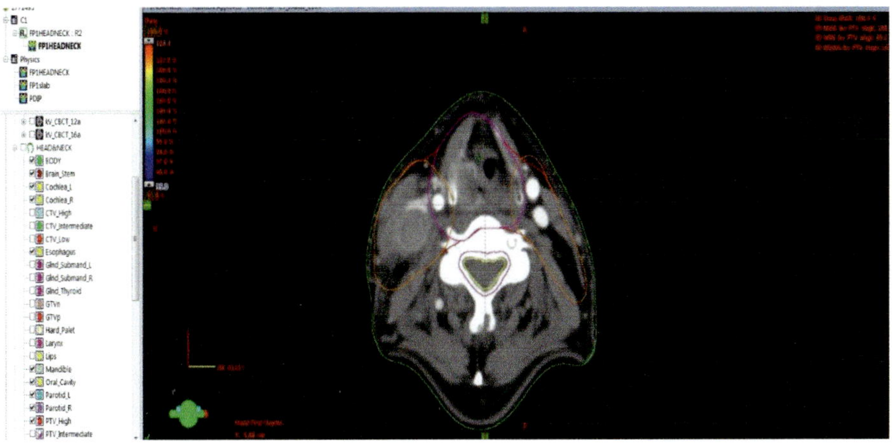

Fig. 12.2 Contouring of primary and nodal regions in a stage IV hypopharyngeal cancer [Courtesy: Department of Radiation Oncology, Manipal Hospital, Delhi]

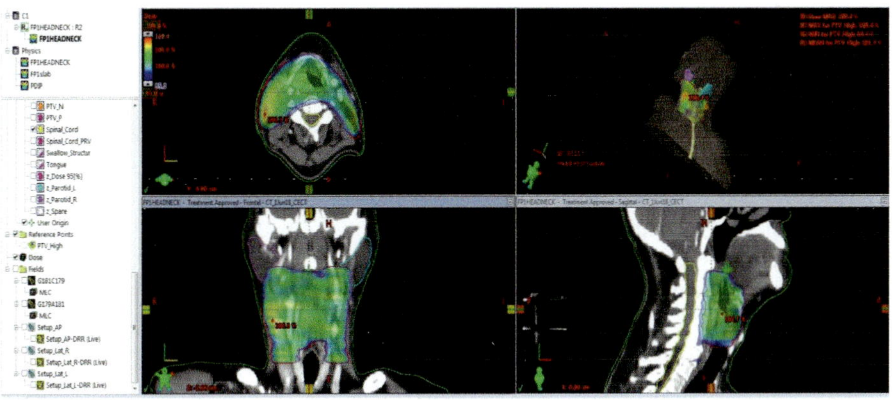

Fig. 12.3 Dose plan generated with VMAT technique (two arcs) in a stage IV hypopharyngeal cancer [Courtesy: Department of Radiation Oncology, Manipal Hospital, Delhi]

microscopic nodal areas. Most published studies and clinical practice of chemoradiotherapy, either induction or concomitant and single or multiple drug regimen, utilize the standard RT course of 6–7 weeks [1, 3, 7, 8, 11, 12, 16, 23, 24]. Altered fractionation, such as hyperfactionation, accelerated fractionation, or hypofractionation, is practiced in a selective manner in clinical trial settings [20, 28, 29]. According to NCI, US recommendation, altered fraction radiotherapy, in patients who are unsuitable for chemoradiotherapy, should be the choice of definitive radiotherapy. In the current practice with IMRT or VMAT, at our institution (Figs. 12.2 and 12.3), a mild hypofractionated regimen of 66 Gy in 30 fractions (5 fractions per week, in 6 weeks) is delivered to the PTV which includes the primary tumor and high-risk nodal region, and the low-risk nodal area receives 54 Gy in 30 fractions (over 6 weeks) simultaneously.

12.4 Recommendations and Strategies for Larynx Preservation

The nonsurgical approaches, described as four options in this chapter, are aimed at laryngeal preservation (LP) in locoregionally advanced HPC. However, Lefebvre (2010) has proposed that a few factors should be kept in mind to offer the nonsurgical therapy to the patients:

1. Definition of larynx preservation varies in different studies from "larynx in place" to the composite definition of "larynx in place without tumor, without feeding tube and without tracheotomy."
2. It should also be noted that, to date, no nonsurgical approach has provided a superior survival effect to that seen with total laryngectomy followed by postoperative radiotherapy.
3. The addition of chemotherapy to radiotherapy has allowed larynx preservation in patients who would, not too many years ago, have been candidates for total laryngectomy.

Hence, the anatomical preservation of larynx, after chemoradiotherapy or bioradiotherapy, should carefully assess and record the posttreatment laryngeal function, swallowing, and quality of life (QOL).

According to the present literature, LP guidelines are currently available and should be routinely followed by institutions and centers, when they undertake the nonsurgical approaches in HPC [30–32].

The evaluation of laryngeal and swallowing functions can potentially add to the improvements in the treatment outcomes after nonsurgical therapy in HPC. According to the guidelines and research in this area, laryngoesophageal dysfunction-free survival (LEDFS) [33] and TALK score [34] are some of the tools for measurement and evaluation while choosing the LP strategy.

LEDFS includes the following factors, which negatively impact the aim of nonsurgical therapy: post-therapy total or partial laryngectomy and tracheostomy/feeding tube within 2 years or later, besides death and local relapse [33]. The TALK score consists of tumor (T) stage, serum albumin (A) level, alcohol/liquor (L) intake, and Karnofsky (K) performance status [34].

Criteria for choosing larynx preservation approach in locoregionally advanced HPC:

1. Patients who are routinely suitable
   - T2–T3 tumors, N0–N1 nodal status
   - Able to swallow foods and the speech is reasonably preserved
2. Relative contraindications
   - T4 tumor, N2b/N2c nodal status
   - Requires a feeding tube
   - Comorbidities (which compromise kidney, lung, and heart functions)

3. Major contraindications
   - T4 tumor with gross soft tissue and cartilage infiltration
   - N3 nodal status
   - Age >70 years, KPS < 70
   - Tracheostomy and feeding tube (both are required for starting CRT/BRT)

12.5 Morbidities Associated with Chemoradiotherapy or Bio-radiotherapy for Laryngeal Preservation in HPC

In recent years, since the beginning of the twenty-first century, the surgical practice for laryngeal and hypopharyngeal cancers has declined, and there is a global surge in the routine practice of nonsurgical therapy [2, 3, 5, 6, 18, 35]. This enthusiasm should be balanced in the clinical practice because there are several morbidities associated with CRT and/or BRT.

Morbidities of different types and grades occur: (1) increased mucosal reaction leading to dysphagia, hoarseness, cough, aspiration, and breathing difficulty; (2) skin morbidities causing pain, restriction in oral and neck functions; (3) hematologic toxicities such as anemia, fever, and need for blood transfusion; and (4) general health decline caused by treatment-related disruption in activities of daily living, fatigue, and loss of appetite that are seen as the main morbidities of currently recommended nonsurgical approaches. A patient undergoing CRT/BRT can have a constellation of these morbidities [3–5, 16, 31, 33, 36, 37]. It is observed that the grade III–IV morbidities which require active medical attention or treatment interruption are in the range of 25–50% [3, 7, 15, 16, 36, 37]. One study on long-term morbidities showed that the overall pharyngeal dysfunction, laryngeal dysfunction, and aspiration rates were 36%, 27%, and 25%, respectively [36].

When we consider to avoid the negative impact of loss of speech and compromised swallowing after surgery, similar attention is crucial for the consequential morbidities after nonsurgical therapy. It is imperative to record the morbidities on a longitudinal time frame, because nearly one-third of CRT-treated patients will experience difficulties in daily QOL [38].

12.6 Strategies to Reduce Chemoradiotherapy- or Bio-radiotherapy-Induced Morbidity

12.6.1 Early Nutritional Interventions

Head and neck cancer patients are at high risk of malnutrition in part because of pre-existing unhealthy lifestyles (e.g., alcohol and smoking addiction) and in part due to local tumor interference leading to dysphagia and a reduced food intake. Moreover, cancer therapy (including surgery, radiation, and chemotherapy) can further negatively affect nutritional status and treatment tolerance. Current research in this area strongly argue to favor early and tailored nutritional counseling and intervention which can improve treatment tolerance and influence the clinical outcome [39]. Early nutritional intervention (often neglected) has been shown to maintain body weight, reduces hospital admissions, and is of utmost importance when LP is aimed at in locoregionally advanced HPC.

12.6.2 IMRT Aimed to Reduce Late Dysphagia

The incidence of dysphagia depends on treatment modality, tumor site and stage, patient age, pre-treatment weight loss, pre-treatment swallowing capacity, and habits like smoking and alcohol intake. It is now understood both radiotherapy and chemotherapeutic drugs can induce swallowing dysfunction [3, 26, 27, 36, 37]. Radiation can reduce hyoid bone movement and damage the pharyngeal constrictors, the glottic and the supraglottic larynx, causing dysphagia and aspiration [40]. Anatomical structures known to be involved in development of dysphagia constitute pharyngeal constrictor muscles, upper esophageal sphincter, cricopharyngeus muscle, cervical esophagus, glottic and supraglottic larynx, base of tongue, and the covering hyoid bone [40]. Dose–volume toxicity relationships for these swallowing structures are reported. Reducing mean dose to less than 50 Gy and reducing volume receiving 50 Gy to these structures may be helpful. Radiotherapy outcome data have suggested that compared with the 2-D and 3-D plans, standard IMRT decreases the morbidities of xerostomia, hoarseness, and dysphagia, besides giving higher conformity in target (tumor) dose [3, 25–27, 31, 40]. In order to reduce the acute and late toxicities of CRT and BRT modalities in HPC for the larynx preservation, besides the chemotherapy and targeted drug regimen, the emphasis on 3-D image-based IMRT and VMAT techniques should not be undervalued (Figs. 12.1, 12.2, and 12.3).

12.7 Treatment Outcomes of Laryngeal Preservation with CRT and/or BRT in Advanced HPC

The expected 2-year overall survival (OS) in hypopharyngeal SCC is around 50% in disease stage III and 30% in stage IV. Five-year OS ranges from 35% in stage III to less than 20% in stage IV [2–5, 41]. Current results show that larynx preservation with nonsurgical therapy is in the range of 52–79% at 2–3 years and 35–67% at 5 years (Table 12.1) [7, 16, 17, 21].

12.8 Summary and Conclusion

1. Larynx preservation in carcinoma of hypopharynx is safe and feasible option for locoregionally advanced stage HPC.
2. T4a and N2 disease without massive cartilage invasion may be taken up for larynx preservation after discussion within the multidisciplinary team and with patient.

3. T4 disease with massive cartilage and soft tissue invasion and N3 nodal status are not suitable candidates for larynx preservation.
4. Induction chemotherapy followed by RT and concurrent CRT are current standards for LP.
5. Treatment intensification with TPF-based induction therapy followed by CRT shows promise yet may be associated with poor compliance and increased toxicity.
6. Results within large cohorts and population-based series highlight that for hypopharyngeal carcinomas there is trend away from surgical therapy and that in contrast to laryngeal cancer, survival for hypopharyngeal cancer has improved after larynx preservation.
7. Organ preservation should not be considered synonymous with laryngeal function preservation. Laryngoesophageal dysfunction-free survival (LEDFS), TALK score, and QOL are some of the tools for measurement and evaluation while choosing the LP strategy.
8. Combined modality therapy (CRT or BRT) is associated with increased rate and severity of long-term toxicities particularly dysphagia. Early nutrition supplementation and swallowing sparing IMRT/VMAT have the potential to reduce these morbidities.

References

1. Gupta T, Chopra S, Agarwal JP, Laskar SG, D'cruz AK, Shrivastava SK, Dinshaw KA. Squamous cell carcinoma of the hypopharynx: single-institution outcome analysis of a large cohort of patients treated with primary non-surgical approaches. Acta Oncol. 2009;48:541–8.
2. Petersen JF, Timmermans AJ, van Dijk BAC, et al. Trends in treatment, incidence and survival of hypopharynx cancer: a 20-year population-based study in the Netherlands. Eur Arch Otorhinolaryngol. 2018;275:181–9.
3. Krstevska V. Hypopharyngeal Cancer. In: Agulnik M, editor. Head and Neck Cancer. London: InTech; 2012. ISBN: 978-953-51-0236-6. Available from: http://www.intechopen.com/books/head-and-neckcancer/hypopharyngeal-cancer.
4. Pracy P, Loughran S, Good J, Parmar S, Goranova R. Hypopharyngeal cancer: United Kingdom National multidisciplinary guidelines. J Laryngol Otol. 2016;130(S2):S104–10.
5. Hall SF, Groome PA, Irish J, O'Sullivan B. Radiotherapy or surgery for head and neck squamous cell cancer: establishing the baseline for hypopharyngeal carcinoma? Cancer. 2009;115:5711–22.
6. Takes RP, Strojan P, Silver CE, Bradley PJ, Haigentz M Jr, Wolf GT, Shaha AR, Hartl DM, Olofsson J, Langendijk JA, Rinaldo A, Ferlito A. International Head and Neck Scientific Group. Current trends in initial management of hypopharyngeal cancer: the declining use of open surgery. Head Neck. 2012;34:270–81.
7. Lefebvre JL, Chevalier D, Luboinski B, Kirkpatrick A, Collette L, Sahmoud T. Larynx preservation in pyriform sinus cancer: preliminary results of a European Organization for Research and Treatment of Cancer phase III trial. EORTC Head and Neck Cancer Cooperative Group. J Natl Cancer Inst. 1996;88:890–9.
8. Zelefsky MJ, Kraus DH, Pfister DG, Raben A, Shah JP, Strong EW, Spiro RH, Bosl GJ, Harrison LB. Combined chemotherapy and radiotherapy versus surgery and postoperative radiotherapy for advanced hypopharyngeal cancer. Head Neck. 1996;18:405–11.

9. Department of Veterans Affairs Laryngeal Cancer Study Group, Wolf GT, Fisher SG, Hong WK, Hillman R, Spaulding M, Laramore GE, Endicott JW, McClatchey K, Henderson WG. Induction chemotherapy plus radiation compared with surgery plus radiation in patients with advanced laryngeal cancer. N Engl J Med. 1991;324:1685–90.
10. Lefebvre JL, Andry G, Chevalier D, et al. Laryngeal preservation with induction chemotherapy for hypopharyngeal squamous cell carcinoma: 10-year results of EORTC trial 24891. Ann Oncol. 2012;23:2708–14.
11. Pignon JP, Bourhis J, Domenge C, Designé L. Chemotherapy added to locoregional treatment for head and neck squamous-cell carcinoma: three meta-analyses of updated individual data. MACH-NC Collaborative Group. Meta-Analysis of Chemotherapy on Head and Neck Cancer. Lancet. 2000;355(9208):949–55.
12. Adelstein DJ, Li Y, Adams GL, Wagner H Jr, Kish JA, Ensley JF, Schuller DE, Forastiere AA. An intergroup phase III comparison of standard radiation therapy and two schedules of concurrent chemoradiotherapy in patients with unresectable squamous cell head and neck cancer. J Clin Oncol. 2003;21:92–8.
13. Pignon JP, LeMaitre A, Maillard E, et al. Meta-analysis of chemotherapy in head and neck cancer (MACH-NC): an update on 93 randomized trials and 17,346 patients. Radiother Oncol. 2009;92:4–14.
14. Corvò R. Evidence-based radiation oncology in head and neck squamous cell carcinoma. Radiother Oncol. 2007;85:156–70.
15. Hitt R, López-Pousa A, Martínez-Trufero J, et al. Phase III study comparing cisplatin plus fluorouracil to paclitaxel, cisplatin, and fluorouracil induction chemotherapy followed by chemoradiotherapy in locally advanced head and neck cancer. J Clin Oncol. 2005;23:8636–45.
16. Janoray G, Pointreau Y, Garaud P, Chapet S, Alfonsi M, Sire C, Jadaud E, Calais G. Long-term results of a multicenter randomized phase III trial of induction chemotherapy with cisplatin, 5-fluorouracil, ± docetaxel for larynx preservation. J Natl Cancer Inst. 2015;108(4):djv368. https://doi.org/10.1093/jnci/djv368. 1 April 2016.
17. Lorch JH, Goloubeva O, Haddad RI, Cullen K, Sarlis N, Tishler R, Tan M, Fasciano J, Sammartino DE, Posner MR, TAX 324 Study Group. Induction chemotherapy with cisplatin and fluorouracil alone or in combination with docetaxel in locally advanced squamous-cell cancer of the head and neck: long-term results of the TAX 324 randomised phase 3 trial. Lancet Oncol. 2011;12:153–9. https://doi.org/10.1016/S1470-2045(10)70279-5.
18. Cohen EE, Karrison TG, Kocherginsky M, Mueller J, et al. Phase III randomized trial of induction chemotherapy in patients with N2 or N3 locally advanced head and neck cancer. J Clin Oncol. 2014;32:2735–43.
19. Bozec A, Benezery K, Ettaiche M, Chamorey E, Vandersteen C, et al. Induction chemotherapy-based larynx preservation program for locally advanced hypopharyngeal cancer: oncologic and functional outcomes and prognostic factors. Eur Arch Otorhinolaryngol. 2016;273:3299–306.
20. Bonner JA, Harari PM, Giralt J, Azarnia N, et al. Radiotherapy plus cetuximab for squamous-cell carcinoma of the head and neck. N Engl J Med. 2006;354:567–78.
21. Lefebvre JL, Pointreau Y, Rolland F, Alfonsi M, Baudoux A, et al. Induction chemotherapy followed by either chemoradiotherapy or bioradiotherapy for larynx preservation: the TREMPLIN randomized phase II study. J Clin Oncol. 2013;31:853–9.
22. Owen RD. The problem of hypopharyngeal carcinoma. Proc R Soc Med. 1950;43:157–70.
23. Bataini P, Brugere J, Bernier J, Jaulerry CH, Picot C, Ghossein NA. Results of radical radiotherapeutic treatment of carcinoma of the pyriform sinus: experience of the Institut Curie. Int J Radiat Oncol Biol Phys. 1982;8:1277–86.
24. Ahmad K, Fayos JV. Role of radiation therapy in carcinoma of the hypopharynx. Acta Radiol Oncol. 1984;23:21–6.
25. Huang WY, Jen YM, Chen CM, Su YF, Lin CS, Lin YS, Chang YN, Chao HL, Lin KT, Chang LP. Intensity modulated radiotherapy with concurrent chemotherapy for larynx preservation of advanced resectable hypopharyngeal cancer. Radiat Oncol. 2010;15(5):37.
26. Teoh M, Clark CH, Wood K, Whitaker S, Nisbet A. Volumetric modulated arc therapy: a review of current literature and clinical use in practice. Br J Radiol. 2011;84:967–96.

27. Moncharmont C, Vallard A, Guy JB, Prades JM, Rancoule C, Magné N. Real-life efficacy of volumetric modulated arc therapy in head and neck squamous cell carcinoma. Eur Ann Otorhinolaryngol Head Neck Dis. 2017;134:165–9.
28. Lacas B, Bourhis J, Overgaard J, Zhang Q, Grégoire V, Nankivell M, MARCH Collaborative Group, et al. Role of radiotherapy fractionation in head and neck cancers (MARCH): an updated meta-analysis. Lancet Oncol. 2017;18:1221–37.
29. Overgaard J, Mohanti BK, Begum N, Ali R, Agarwal JP, Kuddu M, Bhasker S, Tatsuzaki H, Grau C. Five versus six fractions of radiotherapy per week for squamous-cell carcinoma of the head and neck (IAEA-ACC study): a randomised, multicentre trial. Lancet Oncol. 2010;11:553–60.
30. Lefebvre JL. Candidates for larynx preservation: the next step? Oncologist. 2010;15(Suppl. 3):30–2.
31. Lagha A, Chraiet N, Labidi S, Rifi H, Ayadi M, et al. Larynx preservation: what is the best non-surgical strategy? Crit Rev Oncol Hematol. 2013;88:447–58.
32. Ang KK. Larynx preservation clinical trial design: summary of key recommendations of a consensus panel. Oncologist. 2010;15(Suppl. 3):25–9.
33. Caudell JJ, Carroll WR, Spencer SA, Bonner JA. Examination of laryngoesophageal dysfunction-free survival as an endpoint in nonsurgical treatment of squamous cell carcinomas of the larynx and hypopharynx. Cancer. 2011;117:4447–51.
34. Sherman EJ, Fisher SG, Kraus DH, Zelefsky MJ, et al. TALK score: development and validation of a prognostic model for predicting larynx preservation outcome. Laryngoscope. 2012;122:1043–50.
35. Rosenthal DI, Mohamed AS, Weber RS, Garden AS, et al. Long-term outcomes after surgical or nonsurgical initial therapy for patients with T4 squamous cell carcinoma of the larynx: a 3-decade survey. Cancer. 2015;121:1608–19.
36. Chen LY, Huang CC, Tsou YA, Bau DT, Tsai MH. Prognostic factor of severe complications in patients with hypopharyngeal cancer with primary concurrent chemoradiotherapy. Anticancer Res. 2015;35:1735–41.
37. Bradley PT, Bradley PJ. Treatment of hypopharyngeal carcinoma with primary chemoradiotherapy: functional morbidity. Curr Opin Otolaryngol Head Neck Surg. 2012;20:89–96.
38. Al-Mamgani A, Mehilal R, van Rooij PH, Tans L, Sewnaik A, Levendag PC. Toxicity, quality of life, and functional outcomes of 176 hypopharyngeal cancer patients treated by (chemo)radiation: the impact of treatment modality and radiation technique. Laryngoscope. 2012;122:1789–95.
39. Bossola M. Nutritional interventions in head and neck cancer patients undergoing chemoradiotherapy: a narrative review. Nutrients. 2015;7:265–76.
40. Eisbruch A, Schwartz M, Rasch C, Vineberg K, et al. Dysphagia and aspiration after chemoradiotherapy for head-and-neck cancer: which anatomic structures are affected and can they be spared by IMRT? Int J Radiat Oncol Biol Phys. 2004;60:1425–39.
41. Newman JR, Connolly TM, Illing EA, Kilgore ML, Locher JL, Carroll WR. Survival trends in hypopharyngeal cancer: a population-based review. Laryngoscope. 2015;125:624–9.

Salvage Surgery in Post-radiotherapy/ Chemoradiation in Carcinoma of the Larynx and Hypopharynx

13

Sudhir Bahadur

13.1 Introduction

Radiotherapy alone is the standard care of treatment for early disease of the larynx and hypopharynx. Similarly, cisplatin-based chemoradiation is an established treatment strategy for organ preservation in select moderately advanced lesions [1–4]. However, nearly 40% of cases are diagnosed with residual or recurrent locoregional disease after chemoradiation [5].

Salvage laryngectomy or neck dissection is usually available as a curative option for select patients of residual or recurrent disease, depending upon whether the disease has failed at the primary (local) site or in form of lymph node metastasis (but no evidence of primary tumour) or at both local and regional sites.

13.2 Diagnosis

Diagnosis of residual or recurrent tumour following radiotherapy or chemoradiation is often difficult and delayed. For laryngeal and hypopharyngeal lesions, mean interval from radiation to detection or recurrence was 14.5–10.6 months, respectively [6]. The clinical features suggesting residual/recurrent pathology include persistence or recurrence of symptoms and physical findings including radiation oedema usually beyond 2 months of completion of radiation/chemoradiation with or without fixation and widening of larynx [7]. Imaging studies including MRI and PET scan are extremely useful in further supporting the clinical suspicion. However, biopsy from the deeper tissues is required to confirm the diagnosis. Often the biopsy taking is difficult and may have to be repeated more than once. Negative biopsies do not exclude the presence of residual or recurrent neoplasm.

S. Bahadur (✉)
Department of Otolaryngology and Head-Neck Surgery, Formerly at All India Institute of Medical Sciences, New Delhi, India

S. Bahadur et al. (eds.), *Carcinoma of the Larynx and Hypopharynx*,
https://doi.org/10.1007/978-981-13-3110-7_13

There is suggestion in literature that the tumour may become larger (higher stage) as compared to initial stage following radiation/chemoradiation. It is because submucosal extent of disease is often underestimated. This fact is complicated by increased incidence of cartilage invasion and spread along the perivascular space and mucous glands [8]. Occasionally, the lesion may continue to grow and present as unresectable disease.

13.3 Re-irradiation

Re-irradiation is currently considered as effective treatment for carefully selected locally recurrent or second primary tumours of the head and neck in previously irradiated field. This has been made possible due to advances in technology (IMRT and stereotaxy) and safety in delivery of high-precision radiotherapy. However, despite several advances there are limitations and still not enough data on the subject.

13.4 Salvage Surgery

It has been estimated that feasibility of salvage surgery for tumour recurrence is generally low; of the patients with locoregional failure without distant metastasis, 27.3% of these could not have salvage surgery and died because of disease progression within a few months [9].

It has been reported that 33–66% of the patients with local and/or regional recurrences after chemoradiation underwent salvage surgery for carcinoma of the larynx and hypopharynx [6] (Figs. 13.1, 13.2, 13.3, 13.4, and 13.5).

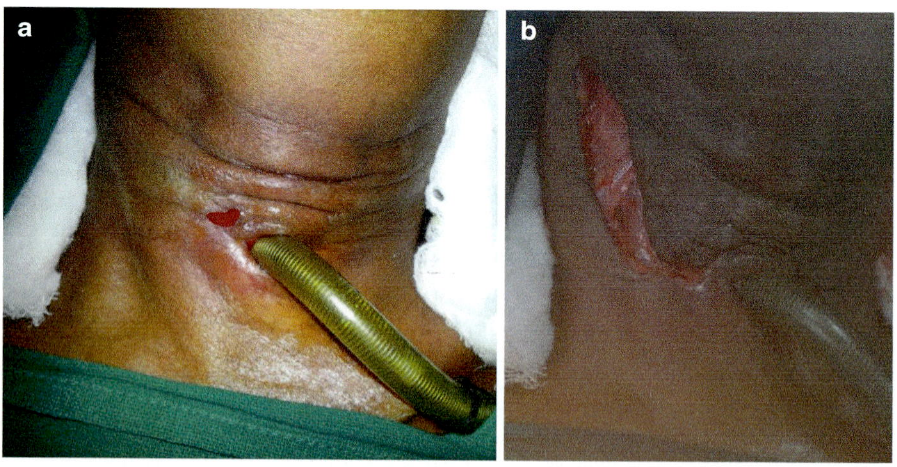

Fig. 13.1 (**a**) Irradiated skin. Preoperative tracheostomy (**b**) Raising of the skin flaps via Apron-collar incision.

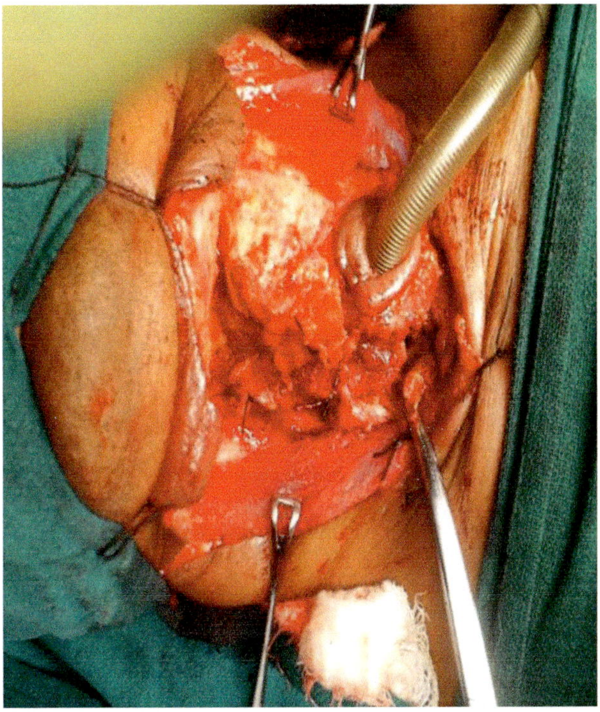

Fig. 13.2 Raising of the skin flaps and skeletonization of the larynx

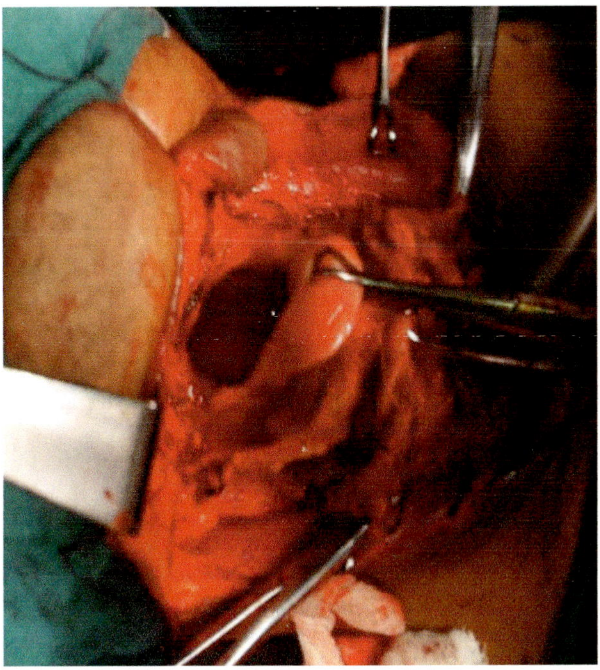

Fig. 13.3 Opening of the larynx

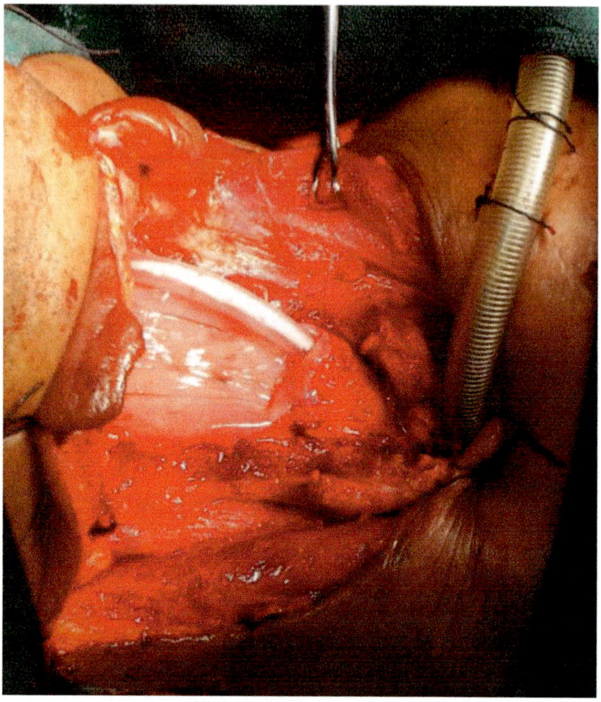

Fig. 13.4 Larynx specimen has been removed. Remaining hypopharyngeal mucosa seen in the picture with Ryle's tube

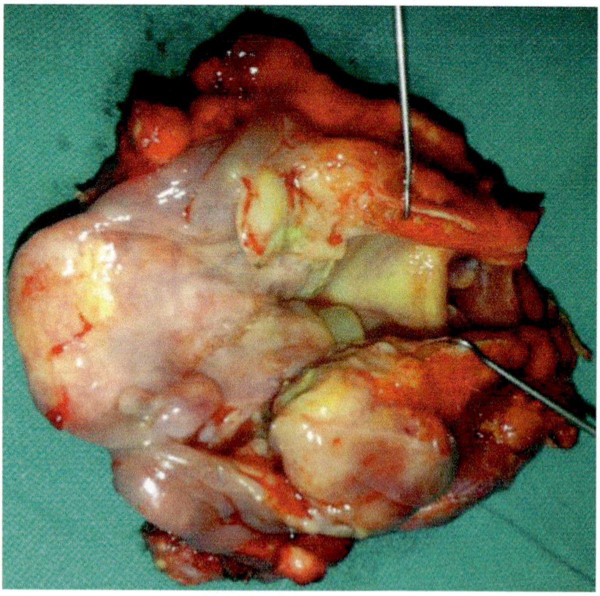

Fig. 13.5 Laryngectomy specimen. Note the grossly oedematous larynx

The extent of salvage surgery is debated in literature. Total laryngectomy with or without a neck dissection is often required for residual or recurrent resectable disease following radiotherapy or chemoradiotherapy failure. Recurrences after radiotherapy are often not salvageable by partial laryngectomy, though it has been described in early lesion [10–12]. Biller et al. defined criteria for vertical hemilaryngectomy after radiation failure [13]. It is suggested that 30–60% patients of T_1 and T_2 lesions can be salvaged with partial laryngectomy [14]. However, the recurrence should correlate with the original primary tumour before radiotherapy in case partial laryngectomy is undertaken. The partial laryngectomy after radiation may lead to persistent laryngeal oedema, delayed decannulation and increased hospital stay.

13.5 Morbidity

It is well known that morbidity of salvage surgery in residual or recurrent disease is relatively high. The development of pharyngocutoneous fistula formation, following total laryngectomy often mars healing of wound, increases the morbidity and prolongs the hospitalisation of the patients. High fistula rates of 11–75% after salvage laryngectomy have been reported by several authors [15–21]. This variation in the rates of fistula formation depend upon the dose of radiation, tumour stage and site of disease and time from initial therapy. The combination of chemoradiation further increases the complication rates [15, 16].

The increase in complications has been blamed on several factors including poor nutrition and immune status [15]. However, the only significant predictor noted has been radiotherapy/chemoradiotherapy; besides, other predictors mentioned include lower postoperative haemoglobin, low albumin level, prior tracheostomy, tobacco and alcohol use, early removal of drains and surgical procedures involving the hypopharynx [20–24]. Whether the interval between chemoradiation and salvage surgery influences the fistula formation remains unclear.

13.6 Prevention

Some authors have proposed the use of elective gastrostomy or creating oropharyngeal fistula to reduce the impact of fistula formation [25, 26].

The pectoralis major myocutaneous flaps have been found to be very useful to cover important structures in the neck with which vascularised tissue from nonirradiated area is raised to minimise the healing problems. Smith et al. [27] reported significant reduction in the fistula rate with the use of pectoralis major myocutaneous flap for reconstruction. Similarly, Sayle et al. [28] reviewed the meta-analysis of 33 studies and found only 10% fistula rate for salvage laryngectomy with 'onlay' flap reinforced closure versus 28% fistula rate with salvage laryngectomy when no flap was used. Likewise, Paleri et al. [29] described in a systemic review of nearly 600 patients, a reduced risk of fistula by one third was noted in patients who had flap reconstruction carried out. Several other authors have also noted the usefulness in significantly reducing the fistula formation from 73% to 13% when the flap was used in subgroup of patients with diabetes, vascular disease or poor nutritional status [30]. Free vascular flaps like radial forearm flaps have also been used to reconstruct the laryngectomy defects to reduce the fistula rate [31, 32].

13.7 Management of Neck Metastasis

In presence of isolated neck metastasis after initial radiation/chemoradiation, a neck dissection is indicated after local recurrence or second primary cancer has been excluded by CT scan and endoscopy. The complication rate is usually low because the pharynx is not opened. The indication of neck dissection is based on clinical and radiological suspicion. The neck dissection may be considered overtreatment particularly if no viable tumour is found on final histopathology. The main issue lies in distinguishing scarred lymph nodes from nodes which contain viable tumour [33]. Positron emission tomography so far does not seem to answer the question [34].

Patients with positive node have a tendency for further regional recurrences and distant metastasis; however, most authors advocate a neck dissection for all patients with N_2 or N_3 resectable disease. However, doing a radical neck dissection versus a selective neck dissection is still a subject of debate.

13.8 Oncologic Outcome

Several authors have commented upon less than satisfactory results following salvage surgery in radiation/chemoradiation failed cases. Parsons et al. [35] noted 5-year local disease control following salvage surgery of 58% versus 70% in previous radiation and chemoradiation failures, respectively. However, the overall survival rate was 27% and 50% in two groups. Several other authors have also reported poor 5-year survival rates of 20–40% [33–35].

In contrast, a few authors have published good 5-year survival rates of 63–86% but mostly in patients with early disease (T_1 and T_2) who underwent salvage surgery following radiation failures [11, 36, 37]. In hypopharyngeal cancer, though, salvage surgery is possible only in a few selected patients but usually with poor outcome [6, 21].

Several authors have commented upon the poor prognostic factors including the aggressive tumour biology in residual and recurrent disease, comorbidity, older age, nodal metastasis with extra capsular spread of disease, and positive surgical margins [5, 23]. It is because of low survival after salvage surgery, particularly in advanced lesions and high complication rate and consequent morbidity, that the advantage of salvage surgery is sometimes questioned [5]. However, in properly selected patients of early to moderate size tumours in younger patients, salvage surgery has an important role to play in treatment of residual or recurrent disease and is an integral part of organ preservation.

13.9 Authors' Comment

Role of radiotherapy in treatment of early tumours of the larynx and hypopharynx resulting in organ preservation is well established. Similarly, several advances have been made in select advanced tumours with chemoradiation to achieve a similar aim. However, a significant number of patients are likely to fail either locally or regionally or both within 2 years of treatment. It is extremely important to carefully follow up these patients at regular intervals and maintain high index of suspicion for any recurrences. Diagnosis is difficult, and MRI is a useful technique to reinforce the clinical suspicion. Endoscopy and biopsy may have to be done more than once to confirm the diagnosis. The morbidity following salvage surgery is considerable and can be minimised to significant extent by using vascularised flaps from nonirradiated area, e.g. pectoralis major myocutaneous flap from the chest. The rates of pharyngocutaneous fistula formation, thus, can be reduced. Open partial laryngectomy or endoscopic laser surgery is possible in select early lesions of the larynx or hypopharynx with good outcome. However, most recurrences will require total laryngectomy with guarded prognosis based on stage of disease. However, outcome in hypopharyngeal cancer following salvage surgery is poor.

Patients with persistent neck node metastasis (N_1) after radiation/chemoradiation failure need to be treated with modified radical neck dissection or radical neck dissection. Role of selection of neck dissection is debatable. However, in cases with N_1 disease where node has disappeared following treatment may be observed with FDG PET and if the latter is negative can be followed up.

Patients with N_2 or N_3 resectable disease require treatment with radical neck dissection irrespective of type of response to radiotherapy/chemoradiation.

13.10 Quality of Life in Patients After Concurrent Chemoradiotherapy vs Total Laryngectomy

Curative treatment of advanced cancers of the larynx and hypopharynx has traditionally consisted of total laryngectomy with or without pharyngectomy. The morbidity resulting from surgery is considerable in form of permanent tracheostome and loss of speech, though patient can be helped a great deal with vocal rehabilitation.

In the last two decades, however, there has been greater use of sequential or concurrent chemoradiotherapy conserving the pharyngo-laryngeal organ. Its feasibility and efficacy in organ preservation and oncologic control have received sufficient attention in literature [1, 38–40].

In early years, most authors believed that not sacrificing the larynx was good enough to maintain quality of life without appreciating that toxic effects of chemotherapy and radiotherapy itself may impair the quality of life. There are a few studies which have assessed the long-term quality of life issues after total laryngectomy and after chemoradiation [41–44]. These studies mentioned significant increase in acute and late toxic effects compared with conventional radiotherapy alone. In acute stage, nausea, haematopoietic toxic reactions and severe mucositis are important features, whereas long-term problems include compromised oral functioning, swallowing, soft tissue fibrosis and discomfort and pain.

Guibest et al. [45] used the EORTC QOL questionnaire comprising a generic (QLQ-C30) [43] and head and neck cancer-specific sectran (QLQ-H&N35) [44]. It was observed that by combining the two sections, much more useful information could be gained for assessment of QOL. It was shown that patients managed by sequential or concurrent chemoradiotherapy showed greater symptoms of dry mouth and thick saliva than those undergoing postoperative radiotherapy following surgery probably due to accumulation of toxicity.

The literature contains contradictory reports regarding quality of life following chemoradiation or laryngectomy. The former (chemoradiation group) was found to be associated with significantly better QOL [46], whereas several authors have not found any significant difference in the two groups [42, 45–48]. Some authors have also demonstrated preservation of overall quality of life despite the loss of laryngeal function [42]. Nevertheless, physical change in self-image, difficulty in communication and social isolation are some of the issues following total laryngectomy which may impair quality of life [49].

13.11 Voice and Swallowing

Post-radiation xerostomia, fibrosis oedema and mucositis may have a negative effect on both voice and swallowing. Besides, a significant number of patients in concurrent chemoradiation group demonstrate difficulty in swallowing. Forastiere et al. [39] noted that 3% of patients in this group could not swallow, requiring regular dilatation or PEG or gastrostomy 1 year after treatment with chemoradiation. Also, nearly one fourth cases in this group were only able to swallow soft food or liquids. Similarly, a small number of cases were on permanent tracheostomy. These issues, though occurring in significant minority of patients in concurrent chemoradiotherapy group, impair the functional results and thus quality of life of patients.

Significantly, several authors did not observe any difference between treatment groups with regard to voice and swallowing disorder [45, 50, 51]. Several factors may explain this phenomenon. It could be due to effectiveness of vocal rehabilitation following laryngectomy. Another reason for absence of differences in two groups could be because QOC was assessed in these studies 1 year after treatment was over and that probably allowed patients to recover from acute side effects [44]. However, QOL is impaired to varying degree in almost all patients whether treated by medical or surgical management affecting different aspects [9]. Despite this, presumption persists that post-treatment QOL is generally better following chemoradiation than with surgery [41].

There is growing evidence that suggests that though organ sacrifice may have detrimental functional effect, patients often get rehabilitated or adapt much better than was anticipated and overall QOL is usually maintained [42, 52, 53]. Besides it is not commonly recognised that preservation of a nonfunctional organ (larynx) is of little value [41] and as such significantly impairs the quality of life.

References

1. Forastiere AA, Coepfert H, Maor M, et al. Concurrent chemo-therapy and radio-therapy for organ preservation in advanced laryngeal cancer. N Engl J Med. 2003;349:2091–8.
2. Wolf GT, Hong WK. Induction chemotherapy for organ preservation in advanced laryngeal cancer: is there a role? Head Neck. 1995;17:279–83.
3. Lefebvre JL, Chevalier D, Luboinski B, et al. Larynx preservation in pyriform sinus cancer; preliminary results of a European Organisation for research and treatment of cancer phase III trial. EURTC Head and Neck Cancer Co-operative Group. J Natl Cancer Inst. 1996;88:890–9.
4. Lefebvre JL, Rolland F, Tresselar M, et al. Phase III randomized trial on larynx preservation comparing sequential versus alternating chemotherapy and radiotherapy. J Natl Cancer Inst. 2009;101:142–52.
5. Van-Der Putten L, De Bree R, Doornaert PA, et al. Salvage surgery in post-chemo-radiotherapy laryngeal and hypopharyngeal carcinoma: outcome and review. Acta Otorhinolaryngol Ital. 2015;35:162–72.
6. Sandro J, Stoeckli SJ, Pawlik AB, Margereta L, et al. Salvage surgery after failure of non-surgical therapy for carcinoma of the larynx and hypopharynx. Arch Otolaryngol Head Neck Surg. 2000;126:1473–7.
7. Bahadur S, Amatya RC, Kackar SK. Enigma of post-radiotherapy oedema in diagnosis of residual or recurrent disease of larynx and pyriform fossa. J Laryngol Otol. 1985;99:763–5.
8. Brandenburg JH, Condon KG, Frank W. Coronal sections of larynges from radiation therapy failures: a clinical pathologic study. Otolaryngol Head Neck Surg. 1986;95:213–8.
9. Suzuki K, Hayashi R, Ebihara M, et al. The effectiveness of chemo-radiation therapy and salvage surgery for hypopharyngeal squamous cell carcinoma. Jpn J Clin Oncol. 2013;43:1210–7.
10. Supriano G, Pellini R, Romano G, et al. Supracricoid partial laryngectomy as salvage surgery after radiation failure. Head Neck. 2002;24:759–63.
11. Nibu K, Kamata S, Kawabata K, et al. Partial laryngectomy in treatment of radiation failure of early glottic carcinoma. Head Neck. 1997;19:116–20.
12. Lydiatt WM, Shah JP, Lydiatt KM. Conservation surgery for recurrent carcinoma of the glottic larynx. Am J Surg. 1996;172:662–4.
13. Biller HF, Barnhill FR, Ogura JH. Hemilaryngectomy for radiation failure for carcinoma of vocal cord. Laryngoscope. 1970;80:249.
14. Walters GW, Patel SG, Rhys-Evans PH. Partial laryngectomy for recurrent laryngeal carcinoma. Clin Otolaryngol Allied Sci. 2000;25:146–52.
15. Ganly I, Patel S, Matsuo J, et al. Post-operative complications of salvage total laryngectomy. Cancer. 2005;103:2073–81.
16. Weber RS, Berkey BA, Forastiere A, et al. Outcome of salvage total laryngectomy following organ preservation therapy. The radiation therapy oncology trial 91-11. Arch Otolaryngol Head Neck Surg. 2003;129:44–9.
17. Sarkar S, Mehta SA, Tiwari J, et al. Complications following surgery for carcinoma of the larynx and pyriform fossa. J Surg Oncol. 1990;43:245–9.
18. Johanson IV, Overgaard O, Elbrond O. Pharyngocutaneous fistula after laryngectomy Influence of previous radiotherapy and prophylactic metronidazole. Cancer. 1988;61:673–8.
19. Bahadur S, Amatya RC, Kacker SK, Madan N. Etiology and management of pharyngocutaneous fistulae following laryngectomy. Indian J Otolaryngol. 1985;37:1–3.
20. Davidson J, Keane T, Brown D, et al. Surgical salvage after radiotherapy for advanced laryngopharyngeal carcinoma. Arch Otolaryngol Head Neck Surg. 1997;123:420–4.

21. Lavalle RJ, Maw AR. The etiology of post-laryngectomy pharyngocutaneous fistulae. J Laryngol Otol. 1972;86:785–93.
22. Leon X, Qner M, Orns CL, et al. Results of salvage surgery for local or regional recurrence after larynx preservation with induction chemotherapy and radiotherapy. Head Neck. 2001;23:733–78.
23. Tan HK, Giger R, Auperin A, et al. Salvage surgery after concomitant chemo-radiation in head and neck squamous cell carcinomas – stratification for post-salvage survival. Head Neck. 2010;32:139–47.
24. Paydarfar JA, Birkmeyar NJ. Complications in head and neck surgery: a meta-analysis of post-laryngectomy pharyngocutaneous fistula. Arch Otolaryngol Head Neck Surg. 2006;132:67–72.
25. Panje WR, Namon AJ, Vokes E, et al. Surgical management of the head and neck cancer patient following concomitant multimodal therapy. Laryngoscope. 1995;105:97–101.
26. Lee JH, Marchtay M, Unger LD, et al. Prophylactic gastrostomy tubes in patients undergoing intensive irradiation for cancer of the head and neck. Arch Otolaryngol Head Neck Surg. 1998;124:871–5.
27. Smith TJ, Burrage KJ, Ganguli P, et al. Prevention of post laryngectomy pharyngocutaneous fistula: the Memorial University experience. J Otolaryngol. 2003;32:222–5.
28. Sayles M, Grant DG. Preventing pharyngocutaneous fistula in total laryngectomy: a systematic reviewed and meta-analysis. Laryngoscope. 2014;124:1150–63.
29. Paleri V, Drinnan M, Van den Brackel MW, et al. Vascularized flaps to reduce fistula following salvage total laryngectomy: a systemic review. Laryngoscope. 2014;124:1848–53.
30. Righini C, Lequeux T, van den Burg CD, et al. The pectoralis myofascial flap in pharyngolaryngeal surgery after radiotherapy. Eur Arch Otolaryngol. 2005;262:357–61.
31. Tsou YA, Hua CH, Lin MH, et al. Comparison of pharyngocutaneous fistula between patients following by primary laryngopharyngectomy and salvage laryngopharyngectomy for advanced hypopharyngeal cancer. Head Neck. 2010;32:1494–500.
32. Withrow KP, Rosenthal EL, Gourin CG, et al. Free tissue transfer to manage salvage laryngectomy defects after organ preservation failure. Laryngoscope. 2007;117:781–4.
33. Relic A, Scheich M, Stapf J, et al. Salvage surgery after induction chemotherapy with paclitaxel/cisplatin and primary radiotherapy for advanced laryngeal and hypopharyngeal carcinoma. Eur Arch Otolaryngol. 2009;266:1799–180.
34. Brokovich VS, Miller FR, Karnad AB, et al. Role of positron emission tomography scans in the management of the N Positive neck in head and neck carcinoma after radio-therapy. Laryngoscope. 2006;116:855–8.
35. Parsons JT, Mendelhall WM, Stringer SP, et al. Salvage surgery following radiation failure in squamous cell carcinoma of the supraglottis larynx. Int J Radiat Oncol Biol Phys. 1995;32:605–9.
36. McLaughlin MP, Parson JT, Fein DA, et al. Salvage surgery after radiotherapy failure in T_1-T_2 squamous cell carcinoma of the glottis larynx. Head Neck. 1996;18:229–35.
37. Chambell BH, Goepfert H. Partial laryngectomy as a salvage procedure for radiation failure. In: Kagan AR, Miles J, editors. Head and neck oncology clinical management. New York: Pergamon Press Inc; 1989. p. 91–5.
38. The Department of Veterans Affairs Laryngeal Cancer Study Groups. Induction chemotherapy plus radiation compared with surgery and radiation in patients with advance laryngeal cancer. N Engl J Med. 1991;324:1685–90.
39. Posner MR, Hershock DM, Blajman CR, et al. Cisplatin and fluorouracil alone or with decetaxel in head and neck cancer. N Engl J Med. 2007;357:1705–15.
40. Lefebvre JL. What is the role of primary surgery in the treatment of laryngeal and hypopharyngeal cancer? Arch Otolaryngol Head Neck Surg. 2000;126:285–8.
41. Lefebvre JL, Latigau E. Preservation of form and function during management of cancer of larynx and hypopharynx. World J Surg. 2003;27:811–6.
42. Hanna E, Sherman A, Cash D, et al. Quality of life for patients following total laryngectomy vs chemo-radiation for laryngeal preservation. Arch Otolaryngol Head Neck Surg. 2004;130:875–9.

43. Aaronson NK, Ahmedzai S, Bergman B, et al. European organisation for research and treatment of Cancer QLQC30: a quality of life instrument for use in international clinical trials in oncology. J Natl Cancer Inst. 1993;85:365–76.
44. Bjordal K, Hammerlid E, Abiner Almqvisr M, et al. Quality of life in head and neck cancer patients: validation of the European Organisation for Research and Treatment Cancer Quality of life Questionnaire. H & N 35. J Clin Oncol. 1999;17:1008–19.
45. Guibert M, Lepage B, Woisard V, et al. Quality of life in patients treated for advanced hypopharyngeal or laryngeal cancer. Eur Ann Otolaryngol Head Neck. 2011;128:218–23.
46. Boscolo-Rizzo P, Maranato F, Marchiori C, et al. Long term quality of life after total laryngectomy and post operative radiotherapy versus concurrent chemo-radiotherapy for laryngeal preservation. Laryngoscope. 2008;118:300–6.
47. Trivedi NP, Swaminathan DK, Thanakappan KK, et al. Comparison of quality of life in advanced laryngeal cancer patients after concurrent chemoradiotherapy vs total laryngectomy. Otolaryngol Head Neck Surg. 2008;139:702–7.
48. El-Deiry M, Funk GF, Nalwa S, et al. Long term quality of life for surgical and non-surgical treatment of head and neck cancer. Arch Otolaryngol Head Neck Surg. 2005;131:879–85.
49. Ramirez MJ, Ferriol EE, Domenech FG, et al. Psychosocial adjustment in patients surgically treated for laryngeal cancer. Otolaryngol Head Neck Surg. 2003;129:92–7.
50. Terrel JE, Fisher SG, Wolf GT, The Veterans Affairs Laryngeal Cancer Study Group. Long term quality of life after treatment of laryngeal Cancer. Arch Otolaryngol Head Neck Surg. 1998;124:854–971.
51. Deleylannis FW, Weymuller EA Jr, Coltrera MD, et al. Quality of life after laryngectomy: are disabilities important? Head Neck. 1999;21:319–24.
52. Morton RP, Izzard ME. Quality of Life outcomes in head and neck cancer patient's. World J Surg. 2003;27:884–9.
53. de Graeff A, de Leepw JR, Ross WJ, et al. Long term quality of life of patients with head and neck cancer. Laryngoscope. 2000;110:98–106.

Surgical Complications and Management

14

Sudhir Bahadur

14.1 Introduction

The complications following major surgery are not uncommon, and these often produce considerable morbidity, prolonged hospital stay, delayed access to postoperative adjuvant treatment and even mortality. It is important for the surgeon to be aware and inform the patient and relatives accordingly. While it may not be possible to discuss all the complications, it is still useful to mention the common general and specific complications that might occur in the intra- or postoperative period. General complications relate to risk of undergoing any major surgery, whereas, the specific ones relate to the particular surgical procedure [1, 2]. A complication can thus be described as an adverse event which affects recovery of the patient.

Most patients of carcinoma of the larynx and hypopharynx have a history of tobacco intake in the form of smoking and usually associated with alcohol consumption. These are thus likely to be associated with cardiovascular and respiratory ailments, and these comorbidities are likely to produce an effect on the recovery as well as on the prognosis [1–4]. The anaesthetist involved should be consulted preoperatively, and he may suggest further medical attention, if required.

14.2 Management

The development of medical complication is associated with prolonged hospital stay and increased mortality [5]. Similarly, attention should be paid to the comorbidities to reduce the surgical complication rates [6].

S. Bahadur (✉)
Department of Otolaryngology and Head-Neck Surgery, Formerly at All India Institute of Medical Sciences, New Delhi, India

S. Bahadur et al. (eds.), *Carcinoma of the Larynx and Hypopharynx*,
https://doi.org/10.1007/978-981-13-3110-7_14

14.2.1 Cardiovascular

Patients may be classified into low-, medium- or high-risk cases based on number of risks present. The rate of DVT and subsequent pulmonary embolism in the head and neck surgery is low (less than 1%) [7].
Ischaemic heart disease is common in patients of carcinoma of the larynx and hypopharynx because of previous history of smoking. Myocardial infarction may occur in the postoperative period due to imbalance between myocardial oxygen supply and demand in presence of pre-existing coronary artery disease. Therefore, preoperative assessment and optimization are necessary. The myocardial infarction usually occurs 1–4 days after surgery when effects of anaesthesia decline and perioperative pain and fluid shifts occur [8].

14.2.2 Respiratory

14.2.2.1 Pneumonia

Most patients because of previous exposure to smoking suffer from chronic obstructive pulmonary disease [9]. It is important to optimize the lung functions preoperatively with chest physiotherapy, antibiotics and bronchodilators, if necessary. The tracheostomy if carried out for respiratory obstruction may also increase chances of postoperative pneumonia. Likewise, major surgical procedures on the thorax and abdomen as required for total laryngopharyngo-oesophagectomy may also impair chest function and predispose to pneumonitis.

14.2.2.2 Aspiration

Aspiration can be a serious complication in patients undergoing partial laryngectomy, particularly the supraglottic laryngectomy. Since most patients are in the middle and elderly age groups and have been exposed to smoking and thus may have poor chest status, preoperative evaluation and assessment should be carried out before planning conservation surgery.

14.2.2.3 Pneumothorax

The pleura may be injured during surgery while performing dissection low in the neck or during surgery like total laryngopharyngo-oesophagectomy. Pneumothorax produces compromise on respiratory and circulatory systems and results in difficult breathing and decrease in oxygen saturation. The pneumothorax if considered > 15% on chest X-ray should be considered for chest tube drainage [10].

14.2.3 Nutrition

All patients should be assessed preoperatively as well as postoperatively to monitor nutrition level in order to ensure good wound healing and minimal complications.

Various measures noted include weight, body mass index (BMI) and skinfold measurements (e.g. triceps) and noting the serum albumen and lymphocyte count [2]. Dietician should be consulted beforehand.

14.2.4 Specific Metabolic Complications

14.2.4.1 Shock

Shock should be avoided in the postoperative period because it can lead to adverse results. If it does happen, it should be diagnosed early so that prompt action can be taken. In the state of shock, the circulation is not able to meet the metabolic requirements of the body. It can be either due to lack of circulating fluid (hypovolaemic shock) or due to failing heart (cardiogenic shock) or due to increased metabolic needs of the body (septic shock) [2]. Early management includes giving oxygen and infusion with isotonic crystalloids. Ringers: lactate or normal saline is the initial fluid requirement, 1–2 L given as the initial rapid bolus. Total amount of fluid given is roughly 3 ml for each ml of blood loss [11]. It is extremely important to measure the urinary output to monitor tissue perfusion (about 30–50 ml/h for most adults). Besides, mental state, peripheral perfusion, pulse and blood pressure should be constantly monitored. Blood transfusion should be considered based upon the estimate of blood loss. Patients who do not respond to crystalloid fluids of 1–2 L may be considered for central venous pressure (CVP) catheter [2].

Septic shock is defined as sepsis along with persistent hypotension despite fluid transfusion and still producing tissue hypoperfusion [12]. Postoperative infection may lead to either localized lesion or extensive systemic inflammatory response syndrome (SIRs). Patients in elderly age group with comorbidities or immune-compromised conditions or on chemotherapy or with liver or kidney disease or HIV patients are vulnerable for development of SIRs.

Complications of septic shock include central nervous system dysfunction, adult respiratory distress syndrome (ARDS), liver failure, acute renal failure (ARF) and disseminated intravascular coagulation (DIC). The reported mortality rate is high. Therefore septic shock should be diagnosed early and treated aggressively in the intensive care unit for regular monitoring. Broad-spectrum antibiotics are given parenterally to cover gram-positive, gram-negative and anaerobic bacteria.

14.2.4.2 Calcium Level

The estimation of calcium levels is important after total thyroidectomy or even after laryngectomy. The incidence is higher in patients receiving radiotherapy either preoperatively or postoperatively. Postoperatively monitoring of serum calcium and thyroid function test is required in patients undergoing total laryngopharyngo-oesophagectomy for extensive hypopharyngeal cancers and in whom total thyroidectomy is part of surgery. These patients need to be observed for evidence of hypocalcemic tetany, and urgent measures need to be taken to correct serum calcium levels.

14.2.4.3 Electrolyte Disturbances

The most common electrolyte change in the postoperative period is hyponatremia characterized by mental changes and depression. It is usually dilutional, through it may be related to secretion of antidiuretic hormone.

14.2.5 Bleeding

Postoperative haemorrhage has been usually classified as immediate (primary), reactionary (within 24 h) or secondary (within 5–10 days). It is important to ensure there is complete haemostasis obtained at the end of surgery. Reactionary haemorrhage is attributed to the opening of the vessel in spasm or slippage of inadequately applied tie or clip to the vessel as blood pressure rises after anaesthesia.

It is important to diagnose the problem early so that patient can be returned to the operation theatre, wound opened and bleeding controlled. In the meantime, resuscitative measures, including the replacement of fluids and blood transfusion, should be arranged.

Immediate measures include assessing the full blood count, coagulation factors and electrolytes. An assessment should be made for the need of blood transfusion, Vit K (in case of elevated PT), protamine sulphate (if heparin-overdose) and clotting factors or fresh frozen plasma.

The major vessels with potential source for bleeding during and after neck dissection are the carotid artery and branches of external carotid, the thyro-cervical trunk, transverse cervical artery and the internal jugular vein. The bleeding following the major surgery may manifest in the form of swelling at the local site or the ongoing filling of the surgical drain. Drainage may also fail if the drain becomes blocked by a clot or the vacuum seal fails.

14.2.6 Hematoma

It is important to avoid the postoperative hematoma by careful haemostasis and closed suction drains. Ongoing bleeding manifested by expanding haematoma will indicate immediate return to the theatre.

The wound is reopened and saline irrigation is carried out. Bleeding points are then identified and controlled. However, if haematoma is not expanding and is small to moderate (due to nonfunctional drains), haematoma can be drained in the minor OT and pressure bandage applied for 24–48 h.

Secondary haemorrhage commonly occurs 5–10 days after surgery and is usually due to infection and thus treated with antibiotics. Re-exploration of the wound may be required to control the bleeding.

14.2.7 Internal Jugular Vein Injury

The vein has to be handled with care while simultaneously protecting the vagus, hypoglossal and accessory nerves. A large accidental rent in the vein should be repaired with a running 6-0 nylon suture. However, the possibility of air embolism should be kept in mind and measures to be taken accordingly.

14.2.8 Air Embolism

An air embolism can occur when a large vein is inadvertently injured, and significant amount of air enters into the open vein by negative pressure and passes into the right atrium leading to tamponade of the heart and even prove fatal. It is characterized by clinical cyanosis, hypotension and loud churning noise over the precordium and disappearance of peripheral pulse [11, 12].

The patient should be placed in left Trendelenburg position as soon as venous injury occurs to minimize the risk of air embolism. The other measures in management include direct pressure, stopping nitrous oxide from anaesthesia circuit increasing the venous pressure. The rent should be identified and vein carefully repaired.

14.2.9 Carotid Blow Out

The incidence of carotid artery rupture occurs in 3–4% of patients undergoing neck dissection [13]. Intraoperative repair in stable patients can be performed with nylon sutures with or without shunting. In select patients of tumour invasion, carotid resection with replacement by saphenous vein or synthetic graft can be carried out with the help of a vascular surgeon. However, it is important to preoperatively assess these patients carefully on the MRI.

Risk factors for postoperative carotid artery rupture due to arterial wall necrosis, include previous radiotherapy, flap necrosis and pharyngocutaneous fistula formation. Most patients have prodromal bleeding or warning signals usually 48 h before the actual rupture of the vessel. It is important to surgically intervene at this stage and take the patient to theatre; debridement of the wound (wound toilet) and placement of a vascularised tissue hike myocutaneous flap from the nonirradiated area to cover the carotid and the wound may help avert the carotid blow out. The patient is simultaneously resuscitated with adequate fluids, and blood transfusion and proper antibiotics are administered.

However, in situations of impending or acute carotid blow out, immediate resuscitative measures are taken, and the airway is secured with cuffed tracheostomy tube. Apart from large volume of saline infusion, 4–6 units of blood are tested and crossmatched. If radiology facilities exist, patient can be referred for angiography which is both diagnostic and therapeutic [13, 14]. Temporary balloon test may also be carried out which will reveal adequacy of contralateral carotid artery to the circle of Wills. If assessed, adequate, ligation or embolisation of the ipsilateral vessel can be done with a lower risk of neurological deficit. On the other hand, if collateral supply is insufficient, the options will include stenting or arterial bypass surgery [2]. However, in situations where intervention radiology is not available, surgical intervention will include debridement of the wound and ligation of the vessel with a transfixation suture through healthy portion of the vessel wall with a reported median mortality rate of 40% and neurological complication rate of 9–84% (median 60%) [13].

14.2.10 Chyle Leak

Incidence of chylous fistula is approximately between 1% and 5.8% following neck dissection, mostly on the left side.

The thoracic duct is located behind the left common carotid artery and the vagus nerve. It then arches upwards, forwards and laterally behind the internal jugular vein. It comes in relation with scalene anterior muscle and phrenic nerve and opens into internal jugular vein, subclavian vein or their junction. Thoracic duct usually receives multiple minor lymphatic channels at its upper end, each of which may need to be ligated [14].

Chyle leak is identified as clear fluid intraoperatively and is confirmed by increased flow on valsalva manoeuvre by the anaesthetist who changes the ventilatory circuit to manual and closes the expiratory valve which increases circuit pressure to about 30 mmHg.

Usually, it is not necessary to identify the vessel (duct) as it is very fragile and surrounded by fatty tissue and prone to injury. However, if the leak is identified during surgery, the thoracic duct is ligated along with the surrounding tissue with a non-absorbable suture without going through the vessel wall. In case this procedure fails, fibrin sealant or vicryl mesh may be applied; muscle flaps have been used in severe cases.

Chylous fistula should be suspected in case milky fluid appears in the postoperative period from the neck drain. It may be confirmed either by assessing triglycerides greater than 100 mg/dl or chylomicrons more than 4% in the fluid. Most surgeons favour initial medical management including the fat-free diet and pressure dressing and aspiration of collection under the skin flap. Persistent chyle leak can cause nutritional, immunological and electrolyte imbalance. The collection of fluid can also cause necrosis of the skin flaps and can result in infection.

Indications of re-exploration include complications such as flap necrosis, declining general condition and high-output leak (>300 ml/day) [2, 14]. Identifying and ligating the duct may be difficult due to friable tissue; patient may be placed in the Trendelenburg position, and with continuous positive pressure, ventilation can help locate the duct. Sometimes, the use of operating microscope may also be useful.

14.2.11 Local Infection

Surgical site infection has been described as the most frequent complication with significant rates close to 20% [15–17].

Usually local wound infection is rare after clean procedures such as neck dissection where mucosa has not been opened, and many surgeons may not even advocate prophylactic antibiotics in such situations.

However, in clean contaminated procedures such as total laryngectomy where pharyngeal mucosa has been opened, prophylactic use of antibiotics is indicated. There is some debate whether a single intraoperative dose of broad-spectrum antibiotic followed by 24–48 h of the same drug is as effective as 5–7 days treatment.

There is evidence in literature that short course of antibiotics is as effective, though, in Indian context 5–7 days of antibiotic therapy is preferred.

Various preoperative risk factors have been described that increase the infection rate. These have been classified according to patient factors, tumour factors and type of surgical procedure.

(a) Patient factors include nutritional deficiency, diabetes, tobacco and alcohol consumption and poor oro-dental hygiene.
(b) Tumour factors include stage, site and prior treatment with radiotherapy or chemoradiation and preoperative tracheostomy.
(c) Surgical procedure performed – intraoperative risk factors include whether partial or total laryngectomy or total laryngopharyngo-oesophagectomy with or without a neck dissection has been performed.

Another source of wound infection is methicillin-resistant *Staphylococcus aureus* (MRSA) complicating postoperative recovery [2, 19]. Likewise, elderly patients with a septic focus or who stay in intensive care unit for prolonged periods are particularly vulnerable. Strict patient isolation, hygiene and help from microbiology department are extremely important.

14.2.12 Pharyngocutaneous Fistula

The development of pharyngocutaneous fistulae following laryngectomy or laryngopharyngectomy is common morbid complications which adversely affect the wound healing and recovery of the patient. Its incidence has been reported to vary widely from 5% to 75%. The incidence is significantly higher in patients undergoing salvage surgery following chemoradiation failure (60–65 Gy) [18]. The dose of radiotherapy and time interval between radiotherapy and subsequent surgery probably play an important part in the fistula formation. It is mentioned that patients treated with preoperative radiotherapy (50–55 Gy) and total laryngectomy as a part of combined treatment do not suffer from higher fistula than patients undergoing primary surgery.

Besides, other risk factors include preoperative tracheostomy, low postoperative haemoglobin level, poor nutrition, low albumin, comorbidities and local haematoma [17, 19].

The postoperative sepsis usually associated in previously irradiation cases has been noted to be an important factor. *Pseudomonas aeruginosa*, *Staphylococcus pyogenes* and *E. coli* are found to be common organisms [18, 19]. It is important to administer proper antibiotics after culture and sensitivity are obtained, and minor wound toilet may be carried out if necessary. Nasogastric tube (or PEG) feeding is continued. Nearly 50–80% fistulae heal spontaneously within 6–8 weeks, and only 20–30% of these will require surgical repair (Fig. 14.1a, b). It is useful to remember that pharyngocutaneous fistula may fail to heal because of residual or recurrent tumour or because of extensive fistula with mucosal dehiscence or poor general condition of the patient. Once these issues have been addressed and wound is healthy, repair can be attempted. Three types of fistulae requiring surgical repair have been described:

1. Where local mucosa is present but overlying skin is deficient.
2. Where local mucosa is deficient but overlying skin is present.
3. Where both mucosa and overlying skin are deficient.

Pectoralis major or latissimus dorsi myocutaneous flaps are the most used flaps, for repair of fistulae though free flaps can also be used [20].

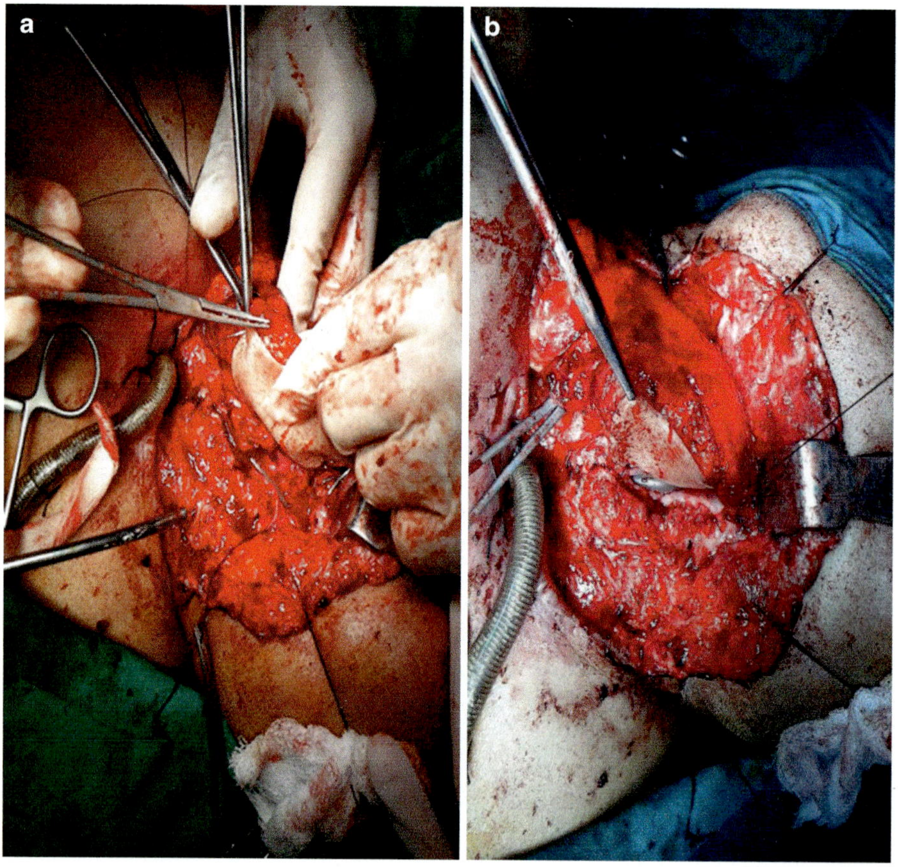

Fig. 14.1 (**a**, **b**) Repair of type 2 fistula (where mucosa is deficient) with PMMF. The muscle also provides protection to the carotids. Ryle's tube can be seen

14.2.13 Neurological

The following nerves are at risk during neck dissection: marginal mandibular nerve, vagus, accessory, hypoglossal, brachial plexus phrenic, superior laryngeal, the sympathetic chain and recurrent laryngeal nerve. It is important to have good anatomic knowledge and awareness of the variations of intraoperative nerve monitoring which is becoming popular with surgeons to avoid nerve injury.

14.2.14 Increased Intracranial Pressure

The intracranial pressure (ICP) rises three times when one internal jugular vein is divided as in a classical radial neck dissection. However, the pressure will rise five-fold when both veins are ligated simultaneously, and therefore, most surgeons either prefer to preserve vein or on one side perform staged neck dissection (with interval of 3 weeks).

Clinical features [2] include restlessness and headache, rise in blood pressure, facial swelling and cyanosis.

Management guidelines to reduce the risk of raised intracranial pressure include avoidance of tight dressing around the neck, avoidance of hyperextension of the neck and nursing the patient in upright position.

Treatment includes inducing an osmotic diuresis using intravenous mannitol, 200 ml of 25% initially.

14.2.15 Airway

Airway obstruction should be anticipated particularly in advanced carcinoma of the larynx and hypopharynx. An elective tracheostomy should be considered prior to surgery if there is compromise of the airway.

Following laryngectomy, tracheostomy after care in the ward or in ICU is extremely important. Later at time of hospital discharge, patient should be instructed to take care and change the tracheostomy tube independently.

14.3 Authors' Comment

Most complications following major surgery impact the morbidity and hospital stay, delay the postoperative treatment and may even produce mortality. Therefore, it is important for the surgeon to be aware of these complications and attempts to minimize these and at the same time keep the patient informed accordingly. It is well known that most patients are in the middle or elderly age group and have been exposed to smoking for long periods and are thus vulnerable to develop cardiac and chest complications subsequently. It is extremely useful to optimize these patients with regard to their medical condition with colleagues from anaesthesia preoperatively. Similarly, careful tissue handling at the time of surgery will reduce the chances of any complication.

If any vessel injury or chylous leak occurs, it should be immediately repaired intraoperatively. Postoperatively, vigil should be maintained for any haematoma formation, airway obstruction (tracheostomy care) and respiratory and cardiac complications. It is useful to administer suitable antibiotics in patients undergoing partial or total laryngectomy where the pharyngeal mucosa has been opened.

However, special care need to be taken for salvage surgery in previously radiation-failed cases with regard to skin incision, tissue care and raising the vascularised flap to minimize the incidence of pharyngocutaneous fistula and for carotid protection [21].

References

1. Goirala A, Bahadur S. Surgical complications in cancers of the upper aerodigestive tract. Indian J Otolaryngol. 1991;43:186–9.
2. Ah-See K, Supria M. Complications and their management. In: Walkinson JC, Gilbert RW, editors. Stell & Maran's text book of head and neck surgery and oncology. 5th ed. London: Hodder Arnold; 2012: p. 195–213.
3. Farwell DG, Reilly DF, Weymuller EA, et al. Predictors of perioperative complications in head and neck patients. Arch Otolaryngol Head Neck Surg. 2002;128:505–11.
4. McCullock TM, Jensen NF, Girod DA, et al. Risk factors for pulmonary complications in the post-operative head and neck surgery patient. Head Neck. 1997;19:372–7.
5. Bhattacharya N, Fried MP. Benchmarks for mortality, morbidity and length of stay for head and neck surgical procedures. Arch Otolaryngol Head Neck Surg. 2001;127:127–32.
6. Ferrier MB, Spuesens EB, Le Cessie S, et al. Co-morbidity as a major risk factor for mortality and complications in head and neck surgery. Arch Otolaryngol Head Neck Surg. 2005;131:27–32.
7. Moreano EH, Hutchison JL, McCulloch TM, et al. Incidence of deep vein thrombosis and pulmonary embolism in otolaryngology – head and neck surgery. Otolaryngol Head Neck Surg. 1998;118:777–84.
8. Grayburn PA, Hillis LD. Cardiac events in patients undergoing non-cardiac surgery. Ann Int Med. 2003;138:506–11.
9. Rao MK, Reilley TC, Schuller DE, et al. Analysis of risk factors for post-operative pulmonary complications in head and neck surgery. Laryngoscope. 1992;102:45–7.
10. Baumann MH, Strange C, Heffner JE, et al. Management of spontaneous pneumo-thorax: an American College of Chest Physicians Delphi Consensus statement. Chest. 2001;119:590–602.
11. American College of Surgeons Committee on Trauma. ATLS advanced trauma life support for doctors. 7th ed. Chicago: American College of Surgeons; 2004.
12. ACCP. American College of Chest Physician/Society of Critical Care Medicine. Consensus conference: definition for sepsis, and organ failure and guidelines for the use of innovative therapies in sepsis. Crit Care Med. 1992;20:864–72.
13. Cohan J, Rad I. Contemporary management of carotid blow out. Curr Opin Otolaryngol Head Neck Surg. 2004;12:110–5.
14. Robbins K, Samant S, Ronen O. Neck dissection. In: Cummings CW, Hanghey BH, Thomas JR, editors. Cummings otolaryngology: head and neck surgery. 5th ed. Philadelphia: Mosby Elsevier; 2010.

15. Park SY, Kim MS, Eom JS, et al. Risk factors and etiology of surgical site infection after radical neck dissection in patients with head and neck cancer. Korean J Int Med. 2016;31:162–9.
16. Hirakawa H, Hasegawa Y, Hanai N, et al. Surgical site infection in clean contaminated head and neck cancer surgery: risk factors and prognosis. Eur Arch s. 2013;270:1115–23.
17. Renel N, Lefebvre D, Fournier C, et al. Risk factors for wound infection in head and neck cancer surgery: a prospective study. Head Neck. 2001;23:447–55.
18. Bahadur S, Amatya RC, Kacker SK, Madan NC. Etiology and management of pharyngocutaneous fistulae following laryngectomy. Indian J Otolaryngol. 1985;37:1–3.
19. Cecaho SB, Soares M, Hennques T, et al. Predictive factors for the post laryngectomy pharyngocutaneous fistula development systemic review. Braz J Otolaryngol. 2014;80:167–77.
20. Tandon DA, Bahadur S, Bhendwal S. Repair of post laryngectomy pharyngocutaneous fistulae by muscle flaps. Indian J Otolaryngol Head Neck Surg. 1996;48:249–51.
21. Kakani RS, Tandon DA, Bahadur S. Role of pectoralis major flap in carotid artery protection. Indian J Otolaryngol Head Neck Surgery. 1995;47(4):288–92.

15 Anaesthetic Complications

Anjali Kochhar

15.1 Difficult Airway

Incidence of difficult airway is significantly higher in patients having airway tumours compared to general population. History of previous radiotherapy or surgery increases the level of difficulty. Detailed history, clinical examination, nasal endoscopy and radiological investigations like CT and MRI are useful tools to assess the airway and plan airway management. Management largely depends on the site and size of the tumour.

When patient presents with features of airway obstruction like stridor and dyspnoea, a detailed assessment may not be feasible. Airway management needs to be carefully planned based on clinical assessment and urgency of the situation. If it is not feasible to secure airway by conventional means (direct laryngoscopy), tracheostomy is done under local anaesthesia [1].

For elective procedures, management options include conventional laryngoscopy and intubation, fibre-optic intubation or elective tracheostomy [2]. It is of paramount importance to maintain oxygenation and ventilation. In anticipated difficult cases, temporary cricothyroidectomy or jet ventilation using a trans-tracheal catheter under local anaesthesia can be used to provide ventilation till airway is secured. Apnoea time can also be increased by using *Trans-nasal Humidified Rapid Insufflation Ventilatory Exchange* (THRIVE) using high flow oxygen delivery systems [3].

Extubation in a patient with difficult airway is more challenging than intubation. A difficult airway to begin with becomes much more difficult to manage after surgery due to oedema and distortion of the airway [4]. At the time of extubation, all the equipment required for difficult intubation should be kept ready, and it should be attempted by experienced anaesthesiologist and in the presence of

A. Kochhar (✉)
Department of Anaesthesiology, Hamdard Institute of Medical Sciences and Research, Jamia Hamdard, New Delhi, India

S. Bahadur et al. (eds.), *Carcinoma of the Larynx and Hypopharynx*,
https://doi.org/10.1007/978-981-13-3110-7_15

surgeon. It is worthwhile to use an airway exchange catheter and extubation done over it, leaving the catheter in place.

After major head and neck cancer surgery, it is recommended to keep the endotracheal tube in situ overnight. It also helps if any complication like bleeding or hematoma occurs and patient requires re-exploration. Tracheostomy care is ensured, and it should be collective responsibility of surgical and anaesthesia team [5].

15.2 Intraoperative Complications

15.2.1 Obstruction/Disconnection of Endotracheal Tube

As head end is not accessible to the anaesthesiologist, it is important to use flexometallic tube and carefully fix it to prevent any kinking or disconnection. Kinking of the tube can lead to increased airway pressures and barotrauma. Disconnection of the tube can cause rapid desaturation. If not timely recognized, hypoxia and cardiac arrest may ensue.

15.2.2 Blood Loss

As major laryngeal surgery may be associated with significant blood loss, extensive procedures require invasive blood pressure monitoring using intra-arterial line. Large bore cannulae are secured, and a central venous line is established either in the antecubital vein or femoral vein. The blood is cross-matched and kept ready. Induced hypotension is used to minimise blood loss. Anaesthetic agents (inhalational agents, remifentanil) or pharmacological drugs (Sodium nitroprusside, metoprolol, and dexmedetomidine) are used to reduce systolic arterial pressure to 85–90 mmHg. Blood transfusion is advocated when blood loss exceeds maximum allowable loss.

15.2.3 Hypothermia

Severe hypothermia can lead to arrhythmias, bleeding diathesis and delayed recovery from anaesthesia. Shivering on emergence increases oxygen demand of the patient and along with peripheral vasoconstriction can compromise blood flow to the newly constructed flap. Temperature monitoring should be instituted at the beginning of the surgery, and care must be taken to prevent hypothermia by using warm intravenous fluids, warming blankets or forced air warmers.

15.2.4 Carotid Sinus Reflex

Stimulation of baroreceptors can lead to arrhythmia and changes in blood pressure. Carotid sinus stimulation can lead to profound bradycardia and arrest. In case of bradycardia, surgeon is informed to release the pressure, and atropine is administered. Local infiltration of the area with lignocaine is beneficial in preventing recurrent reflex.

15.2.5 Air Embolism

It is a rare but potential complication that can occur as surgery is done in head-up position and major vessels are open, increasing the risk of air entry. To diagnose this complication, end-tidal carbon dioxide monitoring is a useful tool. Management is supportive and includes flushing the site with saline, 100% oxygen, Trendelenburg or left lateral position along with aspiration of air from the central line.

15.3 Postoperative Complications

15.3.1 Airway Complications

In the postoperative period, airway obstruction is likely to occur due to airway oedema and distortion. For minimising this risk, preventive steps are taken which include nursing in head-up position, i.v. steroids and nebulisation with adrenaline. If features of airway obstruction appear, airway must be secured by either intubating the trachea or by doing a tracheostomy.

Airway compromise may also be caused by neck hematoma secondary to haemorrhage. Airway must be secured well in time before anatomy is distorted by rapidly enlarging hematoma.

Other causes of desaturation may be obstruction of endotracheal or tracheostomy tube by secretions or blood clots. Frequent suctioning is required to avoid this complication.

Loss of airway can occur due to accidental decannulation of fresh tracheostomy. Patient may rapidly desaturate and become hypoxic. In such a scenario, call for help is made and mask ventilation initiated. If mask ventilation is found to be adequate, patient can be repositioned on a shoulder roll, and attempt is made to reposition the tube using tracheal dilator or cricoid hook. If the attempt fails, intubation can be attempted via oral route and patient can be taken to theatre. Intubation by oral route can cause damage to suture line in partial laryngectomy and tongue resections. It is not feasible option in a total laryngectomy patient.

15.3.2 Pulmonary Complications

Pulmonary complications include exacerbation of the pre-existing disease, pneumonia, pulmonary oedema and respiratory distress.

Patients having head and neck cancers are usually smokers and have co-existing chronic obstructive pulmonary disease and need a thorough evaluation in the preoperative period using chest X-rays, pulmonary function tests and arterial blood gas analysis, wherever indicated.

Preventive strategies include advice to quit smoking, bronchodilator therapy in those with reversible obstruction and antibiotic therapy in patients with suspected infection.

Other factors associated with pneumonia include aspiration and presence of tracheostomy in the postoperative period [6, 7]. Aspiration-associated pneumonia is more often seen with advanced oral and hypopharyngeal carcinoma.

Management of pneumonia includes monitoring of the patient, administration of humidified oxygen by facemask, antibiotics and chest physiotherapy.

Development of pulmonary complications increases rate of admission in intensive care unit and the length of hospital stay and increased healthcare cost.

15.3.3 Systemic Complication

Patients with long-standing alcohol consumption have anaemia and neurological issues; liver enzymes are deranged with alteration in drug metabolism. Alcohol withdrawal is precipitated in the postoperative period.

Cardiac diseases are common and require thorough preoperative evaluation and optimisation. Investigations that can delay the surgery without affecting outcome are not recommended, but it is important to continue all cardiac medications before surgery except the ones interfering with blood clotting. In patients with recent stents, risk of delay in surgery or bleeding should be weighed against risk of stent thrombosis.

Postoperative delirium, electrolyte imbalance and urological complications are more frequently encountered in elderly patients.

15.3.4 Death

Medical complications like cardio-genic shock, pulmonary embolism, septicaemia and multi-organ failure can lead to death. Elderly patients are at higher risk due to long standing smoking history, higher incidence of associated cardio-vascular diseases and poor nutrition.

In a nationwide survey conducted in England, mortality was found to be related to patient factors like increasing age and associated medical illness. Procedure-related factors were emergency surgery, presence of tracheotomy, free flap reconstruction and development of medical complications [8]. Patients with laryngo-pharyngeal cancers are particularly at higher risk as it has been found that these patients belong to lower socio-economic status with higher incidence of associated medical illness and higher chances of undergoing emergency surgery [9, 10].

15.4 Special Consideration

15.4.1 CPR in a Patient with Stoma

Post laryngectomy patient with a permanent stoma (laryngectomee) may be partial neck breather or total neck breather. Partial neck breather patient has communication between their lungs and mouth and nose, whereas total neck breathers can breathe through stoma only.

A laryngectomee may suffer respiratory embarrassment due to stoma obstruction by a mucus plug or foreign body. Cardiac arrest may occur due to other associated medical illnesses. Steps of resuscitation are essentially the same as in other patients, but suction of the stoma should be done before attempting mouth-to-stoma rescue breaths.

Emergency medical personnel may fail to identify specific needs of such patients. Furthermore, laryngectomees may not able to communicate particularly when in respiratory distress or near-arrest situations. Therefore, it is important for laryngectomees to wear bracelets and carry cards or other indications about their medical condition.

References

1. Patel A, Mitchell V. ENT and maxillofacial surgery. In: Ian C, Adrian P, editors. Core topics in airway management. New York: Cambridge University Press; 2005. p. 177–91.
2. Flory S, Appadurai IR. Special considerations in anesthesia for laryngeal cancer surgery. Int J Otolaryngol Clin. 2010;2:185–90.
3. Charters P, Ahmad I, Patel A, Russell S. Anaesthesia for head and neck surgery: United Kingdom National Multidisciplinary guidelines. J Laryngol Otol. 2016;130:s23–7.
4. Garg R, Darlong V, Pandey R, Punj J. Anesthesia for oncological ENT surgeries: review. Internet J Anesthesiol. 2008;20(1):1–8.
5. Coyle MJ, Tyrrell R, Godden A, Hughes CW, Perkins C, Thomas S, et al. Replacing tracheostomy with overnight intubation to manage the airway in head and neck oncology patients: towards an improved recovery. Br J Oral Maxillofac Surg. 2013;51(6):493–6.
6. Madan R, Kairo AK, Sharma A, Roy S, Singh S, Singh L, et al. Aspiration pneumonia related deaths in head and neck cancer patients: a retrospective analysis of risk factors from a tertiary care centre in North India. J Laryngol Otol. 2015;129:710–4.
7. Li L, Yuan W, Zhang S, Wang K, Ruan H. Analysis of risk factors for pneumonia in 482 patients undergoing oral cancer surgery with tracheotomy. J Oral Maxillofac Surg. 2016;74(2):415–9.
8. Nouraei S, Mace AD, Middleton SE, Hudovsky A, Vaz F, Moss C, et al. A stratified analysis of the perioperative outcome of 17,623 patients undergoing major head and neck cancer surgery in England over 10 years. Clin Otolaryngol. 2016;42(1):11–28. https://doi.org/10.1111/coa.12649.
9. Brook I. Urgent care, cardio-pulmonary resuscitation (CPR) and care of laryngectomee during anaesthesia. In: The laryngectomee guide. 2013. p. 141–53.
10. Nouraei SA, Middleton SE, Hudovsky A, Darzi A, Stewart S, Kaddour H, et al. A national analysis of the outcome of major head and neck cancer surgery: implications for surgeon-level data publication. Clin Otolaryngol. 2013;38(6):502–11.

Vocal Rehabilitation Following Laryngectomy

16

Sudhir Bahadur

16.1 Introduction

There have been several advances made in surgical techniques for conservation laryngectomy primarily for early lesions of the larynx providing excellent cure and functional results. Similarly, considerable advances have been made in chemoradiation for organ preservation in select advanced tumours. However, total laryngectomy still remains the gold standard for most advanced carcinoma of the larynx and hypopharynx and following salvage surgery in radiation failed cases. It is well realized that this surgical procedure results in permanent tracheo-stoma and loss of normal voice. Besides, there is loss of nasal function and changes in lung function, apart from increased cough and mucous formation. The swallowing ability is affected as well. These factors directly impact the QOL of these patients [1].

It is therefore extremely important that these patients are suitably rehabilitated both for the loss of speech and also for psychosocial reasons. The livelihood of most patients particularly in the younger age group is also affected, and this subject assumes greater significance. It is also important that patient clearly understands the following facts before surgery:

1. The larynx (voice box) is going to be permanently removed.
2. The patient will be able to speak again with alternative means, whether with the help of oesophageal speech or electronic larynx or treacheo-esophageal shunt prosthesis.
3. The results of surgery are permanent and irreversible.

The team of treating surgeon and speech pathologist can counsel and educate the patient starting from the preoperative period itself.

S. Bahadur (✉)
Department of Otolaryngology and Head-Neck Surgery, Formerly at All India Institute of Medical Sciences, New Delhi, India

S. Bahadur et al. (eds.), *Carcinoma of the Larynx and Hypopharynx*,
https://doi.org/10.1007/978-981-13-3110-7_16

16.2 Alaryngeal Speech

Normally, for speech production, a segment of air column (bellows) is exhaled from the lungs through the vocal cords producing a sound which is later modified by the articulators in the oral cavity and oropharynx to produce speech. However, once the larynx is removed following surgery and also the air column from the lungs is disrupted from the articulators, the speech becomes difficult. The oesophageal speech uses the pharyngeal mucosa as the vibratory surface and oesophagus as the source of air supply, rather than the lungs. Attempts have been made to create surgical shunt in the early 1970s to permit air from the lungs to the pharynx. However, these attempts by several authors such as Staffieri et al. [2] and Conley et al. [3] met with limited success because of aspiration problems. Later, the same principle but utilizing the valve prosthesis in the fistula/shunt (e.g. Blom-Singer, Provox, Gromingen, etc.) improved the outcome significantly and despite the inherent problems is still considered the gold standard in vocal rehabilitation following laryngectomy. The work done by Taub and Spiro [4] is still used as a predictor for development of speech following laryngectomy. The concept of laryngeal transplantation after total laryngectomy is however at an experimental stage [5].

16.3 Oesophageal Speech

Oesophageal speech was the most common mode of alaryngeal communication for several decades. It entails patient injecting air into the oesophagus and then by co-ordinated muscular action; the air is expelled causing cricopharyngeus or pharyngo-oesophageal segment to vibrate producing a sound which can subsequently be articulated into recognizable speech by the articulators in the oral cavity. However, only 25–44% of patients are able to achieve functional speech [6, 7]. The quality of oesophageal speech is dependent upon the motivation and age of the patient and time spent with professional speech trainer.

The patients of laryngeal lesions rather than the hypopharyngeal lesions are able to develop oesophageal speech better mainly because the amount of mucosa resected is larger in the latter. The advantages of oesophageal speech are: (a) it does not require any apparatus, (b) it does not sound mechanical, and (c) and it provides hands-free speech. However, oesophageal speech is rough and breathy, with low pitch and reduced loudness. Patients are able to speak short phrases as compared to lung-powered speech and therefore may not be satisfied with the outcome.

16.4 Artificial Larynx

It is useful for those unable to learn oesophageal speech or do not like to maintain and afford regular change of tracheo-oesophageal prosthesis. It works by applying handheld electronic or pneumatic devices to the side of neck or cheek or less

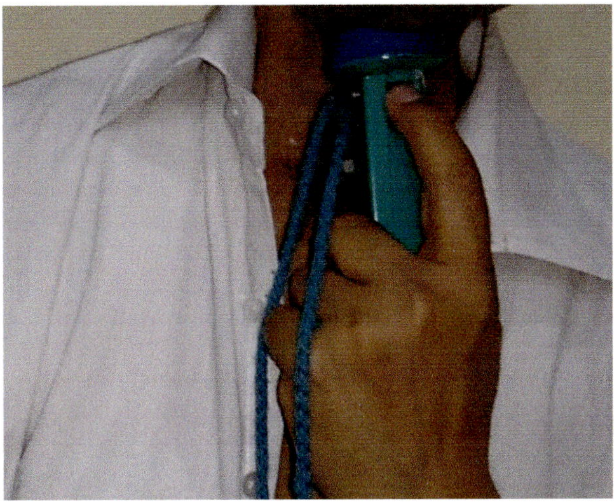

Fig. 16.1 Laryngectomy patient using the artificial electronic larynx

commonly intraorally. The sound vibration is transmitted through the head of electronic device and through tissues in the neck to the oral cavity which is then articulated normally. Early introduction of artificial larynx helps the patient overcome emotional component in the immediate post-operative period without significantly affecting the development of oesophageal speech or TE speech. However, the main disadvantage includes the mechanical, monotonous and robot-like sound quality, maintenance of the device and use of a hand to control it (Fig. 16.1).

16.5 Tracheo-oesophageal Shunt Using Valve Prosthesis

Vocal rehabilitation has improved significantly after the introduction of voice prosthesis by Singer and Blom [8], Blom et al. [9] and Panje [10], and it is considered the gold standard for laryngectomized patients. The technique involves creating shunt between the posterior wall of tracheostoma and upper oesophagus into which later a tracheo-oesophageal prosthesis (one-way silicone valve) is inserted. The air is shunted from the lungs into the oesophagus via the prosthesis, once the stoma is occluded during exhalation. Resulting speech is produced by vibrating mucosa of the pharynx and modified by the articulators in the oral cavity.

The quality of the TE speech is generally excellent. Besides it is intelligible and natural. Also the patient can speak more words per breath compared to oesophageal speech. The main difference, though, is the source of pulmonary air in TEP which sustains the quality of speech in terms of fundamental frequency, words per minute and maximum phonation time [10–14]. The major advantage of TEP is rapid restoration of speech in the post-operative period.

16.6 Primary TEP

It is standard practice to carry out primary tracheo-oesophageal shunt at the time of laryngectomy. The shunt or the puncture site is positioned in the midline, about 10 mm below the mucocutaneous junction on the posterior tracheal wall. The tip of a curved artery forceps is inserted through the pharyngeal defect and advanced into the cervical oesophagus close to the puncture site. An incision is made with the scalpel onto the tip of forceps in the posterior tracheal wall. The forceps is then opened into the tracheal lumen to catch the tip of a 14FG Foley catheter or similar size feeding tube. The latter is than withdrawn through the shunt and placed down into the oesophagus.

The pharyngeal mucosal defect is than closed carefully in the usual way. The pharyngo-oesophagus segment is reconstructed by joining the thyropharyngeus constrictor muscles to the suprahyoid muscles. The tracheostoma is sutured meticulously to the upper and lower skin flaps so as to create adequate size stoma. The neck wound is closed in the usual way with suction drainage. Once the oral feeding has been started, the nasogastric tube is removed and replaced with a suitable tracheo-oesophageal prosthesis within 10–15 days.

However, one has to be careful while dealing with hypopharyngeal tumours because resection may result in less mucosa for repair of the pharynx and, therefore, it is a good idea to mobilize the mucosa from the uninvolved pyriform fossa. Sometimes it is necessary to augment the mucosa, particularly in previously irradiated cases with patch' pectoralis major myocutaneous flap to close the pharynx. Usually transverse mucosal width of 6 cm is necessary for closure to enable good swallowing and adequate tracheo-oesophageal speech [11]. It is important to follow good surgical technique with accurate positioning of tracheostoma and tracheo-oesophageal puncture.

16.6.1 Tonicity Control

Optimal tonicity of pharyngo-oesophageal junction is important for acquiring fluent tracheo-oesophageal speech. A cricopharyngeal myotomy may be performed in the posterior midline, down to submucosal vascular plexus using a scalpel over a 5–6 cm distance between TEP site and the inferior constrictor muscle. Hypertonicity or spasm of these muscles should be avoided which would interrupt the airflow to a varying degree and is the cause of TEP speech failure in significant number of patients [12].

16.6.2 Tracheo-oesophageal Prosthesis

Initially, the voice prosthesis (Blom-Singer, Panje) was designed as non-indwelling. These were simple, cheaper and easier to maintain devices but required certain dexterity. Subsequently in the late 1980s, some low resistance, indwelling voice prostheses (Groningen, Provox) were developed, and these have been preferred. The original

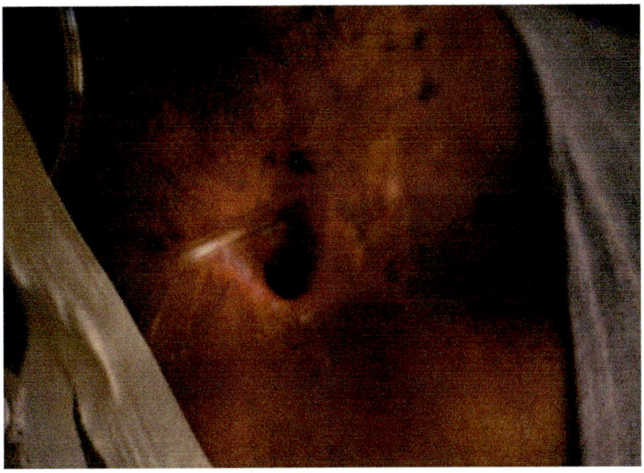

Fig. 16.2 TEP maintained by Ryle's tube

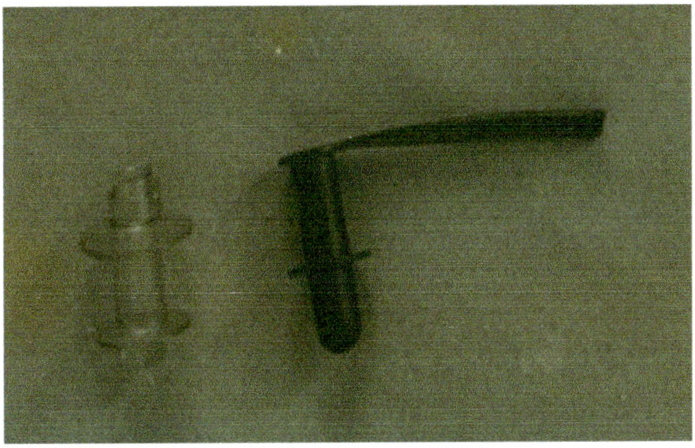

Fig. 16.3 Indigenous voice prosthesis

Provox prosthesis was inserted in the retrograde manner with a special disposable guidewire. But the Provox 2 device can be easily inserted with a simple anterograde fashion with retrograde method still available [13–15]. The advantage of indwelling prosthesis is that it may be cleaned in situ without removal and replaced by an otolaryngologists usually twice a year. It is important to select the voice prosthesis carefully. The factors which are likely to influence the decision include patient's dexterity and willingness to maintain the prosthesis himself, phonatory effort, thickness of the party wall (between posterior wall of the trachea and oesophagus) and durability and cost of the prosthesis [11] (Figs. 16.2, 16.3 and 16.4).

16.6.3 Results and Complications

Results of tracheo-oesophageal speech are excellent, and success rate varies from 70 to 95% [11, 12, 16, 17]. There are several studies available about enhanced quality of life observed [18–20]. The quality of life is positively influenced by level of education and better socio-economic background.

Fig. 16.4 Speech therapist training the patient after the TEP prosthesis (following laryngectomy)

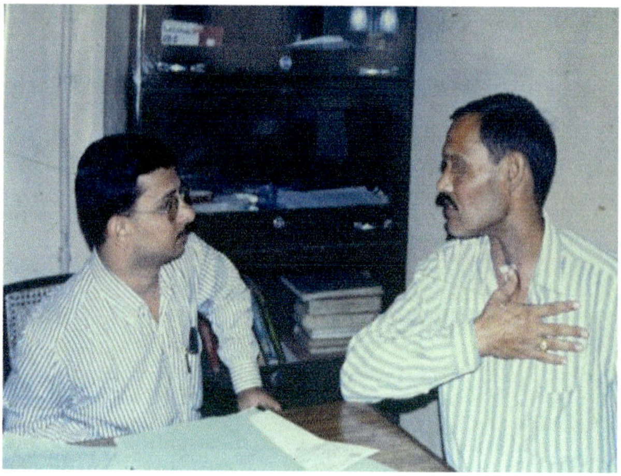

Leakage of fluids through the valve is the commonest indication for replacing the voice prosthesis. The malfunctioning of the prosthesis is generally caused by *candida* deposits on the silicon material. This may occur at varying periods after insertion of the prosthesis. The use of antifungal drugs can influence *candida* growth significantly and contribute to prolong the life of the prosthesis [21]. The reported lifetime of the prosthesis is roughly 4–10 months [22–24].

Leakage outside the prosthesis is also an important cause of replacement of the device. This problem can be solved mostly by downsizing the prosthesis. In case it does not resolve the issue, a possible solution is to temporarily remove the prosthesis and allow the fistula to shrink or a purse string suture may be applied. Local infection can be treated with antibiotics. Rarely, complete closure of tracheo-oesophageal fistula may be required and patient allowed to choose alternate mode of communication, e.g. artificial larynx. Rarely, tumour recurrence may also cause leakage around the prosthesis.

Occasionally, extrusion of prosthesis may occur from the tracheo-oesophageal fistula during cleaning or coughing. If the prosthesis is not replaced immediately, closure of the tract will occur in a few days. A catheter or a nasogastric tube may be used to keep the tract patient until the prosthesis can be replaced. It is well realized that adverse events are unavoidable when using a foreign body in the trachea-oesophageal shunt. However, with increasing realization of problems and their solutions, most adverse events can be managed, and chances of prosthetic vocal rehabilitation are high with excellent voice quality.

In Indian context these are a few studies indicating long-term successful results with prosthetic rehabilitation. The long-term use of prosthetic device with frequent replacement requires for patient to have higher socio-economic status, commitment to use the prosthesis and better educational background [25]. It is therefore recommended in select patients fulfilling the above guidelines and who can come for regular follow-up.

16.6.4 Assessment for Secondary Voice Restoration

Secondary tracheo-oesophageal puncture was originally suggested for patients who failed to develop oesophageal speech. It is still recommended for patients who have failed radiotherapy previously and require total laryngectomy in whom secondary procedure is preferable. It is useful to assess PE segment tonicity before doing secondary TEP.

The assessment of tonicity of PE segment is carried out with videoflouroscopy which is a reliable and accurate method [26, 27]. There are three components of the procedure like modified barium swallow, oesophageal insufflation test and attempted phonation. The modified barium swallow test can rule out presence of spasm of PE segment or a stricture by showing any hold up or delay in passage of barium.
Oesophageal insufflating test (Taub test) simulates airflow to the oesophagus at level of TE shunt. The procedure involves passing a soft rubber catheter transnasally and connecting to the air cylinder under slow flow rate. Patient is asked to count the numbers. An alternate to Taub test was described by Blom et al. [17] in which a catheter passed transnasally into the oesophagus to a distance of about 25 cm and is connected to an adapter placed over the tracheostoma. Thus pulmonary air is transferred to the oesophagus when the patient closes the adapter and attempts to speak.

16.6.5 Surgical Technique

Once the patient has been found suitable, surgical procedure creating the TE shunt is carried out as described by Singer et al. [9] by using the illuminated rigid endoscope. The tip of the endoscope tents the posterior tracheal wall of the stoma, thus facilitating the incision and creation of the shunt. An alternate method has been described by Rhyswan using a long artery forceps alongside the hypopharyngoscope. The artery forceps can been seen and palpated as it tents up the posterior tracheal wall, and an incision can be made and shunt maintained. A TE prosthesis can replace the feeding tube or the catheter in 4–7 days.
Botulinum toxin may be used for chemical neurectomy in cases of failed tracheo-oesophageal speech caused by hypertonicity or spasm [28]. Myotomy may be reserved for cases where botulinum is ineffective.

16.7 Authors' Comment

Total laryngectomy with or without a neck dissection is still an important milestone in treatment of advanced carcinoma of the larynx and following salvage surgery in radiation failed cases. It is understood that surgery results in permanent tracheostome and loss of normal speech, thus impacting the quality life. These patients, therefore, need to be suitably rehabilitated both for the loss of speech and for psychosocial reasons.

There are three modes of vocal rehabilitation mentioned in literature: oesophageal speech, artificial larynx and tracheo-oesophageal prosthetic speech (TEP). The, TEP offers the best methods of communication in terms of quality of speech and its intelligibility in 70–90% cases. It is because the source of pulmonary air in TEP is that quality of speech is sustained. Besides it can be easily carried out at time of initial laryngectomy (primary TEP). However, maintenance and cost are important factors in Indian set-up, as the prosthesis needs to be replaced every 4 to 8 months' time. Thus long-term use of prosthetic device with frequent replacement requires patient to have a higher socio-economic status and commitment to use the prosthesis. It also requires easy access to the medical facility for change of the indwelling prosthesis. Therefore, patient selection is important for advising TEP speech. However, in salvage surgery setting, secondary TEP may be preferred.

Oesophageal speech may still be useful in younger patients who are socio-economically not well off but motivated enough to learn oesophageal speech particularly if training professional is available. Artificial electronic larynx may be considered for elderly patients who lack motivation to learn oesophageal speech or are unwilling to come for regular replacement of prosthesis. Such patients may be advised to use electronic larynx early to overcome psychosocial reason as well.

References

1. Rhys-Evans P, Bloom E. Functional restoration of speech. In: Rhys-Evans PH, Montogomery PG, Gullane PL, editors. Principles and practice of head and neck surgery and oncology. 1st ed. London: Martin Dunitz; 2003. p. 571–602.
2. Stafferi M, Procaccini A, Steiner W, et al. Surgical rehabilitation of speech after total laryngectomy. Laryngol Rhinol Otol. 1978;57:477–88.
3. Conley JJ, de Amesti F, Pierce MK. A new surgical technique for vocal rehabilitation of the laryngectomised patients. Ann Otol Rhinol Laryngol. 1972;67:655–64.
4. Taub S, Spiro DH. Vocal rehabilitation of laryngectomees. Am J Surg. 1972;124:87–90.
5. Birchall MA. Laryngeal transplantation. Br J Surg. 1997;84:739–40.
6. Gates GA, Hearne WN. Predicting Oesophageal speech. Ann Otol Rhinol Laryngol. 1982;91:454–7.
7. Amatya RC, Bahadur S, Kacker SK. Oesophageal speech following laryngectomy. Indian J Otolaryngol. 1985;37:34–5.
8. Singer MI, Blom ED. An endoscopic technique for restoration of voice after laryngectomy. Ann Otol Rhinol Laryngol. 1980;89:529–33.
9. Singer MI, Blom ED, Hamekar RC. Further experience with voice restoration after total laryngectomy. Ann Otol Rhinol Laryngol. 1981;90:498–502.
10. Panje WR. Prosthetic vocal rehabilitation following laryngectomy. Ann Otol Rhinol Laryngol. 1980;89:529–31.
11. Kazi R, Rhys-Evans P, Clarke P. Voice restoration. In: Watkinson JC, Gilebrt R W, editors. Stell and Maran's text book of head and neck surgery and oncology. London: Hodder Arnold; 2012. p. 1079.
12. Nayak U, Kazi R. Voice restoration after total laryngectomy. In: Current science and future prospective. Delhi: Byword; 2009.
13. Hilgers FJM, Schouwenburg PF. A new low resistance, self retaining prosthesis (Provox) for voice rehabilitation after total laryngectomy. Laryngoscope. 1990;100:1202–5.
14. Hilgers FJM, Corndissen MW, Palm AJM. Aerodynamic characteristics of low resistance indwelling Provox voice prosthesis. Eur Arch Otolaryngol. 1993;250:378–80.

15. Hilgers FJM, Ackerstaff AH, Balm AJM, et al. Development and clinical evaluation of second generation voice prosthesis (Provox 2) designed for antigrade and retrograde insertion. Acta Otolaryngol. 1997;117:889–95.
16. Brown DH, Hilgers AJM, Irish JC, Balm AJM. Post laryngectomy voice rehabilitation state of Art at the Millenium. World J Surg. 2003;27:824–31.
17. Blom ED, Singer MI, Hamaker RC. An improved insufflations test. Arch Otolaryngol. 1985;111:211–2.
18. Bozee A, Poissonet G, Chamorey E, et al. Results of vocal rehabilitation using TE. Voice prosthesis after total laryngectomy and their predictive factors. Eur Arch Otolaryngol. 2010;267:751–8.
19. Robertson SM, Yeo J, Dunnet C, et al. Voice, swallowing and quality of life after total laryngectomy. Results of West of Scotland laryngectomy audit. Head Neck. 2012;34:59–65.
20. Monkarbel RV, Dayal PC, Yoo JH, et al. Voice-related quality of life (V-RQOL) outcomes in laryngectomees. Head Neck. 2011;33:31–6.
21. Ameye D, Honraet K, Loose D, et al. Effect of a buccal bioadhesive nystatin tablet on the lifetime of a Provox silicon tracheo-oesophageal prosthesis. Acta Otolaryngol. 2005;125:304–6.
22. Ackerstaff AH, Hilgers FJM, Meeuwis CA, et al. Multi-institutional assessment of the Provox voice prosthesis. Arch Otolaryngol Head Neck Surg. 1999;125:167–73.
23. Aust MR, McCaffrey TV. Early speech results with the Provox prosthesis after laryngectomy. Arch Otolaryngol Head Neck Surg. 1997;123:966–70.
24. Laccourney O, Menard M, Crevier-Buchman L, et al. In situ life time causes for replacement and complication of the Provox voice prosthesis. Laryngoscope. 1997;107:527–30.
25. Thakar A, Bahadur S. Trouble shooting with Tracheo-oesophageal prosthesis. Indian J Otolaryngol Head Neck Surg. 2002;54:27–9.
26. Molvor J, Evans PF, Perry A, Cheesman AD. Radiological assessment of post laryngectomy speech. Clin Radiol. 1990;41:312–6.
27. Perry A. Preoperative tracheo-oesophageal voice restoration assessment and selection criteria. In: Blom ED, Singer MI, Hamekar RC, editors. Tracheo-oesophageal voice restoration following total laryngectomy. San Diego: Singular Publishing Group; 1998. p. 9–18.
28. Lewin JS, Bishop-Leone JK, Forman AD, et al. Further experience with Botox injection for tracheo-oesophageal speech failure. Head Neck. 2001;23:456–60.

Quality of Life

17

Bidhu K. Mohanti

17.1 Introduction

The cancer patient goes through a trajectory of physical symptoms, diagnosis, treatment and survivorship. Quality of life (QoL) assessment is a direct and subject-centred method in the healthcare delivery which is aimed to identify the outcomes, way beyond the standard scales of loco-regional control, disease-free survival, overall survival, morbidities and death.

Health-related QoL indicates the patients' perception of their health. Hence, unlike treatment results assessed by the physicians, QoL measurement is a uniquely subject- or patient-centred approach. It depends not only on disease- and treatment-related factors but also on complex interrelationships of expectations, values and norms, psychologic distress and comparison with other patients.

QoL research has been around for decades and currently is mandatory in cancer clinical trials. Since this is a patient-reported outcome (PRO), the measurement of QoL can give additional valuable information in our routine clinical services. In the 1990s, the World Health Organization (WHO) has defined it as "an individual's perception of their position in life in the context of the culture and value systems in which they live and in relation to their goals, expectations, standards, and concerns" [1]. This chapter introduces methods and challenges of QoL assessment in patients with head and neck cancer, as well as ways to overcome measurement problems and ways to improve their QoL [2].

Patients with head and neck cancer (HNC) report significant and persistent physical, functional and psychosocial problems, including social isolation and delays in

B. K. Mohanti (✉)
Department of Radiation Oncology, Manipal Hospital, New Delhi, India

S. Bahadur et al. (eds.), *Carcinoma of the Larynx and Hypopharynx*,
https://doi.org/10.1007/978-981-13-3110-7_17

returning to work [3]. The disease and its treatments have a disproportionate impact on all aspects of the patient's QoL. However, in the areas of clinical practice and research for HNC patients, the QoL studies are still weak [4].

Larynx and hypopharynx are the two organs intimately related to the voice and swallowing functions. Any disorder or deficit in these two functions carries an adverse impact on daily living.

17.2 Case Scenarios for QoL Assessment

Mr. GKS is 58 years old and works as a supervisor for construction workers in Delhi. He lives with his wife and two college-going children. In the course of his irregular working hours, he got addicted to alcohol and smoking. In the beginning of 2017, he developed persistent hoarseness in voice. Laryngoscopic examination, biopsy of a growth in vocal cord and CT scan showed a diagnosis of laryngeal cancer in stage 2. After receiving the result, he decided to be treated by definitive radiotherapy, with an aim to avoid the surgical removal of a part of his voice box. Six months after the radiotherapy, he is now back at his work and is able to speak smoothly with an occasional hoarseness and dry cough.

Mrs. RW is a 48-year-old housewife with five children. Her husband is a daily wage earner in agriculture. She has to assist her husband on the farming fields. The couple has a regular habit of tobacco chewing. Mrs. RW has chronic anaemia. Two years back, she started with swallowing difficulty and frequent coughs while eating her meals. The tests including a CT scan confirmed a diagnosis of left pyriform sinus carcinoma, T3N1M0. She was treated by surgery and postoperative radiotherapy at a regional cancer centre in Uttar Pradesh. She completed her treatment course and is now on follow-up for a little over 1 year. She complains of pain in the throat and bouts of cough while eating, and the loss of her speech bothers her.

Declaration by Author-Above two cases are anonymised as regards identity and materials, and in order do not require any patient's consent.

Both the patients require attention to their subjective experiences. An adequate approach from the healthcare system to improve the quality of daily living, alongside the periodic assessment of disease status will enhance the survivorship care. There is distinct lack of understanding of the true significance of QOL in the comprehensive care of HNC patients [3, 4]. As more patients will get a disease control or cure on long-term basis, the doctors and nurses should gain the expertise and skills to evaluate the QoL of a patient.

17.3 QoL Assessment Tools for HNC Patients

As explained earlier, the QoL is a subjective experience of the patient. The two main methods of assessment in general are interviews and questionnaires. The preferred method is the self-administered questionnaires, because it gives the opportunity to elicit the patient's responses and as well for the ease of analysis. The presently utilised QoL tools are classified into generic and specific questionnaires. The "generic" is intended to understand the general aspects of a cancer patient, whereas the "specific" probes the more pertinent aspects of a cancer type such as breast, lung, head and neck, etc. The frequently used QoL tools are shown in Table 17.1.

In both clinical and trial settings, the generic and specific questionnaires are used together. Two generic questionnaires, European Organization for Research and Treatment of Cancer Quality of Life Questionnaire (EORTC QLQ-C30) and Functional Assessment of Cancer Therapy (FACT-G) are widely used since the last two decades. The two instruments are aimed to ascertain the patient's QOL related to physical, social, emotional, cognitive and financial aspects of living, along with symptoms and overall health [6, 7]. There is substantial evidence for the reliability, validity and responsiveness of both the EORTC QLQ-C30 and FACT-G in a range of cancer settings, and both are available in a large number of language translations

Table 17.1 Commonly utilised QoL instruments in clinical and research areas

Title	Developed by	Number of items	Note
Specific for cancer patients			
European Organisation for Research and Treatment of Cancer Quality of Life Questionnaire (EORTC QLQ-C30)	EORTC Group (1993) (collaboratively in several culturally diverse areas)	30 short form:EORTC-QLQ-C15	Free of charge for academic and research purposes available at: http://groups.eortc.be/qol/
Functional Assessment of Cancer Therapy (FACT-G)	FACIT group (1993)	27	Different version for the general population available at: http://www.facit.org/FACITOrg/Questionnaires
Specific for HNC patients			
European Organisation for Research and Treatment of Cancer Quality of Life Questionnaire (EORTC QLQ-H&N35)	EORTC group	35	Free of charge for academic users
Functional Assessment of Cancer Therapy, Head and Neck Module (FACT-HN)	FACIT group	39	Free of charge for academic users
University of Washington Quality-of-Life (UW-QOL-R)	Hassan and Weymuller (1993)	10	Available at: http://www.headandneckcancer.co.uk/File.ashx?id=10285
MD Anderson Symptom Inventory–Head and Neck Module (MDASI-HN)	Rosenthal (2007)	28	–

Modified from Ref. [2]

[8]. We have utilised both these tools in our clinical studies [9, 10]. Any of these two generic QoL tools should approximately take 15 min for the completeness of administration or response recording.

In addition to the core questionnaires (EORTC QLQ-C30 or, FACT-G), when the objectives are concerned with the impact of a specific tumour type, treatment or symptom, the specific module which can elicit the relevant aspects should be used. For the HNC patients, the modules which can add to the QOL measurements are EORTC QLQ-H&N35 (35 items) and FACT-HN (39 items).

For example, to measure the QOL of above two patients in the case scenario, EORTC QLQ-C30 should be administered combined with EORTC QLQ-H&N35 or alternatively FACT-G with FACT-HN. The assessment of each patient will require 30–40 min at the outpatient clinic. It has been observed that certain basic principles should be practised for the QoL measurements in the clinical or research setting:

1. The doctor and nurse should be familiar with the generic and specific QoL modules.
2. The patient, and in some situations the surrogate caregiver, should be explained about the nature and objective of QoL assessment in simple language. Consent should be obtained before QoL measurement is carried out.
3. The patient or surrogate should be handed over the questionnaires to read and understand. Whenever possible, the doctor or nurse will be available to clarify any doubt about the different items in a questionnaire.
4. The QoL is a subjective assessment where the patient or surrogate will provide the response to each item without any bias or coercion. The healthcare provider may assist the patient or surrogate in completing the questionnaires.
5. Missing items in the response will be a possibility, when the patient or surrogate may not like to answer an item. However, all efforts and cross-checks should be made for the completeness.
6. The sociocultural context should be respected in carrying out the QoL assessment.
7. Temporal assessments at different times during the disease and treatment trajectory, such as preoperative or baseline before radiotherapy, during/after a treatment course and in follow-up periods, will be valuable to observe the changes in QoL scores and make interventions.
8. The doctors, nurses and other health workers involved for QoL assessment of their patients will be familiar with the scoring system of EORTC or FACT.

At the time of diagnosis and in subsequent encounters during the treatment and follow-up, the HNC patient will have several QoL issues which may not be determined or documented. In the present cancer care delivery, the disease stage, general health status, treatment process, morbidities, recurrence and failures, etc. are given the attention. During the last 25 years, patient QoL whether for curative or palliative approach has been recognised to influence the overall quality of cancer care and survival [4]. More work is needed to improve the clinical utility of these measures in order to link the QOL research to clinical practice [3].

17.4 Treatment Effects

Surgery for cancers of the larynx and hypopharynx was developed in the first half, and subsequently radiotherapy and chemotherapy were integrated in the second half of the twentieth century. The consequences of surgical approaches were recognised in the cured survivors. Physical change and change in self-image, difficulty in communication and social isolation following total laryngectomy may impair quality of life [5]. Alteration in swallowing capacity, aspiration and phonation are the long-term effects of hypopharyngeal extirpation. The rehabilitation following surgery can be augmented by QoL measurements. It is shown that patients can adapt well following the total laryngectomy or pharyngo-laryngectomy. Still several key QoL issues continue to bother the patients [11].

From the early 1990s, chemoradiotherapy (CRT) has advanced as an alternative to surgery and postoperative radiotherapy (S-PORT), in order to achieve cure with organ preservation. The feasibility and efficacy in organ conservation and oncologic control have been demonstrated [12–14]. However, these initial studies, in the last decade of the twentieth century, were not aimed to assess the QoL of patients, trusting that preservation of voice and swallowing is bound to be good for living. In the last 20 years, periodic QoL measurements have shown that radical radiotherapy or chemoradiotherapy for these patients, in stages 3–4, can result in several impairments.

The comparative evaluation between surgery and chemoradiotherapy in cancer of the larynx showed decline in physical function and insomnia, besides the loss of voice, after the laryngectomy. On the other side, chemoradiotherapy resulted in dry mouth, sticky saliva and changes in taste and smell [11].

Subsequent to the findings of VA study, refinements in radiotherapy techniques and chemotherapy regimens have increased the utilisation of CRT in locally advanced laryngeal cancer. The long-term functional larynx preservation rates range from 20 to 50%. In such a scenario of a wide range of voice preservation result, the treating team must have a good understanding to empower the patient about a treatment choice between CRT and S-PORT. Patients, who have severely compromised speech, swallowing, and breathing functions before the initiation of therapy, can have prolonged QoL issues after radiotherapy or CRT. The issues to be identified by periodic QoL assessments after the non-surgical therapies include voice quality, any dietary modification, aspiration, need for tracheostomy and the potential for salvage surgery. The long-term follow-up in the locally advanced T4 laryngeal cancer patients has shown that all these issues are more prominent in the CRT group compared to those treated by S-PORT [15].

In our study, the EORTC QLQ-C30 generic module assessment for the patients who received 70 Gy of conventional radical radiotherapy showed that the radiation-related morbidities of the mucosa, salivary gland and pharynx led to a considerable decline in the physical (PF), social (SF) and emotional (EF) functioning as well as the global health status (GHS) score [9]. This is shown in Fig. 17.1. Such an understanding has helped us in our clinical practice to improve the nutrition and oro-dental health of our patients in pre- and post-therapy phases.

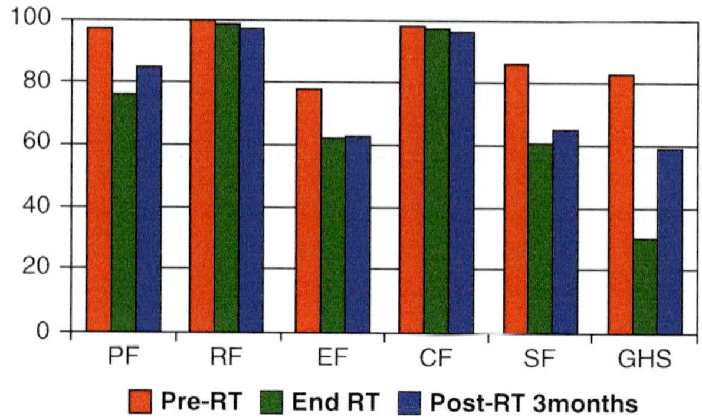

Fig. 17.1 The quality of life (EORTC QLQ-C30) mean scores of five function scales and global health status for head and neck cancer patients, *showing change over time* [9]. *PF* physical function, *RF* role function, *EF* emotional function, CF cognitive function, *SF* social function, *GHS* global health status

The prognosis in hypopharyngeal cancer is considerably poorer compared to cancer of the larynx. These patients are likely to present with both swallowing and speech problems. Since hypopharyngeal cancer occurs in a setting of high alcohol and tobacco abuse and malnutrition, higher morbidities and functional impairments are the consequences of surgery, radiotherapy and chemotherapy. Often the functional losses can become permanent, and the quality of living for a cured patient becomes a matter of daily concern. Total laryngo-pharyngectomy with neck dissection is the standard curative approach in hypopharyngeal cancer. The surgery results in loss of voice and a significant change in the swallowing capacity. Patients experience restriction in neck and shoulder movements, and lingering pain [16]. The QOL measurement before and after surgery should be undertaken to assist the rehabilitation process. Whenever feasible, partial preservation of laryngopharynx, without compromising the oncological result, should be carefully planned.

The advent of CRT for loco-regionally advanced stage 2 to stage 4 patients in the last 20 years, since the EORTC study [13], is reported as a significant milestone in the progress of treatment options for hypopharyngeal cancer. The terms "organ preservation" and "larynx preservation" in particular are frequently unclearly defined or interpreted. Aspiration-free deglutition and voice intelligibility should be measured as key QOL issues after the CRT in cancer of hypopharynx [14]. Besides these two scores, the freedom from neck and shoulder pain, social function and emotional stability are important features to be assessed on a temporal basis in the cancer survivors. Dryness of the mouth, dysphagia and otalgia are the main morbidities from chemoradiotherapy. Reduction in the morbidities and symptom relief should be implemented from the initiation of CRT to improve the QoL.

17.5 Conclusion

In summary, patients diagnosed with laryngeal and hypopharyngeal malignancies face functional challenges unlike many other tumours. The disease and treatments significantly affect the voice, swallowing and associated constitutional aspects of daily living.

When the survival results show equal rates, the trade-off between organ preservation and surgical extirpation requires to be carefully weighed in terms of functional outcomes and QoL issues. Laryngeal and hypopharyngeal cancer patients experience significant impairments after any form of anticancer therapy, be it surgery and postoperative radiotherapy (with or without chemotherapy) or chemoradiotherapy [17]. Traditionally, for the treated patients, outcome parameters such as survival, loco-regional control and morbidities are documented. A complete picture can be obtained about the patient, when QoL assessments are done in conjunction with the standard treatment result parameters.

References

1. Study protocol for the World Health Organization project to develop a Quality of Life assessment instrument (WHOQOL). Qual Life Res. 1993;2:153–9.
2. Singer S, Langedijk J, Yarom N. Assessing and improving quality of life in patients with head and neck cancer. ASCO Educ Book. 2013:e2301–e235. https://doi.org/10.1200/EdBook_AM.2013.33.e230.
3. Ojo B, Genden EM, Teng MS, Milbury K, Misiukiewicz KJ, Badr H. A systematic review of head and neck cancer quality of life assessment instruments. Oral Oncol. 2012;48:923–37.
4. Bjordal K, Bottomley A. Making advances in quality of life studies in head and neck cancer. Int J Radiat Oncol Biol Phys. 2017;97:659–61.
5. Ramírez MJ, Ferriol EE, Doménech FG, et al. Psychosocial adjustment in patient surgically treated for laryngeal cancer. Otolaryngol Head Neck Surg. 2003;129:92–7.
6. Aaronson NK, Ahmedzai S, Bergman B, et al. The European Organization for research and treatment of cancer QLQ-C30: a quality-of-life instrument for use in international clinical trials in oncology. J Natl Cancer Inst. 1993;85:365–76.
7. Cella DF, Tulsky DS, Gray G, et al. The functional assessment of cancer therapy scale: development and validation of the general measure. J Clin Oncol. 1993;11:570–9.
8. Luckett T, King MT, Butow PN, Oguchi M, Rankin N, Price MA, Hackl NA, Heading G. Choosing between the EORTC QLQ-C30 and FACT-G for measuring health-related quality of life in cancer clinical research: issues, evidence and recommendations. Ann Oncol. 2011;22:2179–90.
9. Bansal M, Mohanti BK, Shah N, Chaudhry R, Bahadur S, Shukla NK. Radiation related morbidities and their impact on quality of life in head and neck cancer patients receiving radical radiotherapy. Qual Life Res. 2004;13:481–8.
10. Chawla S, Mohanti BK, Rakshak M, Saxena S, Rath GK, Bahadur S. Temporal assessment of quality of life of head and neck cancer patients receiving radical radiotherapy. Qual Life Res. 1999;8:73–8.
11. Guibert M, Lepage B, Woisard V, Rives M, Serrano E, Vergez S. Quality of life in patients treated for advanced hypopharyngeal or laryngeal cancer. Eur Ann Otolaryngol Head Neck Dis. 2011;128:218–23.
12. The Department of Veterans Affairs Laryngeal Cancer Study Group. Induction chemotherapy plus radiation compared with surgery plus radiation in patients with advanced laryngeal cancer. N Engl J Med. 1991;324:1685–90.
13. Lefebvre JL, Chevalier D, Luboinski B, Kirkpatrick A, Collette L, Sahmoud T. Larynx preservation in pyriform sinus cancer: preliminary results of a European Organization for Research and Treatment of Cancer phase III trial. EORTC Head and Neck Cancer Cooperative Group. J Natl Cancer Inst. 1996;88(13):890–9.
14. Lefebvre JL, Ang KK, Larynx Preservation Consensus Panel. Larynx preservation clinical trial design: key issues and recommendations—a consensus panel summary. Head Neck. 2009;31:429–41.

15. Rosenthal DI, Mohamed AS, Weber RS, Garden AS, Sevak PR, Kies MS, Morrison WH, Lewin JS, El-Naggar AK, Ginsberg LE, Kocak-Uzel E, Ang KK, Fuller CD. Long-term outcomes after surgical or nonsurgical initial therapy for patients with T4 squamous cell carcinoma of the larynx: a 3-decade survey. Cancer. 2015;121:1608–19.
16. Takes RP, Strojan P, Silver CE, Bradley PJ, Haigentz M Jr, Wolf GT, Shaha AR, Hartl DM, Olofsson J, Langendijk JA, Rinaldo A, Ferlito A, International Head and Neck Scientific Group. Current trends in initial management of hypopharyngeal cancer: the declining use of open surgery. Head Neck. 2012;34:270–81.
17. Guibert M, Lepage B, Woisard V, Rives M, Serrano E, Vergez S. Quality of life in patients treated for advanced hypopharyngeal or laryngeal cancer. Eur Ann Otorhinolaryngol Head Neck Dis. 2011;128:218–23.

Printed by Printforce, the Netherlands